Principles of

NASAL

Reconstruction

Principles of
NASAL
Reconstruction

Shan R. Baker, MD
Professor and Chief, Facial Plastic and Reconstructive Surgery
Department of Otolaryngology
University of Michigan Medical Center
Ann Arbor, Michigan

Sam Naficy, MD
Facial Plastic Surgery & Laser Center
Kirkland, Washington

With contributions by **Brian Jewet, MD**
Division of Facial Plastic and Reconstructive Surgery
Department of Otolaryngology/Head and Neck Surgery
University of Miami School of Medicine

Shayne Davidson
Medical Illustrator

Jaye Schlessinger
Medical Illustrator

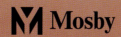

An Imprint of Elsevier Science
St. Louis   London   Philadelphia   Sydney   Toronto

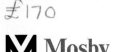
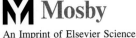

£170

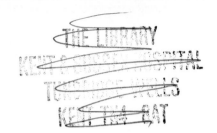

WV 312

A 031058

PRINCIPLES OF NASAL RECONSTRUCTION   ISBN 0–323–01147–0
Copyright © 2002 by Mosby, Inc. All rights reserved.

Notice

Facial Plastic Surgery is an ever-changing field. Standard safety precautions must be followed, but as new research and clinical experience broaden our knowledge, changes in treatment and drug therapy may become necessary or appropriate. Readers are advised to check the most current product information provided by the manufacturer of each drug to be administered to verify the recommended dose, the method and duration of administration, and contraindications. It is the responsibility of the treating physician, relying on experience and knowledge of the patient, to determine dosages and the best treatment for each individual patient. Neither the Publisher nor the editor assumes any liability for any injury and/or damage to persons or property arising from this publication.

The Publisher

Library of Congress Cataloging-in-Publication Data

Principles of Nasal Reconstruction [edited by] Shan R. Baker; Shayne Davidson, Jaye Schlessinger, medical illustrator[s].
p.; cm.
ISBN 0–323–01147–0
1. Nose—Surgery. 2. Rhinoplasty. 3. Flaps (Surgery) I. Baker, Shan R.
[DNLM: 1. Nose—surgery. 2. Reconstructive Surgical Procedures—methods. 3. Skin
Transplantation—methods. 4. Surgical Flaps. WV 312 R311 2002]
RF350 .R43 2002
617.5′23′059—dc21

                                                              2001044975

Acquisitions Editor: Stephanie Donley
Project Manager: Natalie Ware

PI/DNP

Printed in China.

Last digit is the print number: 9 8 7 6 5 4 3 2 1

This book is dedicated to
Catherine, Alexander, and Monica,
the substance of my life.
Shan R. Baker

Preface

Techniques of nasal reconstruction have undergone revolutionary changes over the past two decades. This was primarily related to a series of landmark scientific papers published by Gary Burget, M.D., and Fred Menick, M.D. These papers culminated in the publication of *Aesthetic Reconstruction of the Nose,* which represented a summation of all the techniques these gifted plastic surgeons perfected over the preceding 15 years. This book highlighted the importance of three contemporary principles of nasal reconstruction. The first principle is that of replacing missing tissue with like tissue. For example, nasal lining is replaced with nasal mucosa, upper and lower lateral cartilages are replaced with septal or auricular cartilage grafts, and nasal skin is replaced with adjacent forehead or cheek skin. The second principle is to replace missing portions of the nasal skeleton with cartilage and bone fashioned to precisely replicate the missing part. Burget and Menick also stressed the need to reinforce the nasal skeleton with additional cartilage grafts in the area of the ala and nostril margin to maintain the contour and position of the nostril. The third principle is dividing the topography of the nose into aesthetic units and resurfacing an entire unit with a skin flap if the majority of the skin of the unit is lost. This places scars along contour lines between the units. In the case of the ala, routinely resurfacing the entire ala creates a concentric scar contraction surrounding the ala resulting in a natural convexity of the constructed ala.

The Burget–Menick book brought the art of nasal reconstruction to a level never before attained. It taught the reconstructive surgeon to view the nose as a pattern of light and shadow in variable gradations. It emphasized that contour is the most important feature that distinguishes normal from deformed. It stressed that every effort should be expended to restore a natural contour to the constructed portion of the nose by using thin lining and covering flaps and accurately fabricated structural grafts. Since its publication in 1994, we have used the book as a valuable resource to improve our aesthetic and functional results. The book has established the current standard by which all nasal reconstruction must be measured. So, why publish another textbook on this subject? While the Burget–Menick book tells the surgeon "what" to do, the textbook places less emphasis on "how" to accomplish "what" is required. The purpose of our textbook is to serve as a "working man's" manual for nasal reconstruction by providing the surgeon an accurate, detailed, and well-illustrated step-by-step discussion of the techniques for repairing nasal defects. We hope our book will serve as a valuable supplement to the Burget–Menick book.

Our textbook is divided into three parts. Part One discusses the fundamentals of nasal reconstruction. It provides algorithms to assist the surgeon in selecting the preferred method of restoring internal lining, structural support, and external cover, all of which are governed by the extent of the nasal defect and the availability of resources that can be used for the repair. We hope these algorithms will serve as a valuable reference for the novice surgeon. Part Two represents the "how to" section of the book. It provides detailed step-by-step discussions of techniques used to design, dissect, transfer, and refine flaps and grafts used in nasal reconstruction. It also reviews the prevention and management of complications. In Part Three, each chapter discusses a representative case or cases that demonstrate the application of the principles and techniques described in the earlier chapters. Cases were selected to demonstrate typical complications and limitations confronting all surgeons when reconstructing the nose.

Shan R. Baker, M.D.

Acknowledgments

Although many people have indirectly contributed to the creation of this book, we would like to thank those who had major roles in assisting us in its preparation. Foremost, we are grateful to our patients who through their misfortune of being afflicted with skin cancer have enabled us to learn and perfect reconstructive surgical techniques. A particular gratitude is offered to those patients who have allowed us to publish their photographs in this book. We would like to thank Mary Ellen Garley for assistance with preparation of the manuscript and Karen Chartier for her assistance with procuring photographs. We are grateful to Marcia Stuursma for her friendship, support, and serving as our ambassador to patients and colleagues over an interval that spans nearly the entire career of the senior author. We are most grateful to Kathy Herman-Brown for her unfailing optimisim, unflinching support, and never considering a task too great or too small to perform. Thank you for being such a successful liaison to our patients. Finally, the senior author would like to thank Tim Johnson, M.D., Director of Dermatological Surgery at the University of Michigan, for referral of his patients throughout the many years we have been professionally associated. Without his support and trust, this book would not have been possible.

Contents

PART **III** Representative Cases 223

SECTION **A** Partial Thickness Defects 224

SECTION **B** Full-Thickness Defects 250

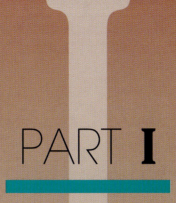

PART **I**

Fundamentals

1

History of Nasal Reconstruction

Brian S. Jewett

Injury and disfigurement of the nose have been well described. Nasal deformity has been attributed to self-infliction, mutilation as a form of punishment, and various disease states.

The first recorded account of mutilation as a form of punishment was in 1500 BC when, in India, Prince Lakshmana deliberately amputated the nose of Lady Surpunakha. King Ravana arranged for the reconstruction of Lady Surpunakha's nose by his physicians, documenting one of the earliest accounts of nasal reconstruction.[1] During the 9th century, Danes slit the noses of Irishmen who could not pay their taxes, and Sixtus Quintus of Rome mandated the amputation of the noses of thieves during the 16th century.[2] In 1769, the Ghoorka King of India ordered the amputation of the nose and lips of all 865 male inhabitants of the captured city of Kirtipoor, Nepal. The king changed the name of the city to Naskatapoor, which means "city without noses."[3] Traumatic amputation of the nose has been established in history as a form of humiliation to such an extent that the practice has insinuated itself into the language of many cultures in the form of idiomatic expressions. For example, in English, the phrase *to lose face* suggests humiliation or embarrassment. In Urdu and Punjabi, the phrase *mera noc kart gaya* is a common expression connoting "you have hurt my feelings," but it literally means "you have cut off my nose."[4]

The repair of nasal defects is the oldest form of facial reconstructive surgery,[5] and the Indian art of total nasal reconstruction represents the first, if not the most important, chapter in the history of plastic surgery.[4]

Early Nasal Reconstruction

The earliest descriptions of total nasal reconstruction come from ancient India during the Vedic period, approximately 3000 BC.[5] The first detailed description of nasal reconstruction is found in the Indian medical treatise *Sushruta Samhita* (700 BC). The operative procedure described was a cheek flap, and it was performed by members of a caste of potters known as Koomas.[6] Vagbhat, a 4th century Indian physician, recounts in greater detail the technique of cheek flap rhinoplasty. He describes the use of topical hemostatic agents, intranasal splints, and leaves. He emphasizes cutting with accuracy, protecting the pedicle, and approximating the edges of the wound carefully.[1] Most of the reconstructions were performed by potters and bricklayers, and advances were made as the tradition was passed down among family members. Surgical equipment included special cements, cotton suture, and ant heads to close wounds.[4]

The first European to record techniques of repairing defects of the nose, lips, and ears by using adjacent tissues was Celsus during the 1st century AD.[7] Paulus Aegineta, a 7th century Greek physician, helped to integrate Eastern medical and surgical practices into Western civilization. He summarized contemporary medical practices in a seven-volume compendium. In the sixth book of the set, he describes the treatment of facial defects by the rearrangement of adjacent healthy tissue.[4]

The Italian Method

In 14th century Italy, Branca de Branca performed a procedure similar to that described in *Sushruta Samhita*.[8, 9] His son, Antonius Branca, went on to describe a new method of nasal reconstruction: the Italian method. This procedure involved transferring a piece of tissue from the arm to the nose in a staged fashion. The operation was tedious, required six stages, and remained a secret within the Branca family. The only contemporary medical text with an accurate report of Branca's procedure is the *Buch der Buendth-Ertznei* (*The Book of Bandage Treatment*), written in 1460 by Heinrich von Pfolspeundt, a knight of the Teutonic Order. The book remained unknown for more than 400 years, hidden in manuscript form in the library of Erfurt University. In the second half of the 19th century, Haeser and Middledorpf discovered it and had it published.[10]

Alessandro Benedetti, professor of anatomy and surgery at Padua University in Italy, was the first to publish results using the Italian method (Fig. 1–1). His publication appeared before Haeser and Middledorpf's book containing the original description by Antonius Branca. Benedetti rebelled against the Greek traditions of teaching anatomy as a blend of science and magic and emphasized teaching through direct observation of facts, with independence of judgment. Benedetti published an eight-volume text on anatomy in 1493. In volume IV, chapter 39, he describes the Italian method of nasal reconstruction[11]:

> At present ingenious men have indicated how to correct nasal deformities. Their method consists in cutting a little piece of flesh from the patient's arm, in the shape of a nose and applying it to the stump. For this they cut the top layer of skin on the arm with a scalpel. Having made a scarification in the nose, if this is needed, or if the nose has been recently cut off, they bind the arm to the head, so that raw surface adheres to raw surface. When the wounds have conglutinated together they take from the arm with a scalpel as much as is needed for the restoration. Blood vessels of the nose supply nourishment to the flap, and finally a covering is obtained, with hairs sometimes growing there after the nature of the arm.

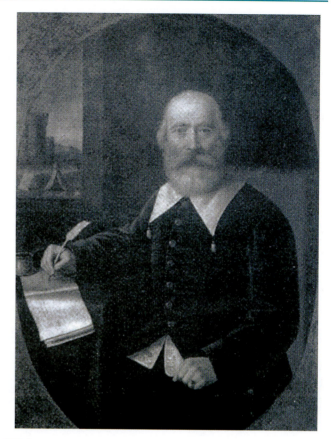

Figure 1–1. Portrait of Alessandro Benedetti, Legnago, Italy.

More than 100 years later, in 1597, Tagliacozzi published *De Curtorum Chirurgia per Insitionem,* which described in detail the Italian method of nasal reconstruction (Fig. 1–2). This was the first text dedicated solely to the subject of plastic surgery. Tagliacozzi reproduced Benedetti's passage in volume I, chapter 19, of his work.[12]

The Indian Method

The origin of using a forehead flap for nasal reconstruction is unclear in history, but the procedure has been performed since 1440 AD by the Mahrattas of Kumar, some Nepalese families, and the Kanghiara family of Kangra, India. The procedure was practiced in secrecy, shared among family members, and it became known as the Indian method.[1, 5]

The first account of the midline forehead flap is found in the *Madras Gazette*, a journal published in Bombay during the 1700s. The article was later reproduced in English in London's *Gentleman's Magazine* (1794), and it fostered the renaissance of nasal reconstructive surgery in Europe.[4] The article describes the fate of Cowasjee, a bullock driver with the English army

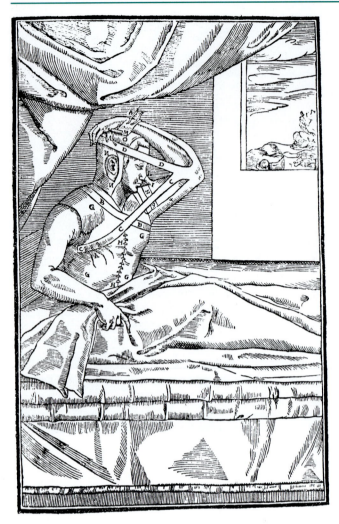

■ **Figure 1-2.** The Italian Method. (From Nichter LS, Morgan RF, Nichter MA: The impact of Indian methods for total nasal reconstruction. Clin Plast Surg 10:635–647, 1983)

in the War of 1792. Cowasjee had been captured by Tipu Sultan, ruler of Mysore, who violently opposed British involvement in southern India. Tipu Sultan cut off food and supplies to the English troops under the command of Cornwallis by attacking the Maharatta bullock drivers who transported needed grains to the British. The Sultan gave rewards for each nose or ear brought back after a raid. Cowasjee lost his hand and nose, and the article describes the operation to restore his nose. The article is signed "B.L.," but the author is assumed to be an English surgeon named Cully Lyon Lucas (Fig. 1–3). The operation was described as follows:

> A thin plate of wax is fitted to the stump of the nose, so as to make it a nose of good appearance. It is then flattened and laid on the forehead. A line is drawn around the wax, and the operator then dissects off as much skin as it covered, leaving undivided a small slit between the eyes. This slit preserves the circulation until

a union has taken place between the new and old parts. . . . Skin is now brought down from the forehead and, being twisted half round, its edge is inserted into the incision, so that a nose is formed with a double hold above, and with its alae and septum below fixed in the incision. A little Terra Japonica is softened with water, and being spread on slips of cloth, five or six of these are placed over each other, to secure the joining. No other dressing but this cement is used for four days. . . . The connecting slips of skin are divided about the twenty-fifth day. . . . The artificial nose is secure and looks nearly as well as the natural one; nor is the scar on the forehead very observable after a length of time.

The English surgeon Carpue learned the procedure and published a book in 1816 called *An Account of Two Successful Operations for Restoring a Lost Nose from Integuments of the Forehead.* His detailed descrip-

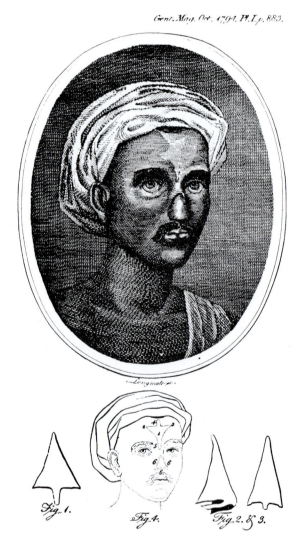

■ **Figure 1-3.** English bullock driver after total nasal reconstruction, as shown in Letter to Editor, London's *Gentlemans Magazine*, 1794. (From Nichter LS, Morgan RF, Nichter MA: The impact of Indian methods for total nasal reconstruction. Clin Plast Surg 10:635–647, 1983)

tion states that the procedure was performed with "an old razor," and lasted about an hour and a half (Fig. 1–4).[13] As Carpue's book circulated throughout Europe, the operation came to be more widely accepted.[14] In 1818, the first book devoted solely to rhinoplasty, *Rhinoplastik,* was published by Carl von Graefe. The book listed 55 articles and books on the subject of rhinoplasty and included Carpue's work.[4] Waren was the first to perform the forehead flap operation in America, and he published his account in the *Boston Medical and Surgical Journal* in 1837.[15]

Internal Lining

As the use of the midline forehead flap became more widespread, it became apparent that the results of reconstructing full-thickness defects without supplying an internal lining were poor. The shape of the nose often became distorted because the skin flap used for reconstruction contracted during the healing process because of the exposed undersurface. Tissues suggested to provide internal linings included skin grafts, nasal mucosa, local flaps, and folding the forehead flap on itself.[16]

During the 19th century, Ernst Blasius, chief of ophthalmologic surgery of Berlin, Johann Friedereich Dief-

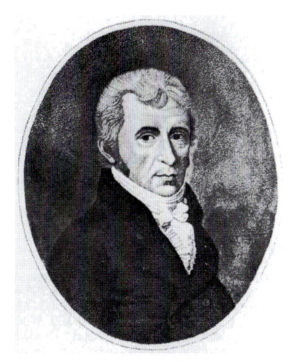

■ **Figure 1–4.** Joseph Carpue (1764–1840), the first European to perform the Indian Method of nasal reconstruction. (From Nichter LS, Morgan RF, Nichter MA: The impact of Indian methods for total nasal reconstruction. Clin Plast Surg 10:635–647, 1983)

fenback, chief of surgery at Munich Hospital, and Natale Petrali of Milan advocated folding the midline forehead flap on itself to provide both external coverage and internal lining. All three surgeons claimed precedence in succeeding with this method of total nasal reconstruction. Based on the date of the first operation to use a folded forehead flap for total nasal reconstruction, the honor goes to Blasius, who performed the procedure in 1838 (Fig. 1–5). Petrali was the first to actually publish an account of this method of reconstruction, in 1842. However, the idea of folding a forehead flap on itself when restoring the lower part of the nose was first suggested by Pierre August Labat of Paris who, in 1834, described using a trilobed forehead flap and turning it inward. Because these surgeons were associated with large teaching hospitals in Europe, the use of midforehead flaps grew in popularity.[8, 17–19]

Using a forehead flap to supply tissue for the internal lining increased the size of the flap required for reconstruction. As flaps increased in size, it became more difficult to pivot the flap 180 degrees in the midline. The awkward but necessary twisting of the flap often compromised the flap's blood supply and made it difficult for the flap to reach the columella. In addition, taking more forehead tissue left large donor-site scars that were unsightly. In 1850, Auvert suggested slanting the flap in an oblique fashion, diagonally across the forehead toward the temporal area. This design provided sufficient length to reach the columella while still allowing the flap to fold on itself. In 1935, Gillies proposed using a design called the up-and-down flap. The pedicle ascended from the origin of the supraorbital vessels on one side and extended to the hair-bearing scalp. The flap then turned downward in an arc to the contralateral supraorbital vessels (Fig. 1–6). Converse, in 1942, described a scalping flap with a longer pedicle that reached to the hair-bearing scalp. This flap left the patient with a hairy pedicle across the eye for weeks prior to division. Ultimately, these flaps caused the patient to live with a large donor-site scar. Patients also experienced significant nasal obstruction secondary to the bulkiness of the tissue, once the forehead flap was folded on itself to provide the lining for the nose.[8]

Other modifications in the design of forehead flaps included extending one limb of the incision inferior to the other, as described by Lisfranc in 1827. Labat curved his incisions proximally, centering the flap over the medial brow and canthus on one side. Both of these modified designs reduced the twist of the pedicle base and brought the flap closer to the recipient site.[9] During the 1930s, Kazanjian was the first to delineate the primary blood supply of the midline forehead flap. He described a precise midline forehead flap that facilitated primary closure of the donor-site wound. This was a major advance in the field, given concerns about the forehead scar that developed after the healing of the

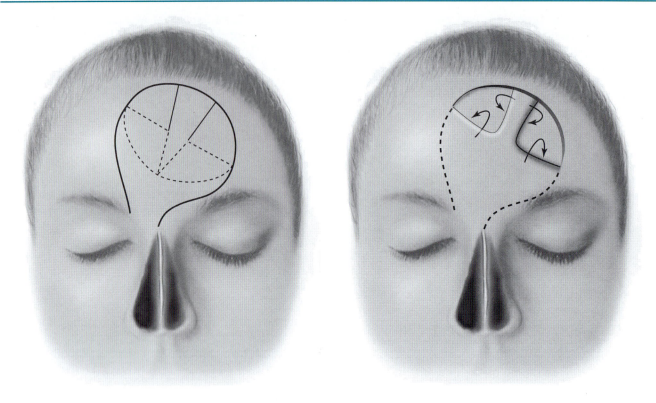

■ **Figure 1-5.** Blasius procedure (1848) for total nasal reconstruction with oval folded flap technique (after Nelaton and Ombredanne, 1904).

site by secondary intention.[20] Kazanjian and Converse illustrated that a gap exists between the paired frontalis muscles, so no compromise of forehead musculature occurs with harvesting of the midline forehead flap.[21] In the 1960s, Millard designed the seagull flap, with lateral extensions for reconstruction of the alae. The extensions were designed to follow the natural creases of forehead wrinkle lines. Incisions for the flap extended below the level of the supraorbital rims to gain extra length and ease of pivoting.[22–24]

While some surgeons were experimenting with larger forehead flaps that could be folded to provide lining, others were exploring the use of adjacent facial tissue as a source for internal lining. In 1874, Volkmann described turning inward portions of residual nasal skin adjacent to the defect to provide internal lining (Fig. 1–7). Thiersch, in 1879, described the transfer of cheek flaps to the nose for internal lining (Fig. 1–8). In 1898, Lossen first applied skin grafts to line the forehead flap. The grafts were placed under the forehead musculature, allowed to heal, and then transferred to the nose as a composite flap. Millard advocated bilateral, superiorly based, hinge melolabial flaps to line the alae and columella.[8] Converse and Casson, in 1969, used a forehead flap for the internal lining and flaps from other donor sites to cover the external nose.[25] Despite the use of adjacent tissue and skin grafts for lining, patients con-

tinued to have difficulty with nasal obstruction. This was due to scar contracture and failure to provide sufficient structural support to the nose. Attempts were made to use cartilage grafts to replace missing nasal framework at the time of forehead flap transfer, but these procedures were often complicated by extrusion or necrosis of the grafts. Insertion of cartilage grafts secondarily was also problematic and often provided little improvement in nasal contour because of contracture of the covering flap.

Surgeons looked to the native nasal mucosa for internal lining. In 1902, de Quervain first used the septum to provide lining and support for the lateral wall of the nose.[26] Kazanjian described a septal flap based on the dorsum. The flap consisted of contralateral mucoperichondrium and was used to line the ala.[21] Gillies described a mucoperichondrial flap based on the caudal septum.[27] Millard described a superiorly based septal flap that was used to reconstruct sidewall defects in amputated, saddle, cleft-lip, and flat noses,[22] and an anteroinferior ipsilateral septal flap for alar lining.[23] Nasal mucosa provided thin, nonobstructive internal lining. The pliability of these lining flaps minimized distortion of the overlying nasal skin. A source of lining tissue independent of the forehead facilitated the design of smaller forehead flaps because they were used solely for external covering.

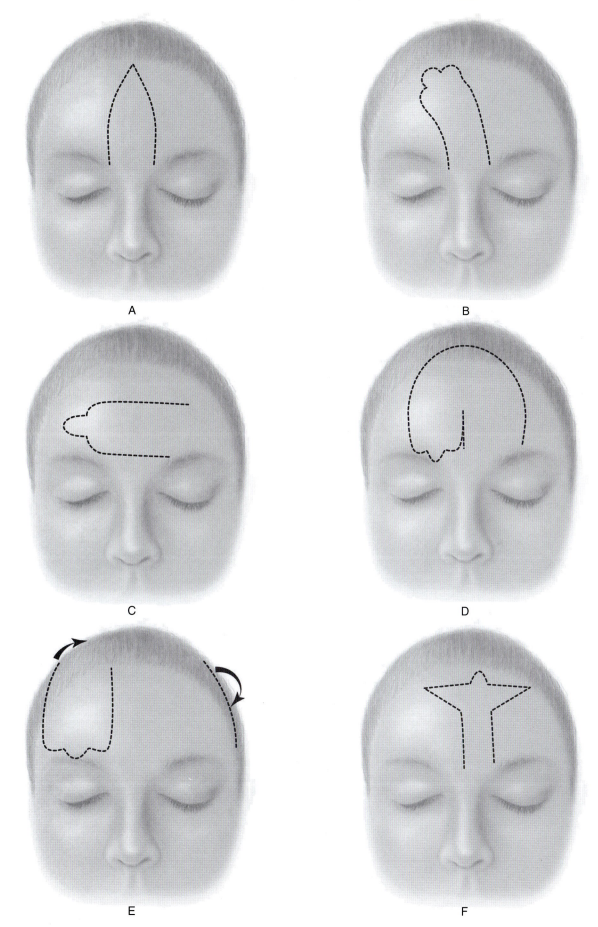

Figure 1-6. Forehead flap designs. *A,* Indian median flap. *B,* oblique flap. *C,* horizontal flap. *D,* Gillies' up-and-down flap. *E,* Converse's scalping flap. *F,* Millard's gull-winged paramedian forehead flap.

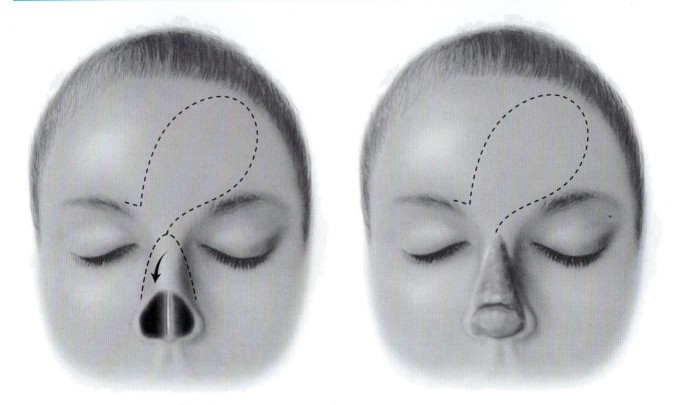

■ **Figure 1-7.** Volkmann's procedure (1874) for total nasal reconstruction, with lining created from remaining nasal skin plus forehead flap for external covering (after Nelaton and Ombredanne, 1904).

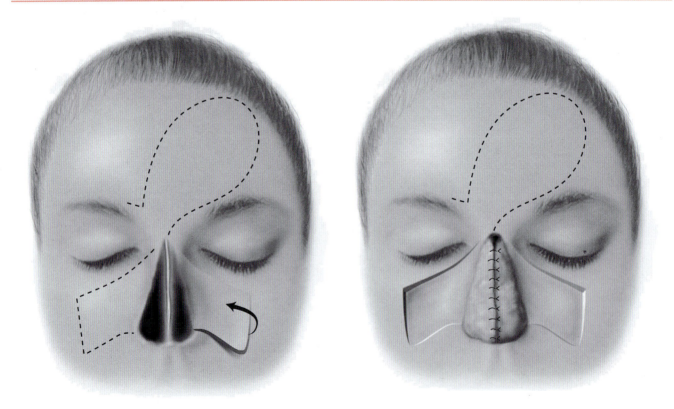

■ **Figure 1-8.** Thiersch's procedure (1879) for total nasal reconstruction with lining created from the cheeks, plus forehead flap used for external covering (after Nelaton and Ombredanne, 1904).

Nasal Framework

It became apparent that addressing deficiencies in the nasal framework was essential to achieving optimal aesthetic and functional outcomes. The choice of tissue to replace the nasal framework has varied over the past two centuries. In 1863, Ollier used a forehead flap with underlying frontal bone.[28a,b] Konig, in 1886, first reported using an iliac bone graft for nasal repair.[29] In 1966, Millard described a refinement of Konig's technique, using a bone graft cantilevered from the nasal process of the frontal bone.[24] The use of costal cartilage has been described by several authors. In 1889, von Mangoldt used costal cartilage for the reconstruction of saddle noses.[30] In 1902, Nelaton placed costal cartilage beneath a forehead flap and subsequently transferred it to the nose as a composite flap.[31] Although costal cartilage, when used as a free graft in the nose, remains intact 4 to 15 years after reconstructive rhinoplasty,[32, 33] warping of the graft may occur.[34] In 1935, Gillies described using composite flaps containing septal cartilage and mucoperichondrium for the repair of defects of the nasal cartilaginous framework.[35, 36] Gillies later used composite chondrocutaneous grafts to provide lining and support for alar defects.[37] Gillies' and Millard's experience with mucosal flaps and septal cartilage grafts was the basis for contemporary approaches to nasal reconstruction.

Skin Coverage

Although forehead flaps became the primary source of skin coverage for sizable nasal defects, methods of using local cutaneous flaps from the nose and cheek were developed to provide coverage for smaller defects. Nasal cutaneous flaps provided good color, thickness, and texture match with the skin at the recipient site, and their donor sites could be closed primarily. The rhombic flap was first described by Limberg in 1963,[38] and various modifications have been reported subsequently.[39–41] Although rhombic flaps are rarely used in nasal reconstruction, they may be helpful in closing small sidewall defects. The original design of the bilobe flap is attributed to Esser, who described it in 1918. The bilobe flap was used for reconstruction of smaller nasal defects, with the original angle of tissue transfer being 90 degrees between each lobe of the flap. These wide angles produced significant standing cutaneous and trap-door deformities of both lobes.[42] Modifications by McGregor[43] and Zitelli[44] were published in 1981 and 1989, respectively. Zitelli emphasized narrow angles of transfer: 45 degrees between each lobe, with total pivotal movement of no more than 90 to 100 degrees.[44] Bilobe flaps continue to be used for repair of small (2 cm or less), centrally located cutaneous defects of the caudal nose (see Chapter 10).

Another nasal cutaneous flap that is used for repair of the nose is the dorsal nasal flap (see Chapter 10). This flap was originally described by Rieger for nasal tip and midnasal wounds. The entire dorsal nasal skin, including a triangular glabellar extension, is elevated and pivoted caudally. The superior aspect of the donor site is closed in a V-to-Y fashion.[45] Refinements of Rieger's design include heminasal flaps that are created by extending an incision directly down the midline of the nose, preserving a lateral base along the nasal-facial sulcus.[46] Problems with alar retraction prompted Cronin to modify the flap by designing a narrower pedicle with a back cut through the medial canthus. He used the flap for defects less than 2.5 cm in diameter.[47] Marchac defined an axial pedicle for the flap using a branch of the angular artery. This allowed even further narrowing of the pedicle and helped to prevent nostril elevation. Marchac emphasized wide undermining of the remaining nasal skin, adjustment of flap thickness along its borders, and modification of the nasal framework to facilitate wound closure.[48, 49] De Fontaine suggested placing the pedicle ipsilateral to the defect during the repair of lateral tip defects, which means no scar occurs across the dorsum. De Fontaine emphasized the use of the flap while still adhering to the principles of nasal aesthetic units.[50] Rohrich used the dorsal nasal flap without a glabellar incision. The flap was based on a broad lateral pedicle, as originally described by Rieger. Rohrich recommended use of the flap for defects smaller than 2 cm wide, located above the tip-defining points, and separated by at least 1 cm from the alar rim.[51]

Cheek flaps used for nasal reconstruction date to the original description in *Sushrata Samhita*. Melolabial flaps may be based superiorly for the repair of nasal alar or sidewall defects. They may also be based inferiorly for the repair of upper lip or columellar defects.[52] Menick introduced the interpolated melolabial flap for the repair of nasal ala defects. Interpolated flaps must be performed in two stages, but they preserve the alar-facial sulcus. When comparing forehead flaps to interpolated melolabial flaps in the reconstruction of alar defects, Arden and colleagues found that melolabial flaps provide an aesthetically superior result.[53] This is probably related to the fact that melolabial flaps have a greater tendency to contract and bulge during wound healing. This ultimately results in a contour that more closely resembles the natural appearance of the ala. Dorsal nasal, bilobe, and interpolated melolabial flaps continue to play important roles in the repair of nasal cutaneous defects.

Recent Developments

During the 1980s and 1990s, Burget and Menick made significant contributions to the art of nasal reconstruction. They stressed the importance of replacing missing nasal tissue with like tissue. Deficiencies in nasal lining were replaced with intranasal mucoperichondrial flaps, and losses of the cartilaginous framework were repaired with septal or auricular cartilage grafts. Cutaneous defects were restored with flaps from the nose, cheek, or forehead. Using these principles, Burget and Menick were able to reconstruct partial- and full-thickness nasal defects, achieving optimal nasal function while closely approximating normal nasal contour and appearance.

Burget and Menick confirmed the safety of extending incisions for the forehead flap below the level of the orbital rim to give the flap added length so that it can reach the nasal tip without entering the hairline.[54–56] They also stressed that the end arterioles of the supratrochlear artery travel just under the dermis, superficial to the muscle, allowing the frontalis muscle to be safely removed from the distal end of the flap.[57] Based on Labat's and Millard's designs of unilateral pedicled flaps, Menick advocated designing the forehead flap so that its central axis is in the paramedian position. This design places the center of the flap directly over the vertical axis of the supratrochlear artery, giving the flap an axial vascular pattern. As a result, the paramedian forehead flap has a more abundant blood supply than its midline counterpart and can be based on a narrower pedicle. The narrow pedicle enables the flap to pivot more easily and to have a greater effective length.[9] Menick's description of the paramedian forehead flap was supported by anatomic studies that better defined the vascular anatomy of the forehead. The supratrochlear artery was consistently found to exit the superior medial orbit 1.7 to 2.2 cm lateral to the midline and to continue its course vertically in a paramedian position, approximately 2 cm lateral to the midline (see Chapter 14). The artery exits the orbit, pierces the orbital septum, and passes under the orbicularis oculi muscle and over the corrugator supercilii muscle. The artery then passes through the frontalis muscle and ascends toward the scalp in a subcutaneous tissue plane. The paramedian flap can be designed with a pedicle as narrow as 1.2 cm.[58–60]

Burget and Menick studied the blood supply of the nasal septum and determined that the septal branch of the superior labial artery was sufficient to support septal mucoperichondrial flaps for lining large, full-thickness nasal defects. They also mobilized the entire septum as a composite flap consisting of a sandwich of cartilage between two layers of mucoperichondrium so as to provide internal lining and structural support for the repair of total nasal defects. They also described the use of bipedicled flaps of residual vestibular skin and soft tissue to line the ala and nostril margin and the use of ipsilateral septal mucoperichondrial flaps to line the caudal one third of the nose.[57] The use of nasal mucoperichondrial flaps to replace nasal lining has become the standard for nasal reconstruction (see Chapters 4 and 11). These flaps are thin, nonobstructive, and sufficiently vascular to nourish cartilage grafts. Their pliability avoids distortion of overlying nasal cartilage and skin.[56]

Burget and Menick also introduced the subunit principle, which divides the nose into units defined by contour lines and zones of transition between nasal skin of varying textures and thicknesses. They advocate placing scars along the junctions of these units so as to hide them in the shadow lines. Flaps are designed to replace topographic units, not defects. Exact templates are created on the basis of the normal contralateral side. In general, when more than half of a unit is missing, the entire unit is resurfaced. Given the advances in aesthetic and functional results obtained by Burget and Menick, the forehead flap has gained popularity. It remains the procedure of choice for total and subtotal nasal reconstructions.[54, 56, 57, 61]

Conclusion

The art of nasal reconstruction is well established in history, dating back to 1500 BC in India. Advances have been made during the past 2 millennia in India, Europe, and America; however, many of the refinements leading to contemporary techniques are attributed to Burget and Menick. Their work has expanded the use of cartilage grafts, mucoperichondrial lining flaps, and forehead flaps to repair smaller nasal defects in which reconstruction by other methods would provide less than optimal aesthetic or functional results. Local flaps remain an important part of the armamentarium of nasal reconstruction, having specific indications depending on the size and location of the nasal defect.

Acknowledgments

The author thanks Larry S. Nichter, M.D., for his assistance and his permission to use various photographs and drawings in this chapter.

References

1. Almast S: History and evolution of the Indian method of rhinoplasty. In Sanvenero-Rosselli G (ed): Transactions of the Fourth International Congress of Plastic and Reconstructive Surgery. Rome, Excerpta Medica Foundation, 1969, p 49.

2. Malz M: Evolution of Plastic Surgery. Baltimore, Williams & Wilkins, 1977.

3. Keegan D: Rhinoplastic Operations. Baltimore, Longod, Baliere, Tindall & Cox, 1900.

4. Nichter LS, Morgan RF, Nichter MA: The impact of Indian methods for total nasal reconstruction. Clin Plast Surg 10:635–647, 1983.

5. Antia NH, Daver BM: Reconstructive surgery for nasal defects. Clin Plast Surg 8:535–663, 1981.

6. Bhishagronta KK (trans): Sushruta Samhita. Calcutta, 1916.

7. Gnudi MT, Webster JP: The Life and Times of Gaspare Tagliacozzi. Milan, Hoepli, 1956.

8. Mazzola RF, Marcus S: History of total nasal reconstruction with particular emphasis on the folded forehead flap technique. Plast Reconstr Surg 72:408–414, 1983.

9. Menick FJ: Aesthetic refinements in use of forehead for nasal reconstruction: The paramedian forehead flap. Clin Plast Surg 17:607–622, 1990.

10. von Pfolspeundt H: In Haeser H, Middledorpf A (eds): Buch der Buendth-Ertznei. Berlin, Reimer, 1868.

11. Furlan S, Mazzola RF: Alessandro Benedetti, a fifteenth century anatomist and surgeon: His role in the history of nasal reconstruction. Plast Reconstr Surg 96:739–743, 1995.

12. Tagliacozzi G: De Curtorum Chirurgia per Insitionem. Venezia, Bindoni, 1597.

13. Carpue JC: An account of two successful operations for restoring a lost nose from the integuments of the forehead. London, Longman, 1816. Reprinted in Plast Reconstr Surg 44:175–182, 1969.

14. McDowell F, Valone JA, Bronn JB: Bibliography and historical note on plastic surgery of the nose. Plast Reconstr Surg 10:149–185, 1952.

15. Waren J: Rhinoplastic operation. Boston Med Surg J 61:69, 1837.

16. Gunter JP: Nasal reconstruction using pedicle skin flaps. Otolaryngol Clin North Am 5:457–480, 1972.

17. Labat L: De la rhinoplastie: Art de restaurer ou de refaire complètement le nez. Paris, Ducessois, 1834.

18. Petrali N: Due parole sull'arte di rifare i nasi. Gazz Mantova 84:5, 1858.

19. Dieffenback JF: Die operative Chirurgie, vol 1. Leipzig, Brockhaus, 1845, p 331.

20. Kazanjian VH: The repair of nasal defects with a median forehead flap: Primary closure of forehead wound. Surg Gynecol Obstet 83:37, 1946.

21. Kazanjian VH, Converse JM: Surgical Treatment of Facial Injuries, Baltimore, Williams & Wilkins, 1949, p 352.

22. Millard DR Jr: Reconstructive rhinoplasty for the lower two-thirds of the nose. Plast Reconstr Surg 57:722–728, 1976.

23. Millard DR Jr: Hemirhinoplasty. Plast Reconstr Surg 40:440–445, 1967.

24. Millard DR Jr: Total reconstructive rhinoplasty and a missing link. Plast Reconstr Surg 37:167–183, 1966.

25. Converse JM, Casson PR: Reconstructive surgery: An integral part of treatment of cancer of the nose. In Gaisford JC (ed): Symposium on Cancer of the Head and Neck, vol 2. St Louis, Mosby, 1969.

26. de Quervain F: Ueber partielle sietliche Rhinoplastik. Zentralbl Chir 29:297, 1902.

27. Gillies HD: Plastic Surgery of the Face. London, Frowde, Hodder, Stoughton, 1920, p 270.

28a. Ollier: Des transplantations périostiques et osseuses sur l'homme, Paris 1862. Gaz Hop 135, 1861; 22, 1862.

28b. Ostéoplastie appliquée à la restauration du nez. Soc Imper de Med de Lyon, 1863.

29. Konig F: Eine neue methode der aufrichtung eingesunkener nasen durch bildung des nasenruckens aus einem haut-periost-knochenlappen der stirn. Verh Dtsch Ges Chir (Berl) 15:41, 1886.

30. von Mangoldt: Correction of saddle nose by cartilage transplantation. McDowell F (trans). Plast Reconstr Surg 46:495, 1970.

31. Nelaton: Discussion sur la rhinoplastie. Bull Mem Soc Chir 28:458, 1902.

32. Sheen JH, Sheen AS: Aesthetic Rhinoplasty. St. Louis, Mosby, 1987, pp 514–519.

33. Ortiz-Monasterio F, Olmedo A, Oscoy LO: The use of cartilage grafts in primary aesthetic rhinoplasty. Plast Reconstr Surg 67:597–609, 1981.

34. Horton CE, Matthews MS: Nasal reconstruction with autologous rib cartilage: A 43-year follow-up. Plast Reconstr Surg 89:131–135, 1992.

35. Gillies H: Experiences with tubed pedicle flaps. Surg Gynecol Obstet 60:291, 1935.

36. Gillies H, Millard DR: The Principles and Art of Plastic Surgery. Boston, Little Brown, 1957, pp 575–576.

37. Gillies HD: A new graft applied to the reconstruction of the nostril. Br J Surg 30:305, 1943.

38. Limberg AA: Design of the local flaps. In Gibson T (ed): Modern Trends in Plastic Surgery. Seven Oaks, England, Butterworth, 1963.

39. Dufourmentel C: La fermeture des pertes de substance cutanée limitées: "le lambeau de rotation en losange." Ann Chir Plast 7:61, 1962.

40. Webster RC, Davidson TM, Smith RC: The thirty-degree transposition flap. Laryngoscope 88:85–94, 1978.

41. Becker FF: Rhomboid flap in facial reconstruction: New concept of tension lines. Arch Otolaryngol 105:569–573, 1979.

42. Esser JFS: Gestielte lokale Nasenplastik mit Zweizipfligem lappen Deckung des Sekundaren Detektes vom ersten Zipfel durch den Zweiten. Dtsch Z Chir 143:385, 1918.

43. McGregor JC, Soutar DS: A critical assessment of the bilobed flap. Br J Plast Surg 34:197–205, 1981.

44. Zitelli JA: The bilobed flap for nasal reconstruction. Arch Dermatol 125:957–959, 1989.

45. Rieger RA: A local flap for repair of the nasal tip. Plast Reconstruct Surg 40:147–149, 1967.

46. Rigg BM: The dorsal nasal flap. Plast Reconstr Surg 52:361–364, 1973.

47. Cronin TD: The V-Y rotational flap for nasal tip defects. Ann Plast Surg 11; 282–288, 1983.

48. Marchac D: Ann Chir Plast Esthet 15:44–49, 1970.

49. Marchac D, Toth B: The axial frontonasal flap revisited. Plast Reconstr Surg 76:686–694, 1985.

50. de Fontaine S, Klaassen M, Soutar DS: Refinements in the axial frontonasal flap. Br J Plast Surg 46:371–374, 1993.

51. Rohrich RJ, Muzaffar AR, Adams WF, et. al.: The aesthetic unit dorsal nasal flap: Rationale for avoiding a glabellar incision. Plast Reconstr Surg 104:1289–1294, 1999.

52. Cameron RR, Latham WD, Dowling JA: Reconstructions of the nose and upper lip with nasolabial flaps. Plast Reconstr Surg 52:145–150, 1973.

53. Arden RL, Nawroz-Danish M, Yod GH, et. al.: Nasal alar reconstruction: A critical analysis using melolabial island and paramedian forehead flaps. Laryngoscope 109:376–382, 1999.

54. Burget GC, Menick FJ: The subunit principle in nasal reconstruction. Plast Reconstr Surg 76:239–247, 1985.

55. Burget GC: Aesthetic restoration of the nose. Clin Plast Surg 12:463–480, 1985.

56. Burget GC, Menick FJ: Nasal reconstruction: Seeking a fourth dimension. Plast Reconstr Surg 78:145–157, 1986.

57. Burget GC, Menick FJ: Nasal support and lining: The marriage of beauty and blood supply. Plast Reconstr Surg 84:189–202, 1989.

58. Shumrick KA, Smith TL: The anatomic basis for the design of forehead flaps in nasal reconstruction. Arch Otolaryngol Head Neck Surg 118:373–379, 1992.

59. Mangold U, Lierse W, Pfeifer G: [The arteries of the forehead as the basis of nasal reconstruction with forehead flaps] [German]. Acta Anat 107:18–25, 1980.

60. McCarthy JG, Lorenc ZP, Cutting-C., et. al.: The median forehead flap revisited: The blood supply. Plast Reconstr Surg 76:866–869, 1985.

61. Menick FJ: Artistry in aesthetic surgery: Aesthetic perception and the subunit principle. Clin Plast Surg 14:723–735, 1987.

2

Anatomic Considerations

Brian S. Jewett

A thorough understanding of nasal anatomy is essential to successful nasal reconstruction. Addressing deficiencies of the external soft-tissue envelope, nasal framework, and internal mucosal lining is an important part of achieving an optimal aesthetic and functional outcome.

The nose is a highly contoured pyramidal structure situated centrally on the face. It is composed of skin, mucosa, bone, cartilage, and intervening supportive tissue, including fat, muscle, and connective tissue. The aesthetically pleasing nose provides a smooth and natural transition from the eyes to the lips. A distorted or deformed nose attracts attention away from the eyes and the lips, thus disrupting the aesthetic harmony of the face. Functionally, the nose is the gateway to the respiratory system. The nose warms, humidifies, and filters the air while allowing inhaled particles to come into contact with olfactory epithelium. Disruptions of normal nasal anatomy can impair nasal function and lead to complaints of nasal obstruction, nasal drainage, and compromised olfaction.

Topographic Analysis

Assessing the external nose requires an appreciation of the relationship between the nose and the rest of the face. In the frontal view, the face is divided into horizontal thirds. The upper third begins at the trichion and ends at the glabella. The middle third extends from the

glabella to the subnasion. The lower third extends from the subnasion to the menton. Nasal height is measured from the radix to the subnasion and should represent 47% of the height of the face from the menton to the radix. In the vertical plane, the face is divided into fifths. Each division equals the horizontal width of a single palpebral aperture. The nasal base, the distance between the alar creases, is ideally equal to the intercanthal distance and represents one fifth of the facial width. The nose occupies the central third of the face in the vertical axis and the central fifth in the horizontal axis and thus should lie precisely in the midline of the face. On the frontal view, a gentle, curved, unbroken line emanates from the eyebrow and courses along the lateral border of the dorsum to end at the tip-defining point. Table 2–1 defines common topographic landmarks often referred to during nasal analysis and evaluation.

A number of geometric measures are used in nasal analysis. The nasofrontal angle is the obtuse angle between a line tangent to the glabella and a line tangent to the tip-defining point, or pronasalae, with both lines originating at the nasion. This angle should measure between 115 and 130 degrees. The nasofacial angle is the angle formed between a line drawn from the nasion to the pronasalae and another line drawn from the nasion to the pogonion. The angle usually measures between 30 and 40 degrees. The nasomental angle is the angle between a line extending from the nasion to the pronasalae and a line extending from the pronasalae to the menton. The nasomental angle usually measures between 120 and 132 degrees. The nasolabial an-

■ **Table 2–1. Nasal Topography**

TOPOGRAPHIC LANDMARK	DESCRIPTION
Trichion	superior margin of forehead at frontal hairline
Glabella	most prominent point in midsagittal plane of forehead
Radix	continuous curve that descends from the superior brow to lateral nasal wall
Nasion	depression at root of the nose corresponds to nasofrontal suture
Sellion	deepest point of nasofrontal angle intersection of forehead slope and the proximal bridge soft-tissue equivalent of nasion
Rhinion	junction of bony and cartilaginous nasal dorsum
Tip-defining point (pronasalae)	anterior-most projection of nasal tip junction of intermediate and lateral crura
Infratip lobule	located caudal to tip-defining point but cephalic to columellar breakpoint
Columellar breakpoint	anterior-most point of soft tissue of nasal columella junction of intermediate and medial crura
Alar groove (supra-alar crease)	crease located at cephalic edge of ala
Alar margin	margin along nostril rim located at caudal aspect of ala
Alar facial sulcus	junctional zone between cheek, upper lip, and alar base represents lateral continuation of alar groove
Nasal facial sulcus	junctional zone between sidewall and cheek
Subnasale	junction of columella and upper lip
Philtrum	midline depression in upper lip
Mentolabial sulcus	point of depression between lower lip and chin
Pogonion	most prominent anterior projection of chin
Menton	lower border of soft-tissue contour of chin
Gnathion	point located at junction of line tangent to pogonion and line tangent to menton
Cervical point	junction of line tangent to anterior margin of neck and line tangent to menton

gle is the angle between the columella and upper lip; ideally it measures between 105 and 115 degrees in females and 90 and 105 degrees in males.

The aesthetic proportions of the ideal nasal shape and size have been established. On the lateral view, the distance from the vermilion border of the upper lip to the subnasale is equal to the distance from the subnasale to the pronasalae.[1] The distance from the alar crease to the midpoint of the nares ideally equals that from the midpoint to the caudal edge of the nasal tip. On the lateral view, a right-angle triangle with the ratios of its sides being 3:4:5, and the vertices being at the nasion, alar-facial sulcus, and tip has been described to illustrate the ideal nasal proportions and size.[2] Figure 2–1 illustrates the standard directional nomenclature.

Aesthetic Units

The nose may be divided into aesthetic units by contour lines that mark zones of transition between nasal skin of differing textures and thicknesses.[3] The aesthetic units include the nasal dorsum, sidewalls, tip lobule, nasal facets, alae, and columella (Fig. 2–2). These units

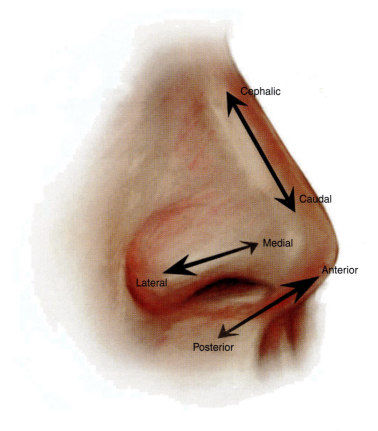

■ **Figure 2–1.** Directional nomenclature of the nose.

are highlighted when incident light is cast on the nasal surface, creating shadows along the borders of each unit and topographic landmark.[3] The framework underlying the nasal skin is primarily responsible for these variations in light reflections. Therefore, precise restoration of the framework is important in the reconstruction of the nose so as to avoid contour irregularities and asymmetries. In addition, repair of nasal skin defects

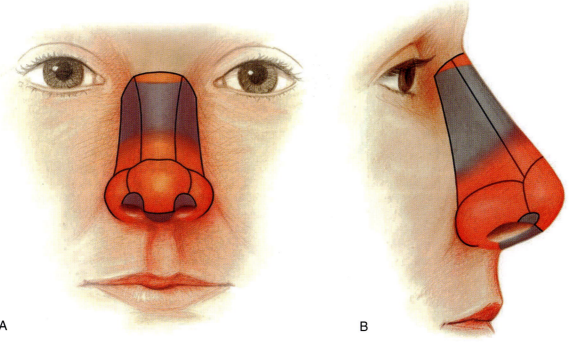

A   B

■ **Figure 2–2.** *A* and *B,* Aesthetic units of nose. Blue represents thin-skinned regions; red represents thicker skinned regions.

with a thin covering flap will help to maintain the definition of aesthetic units and anatomic landmarks.

External Nasal Anatomy

The external nose consists of overlying skin, soft tissue, blood vessels, and nerves. Understanding the variations in skin thickness among the various regions of the nose is an essential aspect of reconstructive nasal surgery. Familiarity with the blood supply is a prerequisite to using local flaps for soft tissue restoration of nasal defects.

■ Skin

Skin thickness varies widely among individuals and among the aesthetic units in any given individual (see Fig. 2-2). Lessard and Daniel analyzed 60 cadaver dissections and 25 patients undergoing septorhinoplasty and found the average skin thickness to be greatest at the radix (1.25 mm) and least at the rhinion (0.6 mm).[4] Skin is thinner and more mobile over the dorsum, whereas it is thicker and more adherent to the underlying nasal framework at the nasal tip and alae (see Fig. 2-2). At the cephalic portion of the nasal sidewalls, the skin is thin; however, caudally it becomes thicker in the vicinity of the alar groove. Despite being thicker at the nasal tip, the skin rapidly transitions to being very thin where it covers the nostril margins and columella. The close approximation of the dermis of the skin lining and covering the nasal facets and nostril margins makes these areas especially vulnerable to notching and contour irregularities after reconstruction.

Sebaceous glands are more numerous in the caudal half of the nose. This is especially true in the non-Caucasian nose, which commonly displays a greater amount of subcutaneous fibrous fatty tissue. This dense layer of tissue, often measuring as much as 6 mm thick, obscures the contour of the underlying alar cartilages in the non-Caucasian nose.[5]

■ Subcutaneous Layer

Four layers compose the soft tissue between the skin and the bony cartilaginous skeleton of the nose: (1) the superficial fatty panniculus, (2) the fibromuscular layer, (3) the deep fatty layer, and (4) the periosteum/perichondrium.[6] The superficial fatty panniculus is located immediately below the skin and consists of adipose tissue with interlacing vertical fibrous septi running from the deep dermis to the underlying fibromuscular layer. This layer is thicker in the glabellar and supratip areas. The fibromuscular layer contains the nasal musculature and the nasal subcutaneous muscular aponeurotic system (SMAS), which is a continuation of the facial SMAS. Histologically, the nasal SMAS is a distinct sheet of collagenous bundles that envelops the nasal musculature. The deep fatty layer located between the SMAS and the thin covering of the nasal skeleton contains the major superficial blood vessels and nerves. This layer of loose areolar fat has no fibrous septae; as a result, immediately below it is the preferred plane for undermining nasal skin. The nasal bones and cartilages are covered with periosteum and perichondrium, which provide nutrient blood flow to these tissues, respectively. The periosteum of the nasal bones extends over the upper lateral cartilages and fuses with the periosteum of the piriform process laterally.[7] Perichondrium covers the nasal cartilages, and dense interwoven fibrous interconnections can be found between the tip cartilages.

■ Muscles

The nasal musculature has been described and classified by Griesman and Letourneau (Fig. 2-3).[8, 9] The greatest concentration of muscle is located at the junction of the upper lateral and alar cartilages. This allows for muscular dilation and stenting of the nasal valve area. All nasal musculature is innervated by the zygomaticotemporal division of the facial nerve.[9]

The elevator muscles include the procerus, the levator labii superioris alaeque nasi, and the anomalous nasi. These muscles rotate the nasal tip in a cephalic direction and dilate the nostrils. The procerus muscle has a dual origin. The medial fibers originate from the aponeurosis of the transverse nasalis and the periosteum of the nasal bones. The lateral fibers originate from perichondrium of the upper lateral cartilages and the musculature of the upper lip. The procerus inserts into the glabellar skin. The levator labii superioris alaeque nasi originates from the medial part of the orbicularis oculi and ascending process of the maxilla and inserts into the melolabial fold, ala nasi, and skin and muscle of the upper lip. The anomalous nasi originates from the ascending process of the maxilla and inserts into the nasal bone, upper lateral cartilage, procerus, and transverse part of the nasalis.[9]

The depressor muscles include the alar nasalis and the depressor septi. These muscles lengthen the nose and dilate the nostrils. The alar nasalis originates from the maxilla above the lateral incisor tooth and inserts into the skin along the posterior circumference of the lateral crura. The depressor septi nasi originates from the maxillary periosteum above the central and lateral incisors and inserts into the membranous septum and the footplates of the medial crura. A minor dilator muscle is the dilator naris anterior, a fanlike muscle originating from the upper lateral cartilage and alar portion of the nasalis before inserting into the caudal margin of the lateral crura and the lateral alar skin.[9]

The compressor muscles rotate the nasal tip in a caudal direction and narrow the nostrils. These muscles

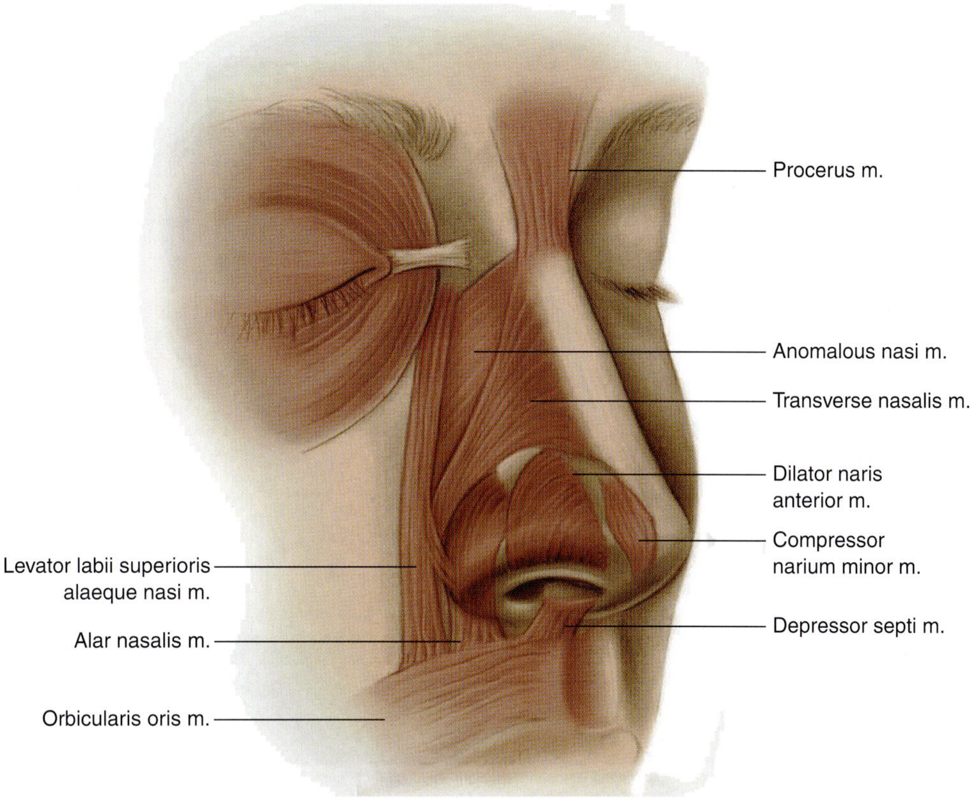

Procerus m.

Anomalous nasi m.

Transverse nasalis m.

Dilator naris anterior m.

Compressor narium minor m.

Depressor septi m.

Levator labii superioris alaeque nasi m.

Alar nasalis m.

Orbicularis oris m.

Figure 2–3. The nasal muscles.

include the transverse portion of the nasalis and the compressor narium minor. The transverse portion of the nasalis muscle originates from the maxilla above and lateral to the incisor fossa. Fibers from the transverse portion insert into the skin and procerus, and some fibers join the alar portion of the nasalis muscle. The compressor narium minor arises from the anterior part of the lower lateral cartilage and inserts into the skin near the margin of the nostrils.[9]

External Blood Supply

Both the internal and the external carotid arteries contribute to the superficial arterial supply of the nose and adjacent area (Fig. 2–4). The angular artery arises from the facial artery and provides a rich blood supply for the melolabial and subcutaneous hinge flaps. A branch of the angular artery, the lateral nasal artery, supplies the lateral surface of the caudal nose. The lateral nasal artery passes deep to the nose in the sulcus between the ala and cheek and is covered by the levator labii superioris alaeque nasi. The artery branches multiple times to enter the subdermal plexus of the skin covering the nostril and cheek.

The dorsal nasal artery, a branch of the ophthalmic artery, pierces the orbital septum above the medial palpebral ligament and travels along the side of the nose to anastomose with the lateral nasal artery. The dorsal nasal artery provides a rich axial blood supply to the dorsal nasal skin and serves as the main arterial contributor to the dorsal nasal flap (see Chapter 10).

The nostril sill and columellar base are supplied by branches of the superior labial artery. A branch of the superior labial artery, the columellar artery, ascends superficial to the medial crura and is transected by a transcolumellar incision during an external rhinoplasty approach.

The nasal tip is supplied by the external nasal branch of the anterior ethmoidal artery as well as by the columellar artery. The anterior ethmoidal artery, a branch of the ophthalmic artery, pierces bone on the medial wall of the orbit at the point where the lamina papyracea of the ethmoid bone articulates with the orbital portion of the frontal bone (the frontoethmoid suture). The vessel enters the ethmoid sinuses to supply the mucosa and sends branches to the superior aspect of the nasal cavity. The external nasal branch of the anterior ethmoidal artery emerges between the nasal bone and the upper lateral cartilage to supply the skin covering the nasal tip. The blood supply of the nasal tip also receives contributions from the lateral nasal artery, a branch of the angular artery.

The venous drainage of the external nose consists of veins with names that correspond to the associated arteries. These veins drain via the facial vein, the pterygoid plexus, and the ophthalmic veins.

External Sensory Nerve Supply

The sensory nerve supply of the nasal skin is supplied by the ophthalmic and maxillary divisions of the fifth cranial nerve (Fig. 2–5). Branches of the supratrochlear

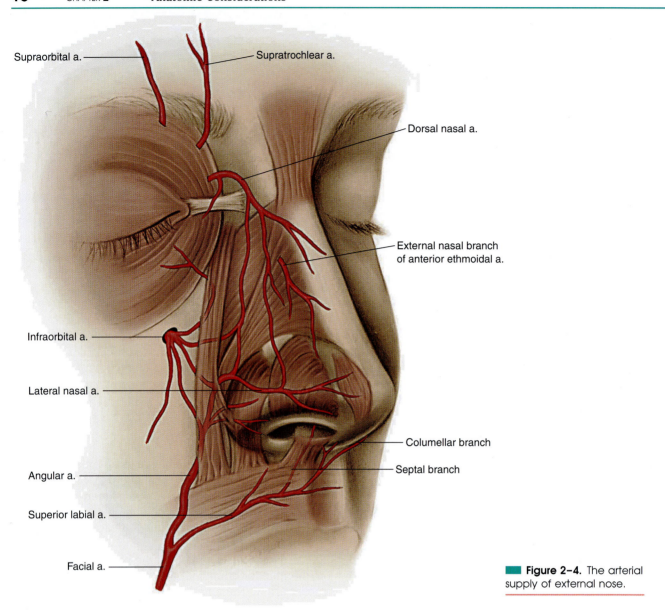

Supraorbital a.

Supratrochlear a.

Dorsal nasal a.

External nasal branch of anterior ethmoidal a.

Infraorbital a.

Lateral nasal a.

Columellar branch

Septal branch

Angular a.

Superior labial a.

Facial a.

Figure 2-4. The arterial supply of external nose.

and infratrochlear nerves supply the skin covering the radix, the rhinion, and the cephalic portion of the nasal sidewalls. The external nasal branch of the anterior ethmoidal nerve emerges between the nasal bone and the upper lateral cartilage to supply the skin over the caudal half of the nose. This nerve is usually transected by soft-tissue elevation during rhinoplasty. The infraorbital nerve provides sensory branches to the skin of the lateral aspect of the nose.

Nasal Skeletal Anatomy

A thorough understanding of the nasal skeleton is essential for proper reconstruction of the nose. When constructing framework grafts, errors in duplicating normal nasal contour may compromise the repair, leading to contour irregularities and functional limitations. The nasal framework consists of both bony and cartilaginous components (Fig. 2–6).

■ Nasal Tip

The caudal third of the nose consists of the lobule (tip), columella, vestibules, and alae. It is structurally supported by paired alar (lower lateral) cartilages, the caudal septum, accessory cartilages, and fibrous fatty connective tissue. The variable configuration of the nasal tip depends on the size, shape, orientation, and strength of the alar and septal cartilages and on the quality and thickness of overlying soft tissue and skin. The alar cartilages are attached to the upper lateral

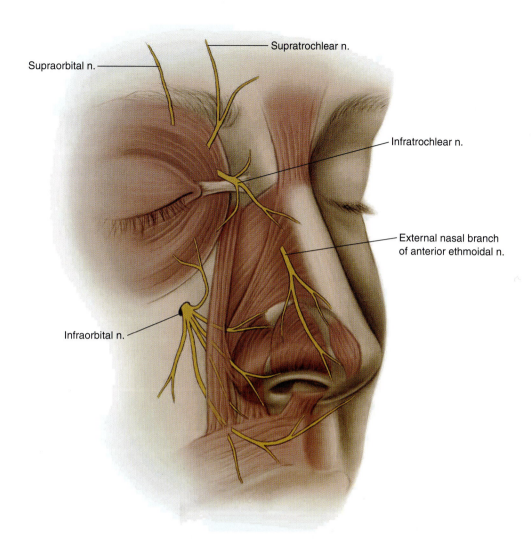

Supraorbital n.

Supratrochlear n.

Infratrochlear n.

External nasal branch
of anterior ethmoidal n.

Infraorbital n.

■ **Figure 2–5.** The sensory
nerve supply of external nose.

cartilages and the septum, and they provide the majority of the support for the tip. The vestibule is bounded medially by the septum and columella and laterally by the alar base. It contains a protruding fold of skin with vibrissae and terminates at the caudal edge of the lateral crus.

The alar cartilage is subdivided into medial, intermediate, and lateral crura (Figs. 2–7 and 2–8). The medial crus consists of the footplate and columellar segments. The footplate is more posterior and accounts for the flared portion of the columellar base. The columellar segment begins at the upper limit of the footplate and joins the intermediate crus at the columellar breakpoint. The breakpoint represents the junction of the tip and the columella. The appearance and projection of the columella are influenced by the configuration of the medial crura as well as that of the caudal septum. Intervening soft tissue between the columellar segments of the medial crura may fill this space; however, in patients with thin skin, the columella may have a bifid

appearance. Columellar asymmetries may be secondary to deflections of the caudal septum or intrinsic asymmetries of the alar cartilages. In the aesthetically pleasing nose, the columella is positioned 2 to 4 mm caudal to the alar margins, and the shape of the nasal base resembles an equilateral triangle. Attractive nostrils are teardrop-shaped, in the opinion of many.

The intermediate crus consists of a lobular and a domal segment. In the majority of noses, the cephalic borders of the lobular segment are in close approximation, and the caudal margins diverge.[10] The intermediate crura are bound together by the interdomal ligament, and lack of intervening soft tissue may give the supratip area a bifid appearance. On a lateral view, the internal structure responsible for the prominence of the tip-defining point, or pronasalae, is the cephalic edge of the domal segment of the intermediate crus. Thus, the shape, length, and angulation of the intermediate crura determine the configuration of the infratip lobule and the position of the tip-defining point. The supratip

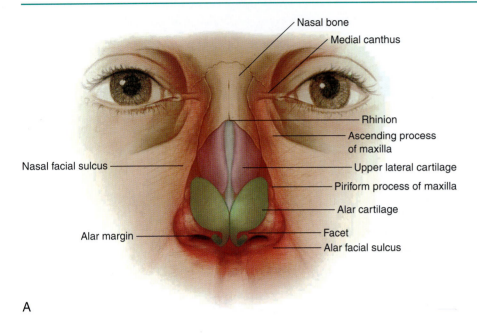

A

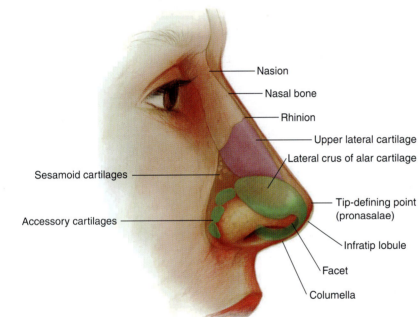

B

■ **Figure 2–6.** *A* and *B*, Nasal framework and soft-tissue relationships.

breakpoint is the junction between the intermediate crus and the lateral crus.

The lateral crus is the largest component of the alar cartilage; it provides support to the anterior half of the alar rim. Resection or weakening of the lateral crus causes a predisposition to alar retraction and notching, an important consideration during nasal reconstruction. Laterally, small sesamoid cartilages are interconnected by a dense, fibrous connective tissue that is contiguous with the superficial and deep perichondrium of the upper lateral cartilage and lateral crus. Inferolaterally, the ala contains fat and fibrous connective tissue but no cartilage. The shape and resiliency of the nostril depend on the dense, fibrous, fatty connective tissue lo-

cated within the confines of the ala, and the integrity of this area should be restored with cartilage grafting when necessary.

■ Cartilaginous Dorsum

The cartilaginous dorsum consists of paired upper lateral cartilages and the cartilaginous septum (see Fig. 2–6). The upper lateral cartilages are overlapped superiorly by the bony framework for a variable distance. The free caudal border of the nasal bones has fibrous connections to the cephalic margin of the upper lateral cartilages. The cephalic two thirds of the cartilaginous dorsum is a single cartilaginous unit. However, caudally

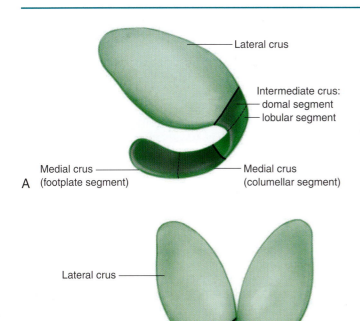

Lateral crus

Intermediate crus:
domal segment
lobular segment

Medial crus
(footplate segment)

Medial crus
(columellar segment)

A

Lateral crus

Intermediate crus
Medial crus

B

Figure 2–7. *A,* Lateral view of alar cartilage. *B,* Frontal view of paired alar cartilages.

there is gradual separation of the upper lateral cartilages from the septum. The lateral borders of the upper lateral cartilages are rectangular in shape and are connected to the piriform aperture by an aponeurosis.[10] The lateral border of the upper lateral cartilage creates a space known as the external lateral triangle. This space is bordered by the lateral edge of the upper lateral cartilage, the extreme lateral portion of the lateral crus, and the edge of the piriform fossa. The space is lined by mucosa and covered by the transverse portion of the nasalis muscle. It may contain accessory cartilages and fibrous fatty tissue that contribute to the lateral aspect of the internal nasal valve. Nasal obstruction may occur as a result of medialization of this space by scar tissue or cartilage grafts used in nasal reconstruction.

■ Bony Dorsum

The bony dorsum consists of paired nasal bones and paired ascending processes of the maxillae (see Fig. 2–6). The bony vault is pyramidal in shape, and the narrowest part is at the level of the intercanthal line. The bony dorsum is divided approximately in half by the intercanthal line, and the nasal bones are much thicker above this level.[11] The sellion is the deepest portion of the curve of soft tissue between the glabella and nasal dorsum, and it marks the level of the naso-

frontal suture line. The nasion is approximately at the level of the supratarsal fold of the upper eyelid. Laterally, the nasal bones articulate with the ascending processes of the maxillae.

Internal Nasal Anatomy

Reconstruction of full-thickness defects of the nose requires restoration of the external skin, the nasal framework, and the internal nasal lining. Failure to address deficiencies in nasal lining may lead to postoperative scarring, contracture, and functional compromise. A brief description of the internal nasal anatomy pertinent to nasal reconstruction follows.

■ Nasal Cavities

The nose is the gateway to the respiratory system. Partitioned by the septum, the nose provides two independent passages between the nostrils and the nasopharynx. Each passage is lined circumferentially with ciliated pseudostratified columnar epithelium. The nasal cavities begin at the limen nasi, which is the junction between the vestibule, lined with squamous epithelium, and the nasal cavities, lined with respiratory epithelium.

Along the lateral aspect of the nasal passages, the turbinates create a complex of mucosally lined peaks and valleys into which drain the ostia of the paranasal sinuses and the nasolacrimal duct. The superior aspect of the hard palate creates the floor of each nasal passage. The nasal roof is the underside of the nasal pyramid; it increases in vertical height anteroposteriorly from the nostril to the skull base. From this point, it decreases in height as it extends posteriorly along the face of the sphenoid to the choanal opening of the nasopharynx. The narrowest portion of each nasal passage is at the caudal margin of the upper lateral cartilage, an area referred to as the internal nasal valve.

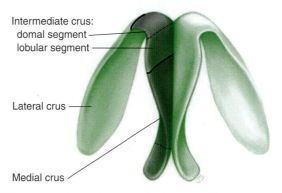

Intermediate crus:
domal segment
lobular segment

Lateral crus

Medial crus

Figure 2–8. Base view of paired alar cartilages.

■ Septum

The septum is constructed of bone posteriorly and cartilage anteriorly. The perpendicular plate of the ethmoid bone forms the bony septum. The cartilaginous septum is a flat plate of cartilage with an irregular quadrilateral shape that articulates with the perpendicular plate of the ethmoid bone, the vomer, and the premaxilla (Fig. 2–9). At the caudal septum, three angles are identified. The anterior septal angle can be palpated by depressing the nasal supratip area. The posterior septal angle is found just above the nasal spine articulation near the lip/nose junction. A midseptal angle is located halfway between the anterior and the posterior septal angles. It is common practice to harvest septal cartilage for use as a cartilage graft in nasal reconstruction. The septum provides support to the nasal dorsum and tip, and a supporting L-shaped strut of caudal and dorsal septum should be preserved to maintain this support.

The cartilaginous septum is covered on both sides by a thin but highly vascular layer of mucoperichondrium. An ideal plane of dissection is located between it and the cartilage. The septal cartilage is, however, dependent on the lining of the mucoperichondrium for its blood supply, and septal cartilage lacking mucoperichondrium on both sides will eventually undergo necrosis. When mucoperichondrium is present on one side of the septal cartilage, the cartilage is likely to survive.

The blood supply to the septum consists of the septal branch of the superior labial artery, branches of the anterior and posterior ethmoidal arteries, and the posterior septal branch of the sphenopalatine artery (Fig. 2–10). Arising from the facial artery, the superior labial artery travels through the orbicularis oris at the level of the vermilion border roll. Lateral to the philtrum and column, it gives off a septal branch that passes almost vertically upward and enters the nasal septum lateral to the nasal spine. It may travel on the cartilaginous septum as a discrete vessel before finally dispersing into the anterior septal vascular plexus. Given this arterial supply, a flap of septal mucoperichondrium can survive based on a 1.3-cm pedicle located in the area between the anterior plane of the upper lip and the lower edge of the piriform aperture. This hinged mucoperichondrial flap may extend from the nasal floor superiorly to the level of the medial canthus and posteriorly to beyond the junction of the cartilaginous septum and the bony septum. Septal flaps based on the septal branch of the superior labial artery may be used to line full-thickness ipsilateral lower nasal vault defects.[12] Dorsally based septal flaps supplied by branches of the anterior and posterior ethmoidal arteries may be used to line full-thickness defects of the contralateral nasal sidewalls.

■ Lateral Nasal Passage

The lateral wall of the nasal cavity contains three turbinates: superior, middle, and inferior. The turbinates are scrolls of bone covered by mucosa. Mucoperiosteal flaps from the inferior and middle turbinates may be used to repair small nasal lining defects. The blood

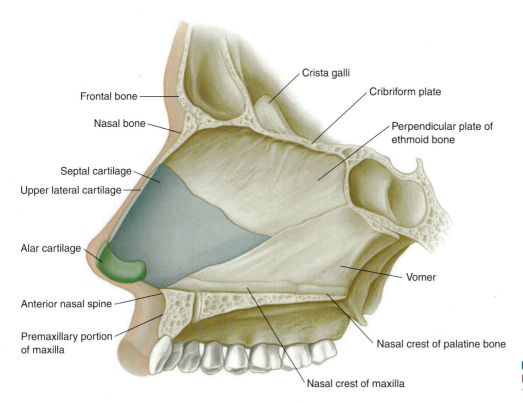

Figure 2–9. Lateral view of left nasal septum.

Crista galli

Cribriform plate

Frontal bone

Perpendicular plate of ethmoid bone

Nasal bone

Septal cartilage

Upper lateral cartilage

Alar cartilage

Vomer

Anterior nasal spine

Premaxillary portion of maxilla

Nasal crest of palatine bone

Nasal crest of maxilla

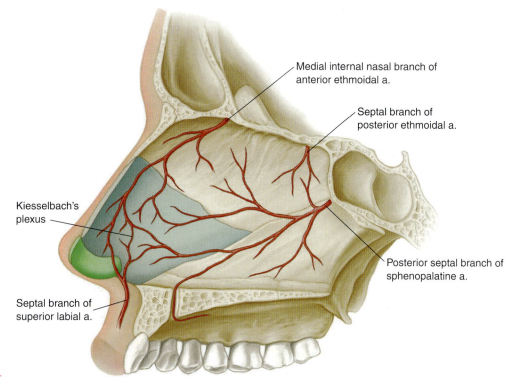

Figure 2–10. Arterial blood supply of left nasal septum.

supply to the lateral nasal passage is derived from branches of the anterior and posterior ethmoidal arteries, the angular artery, and the sphenopalatine artery (Fig. 2–11).

■ Nasal Valve

The internal nasal valve is the cross-sectional area bordered by the septum and the caudal margin of the

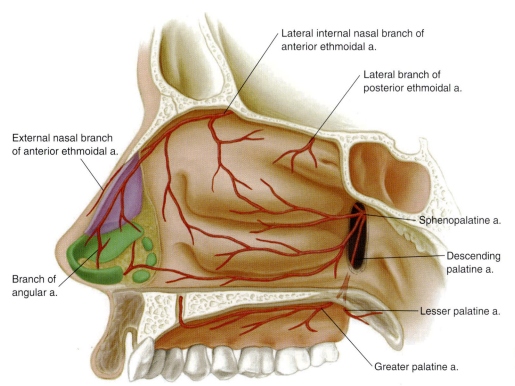

Figure 2–11. Arterial blood supply of right lateral wall of nasal cavity.

inferior turbinate and the upper lateral cartilage. This area may be compromised during tumor resection by the removal or weakening of its structural components. In addition, scar contracture resulting from nasal reconstruction may contribute to partial valve collapse unless preventive measures are performed at the time of surgery. If valve compromise is anticipated, structural cartilage grafts are employed to reinforce the valve.

References

1. Simons RL: Adjunctive measures in rhinoplasty. Otolaryngol Clin North Am 8:17, 1975.

2. Crumley RL, Lancer R: Quantitative analysis of nasal tip projection. Laryngoscope 2:202, 1988.

3. Burget GC, Menick FJ: The subunit principle in nasal reconstruction. Plast Reconstr Surg 76:239, 1985.

4. Lessard ML, Daniel RK: Surgical anatomy of septorhinoplasty. Arch Otolaryngol Head Neck Surg 111:25, 1985.

5. Zingaro EA, Falces E: Aesthetic anatomy of the non-Caucasian nose. Plast Surg Clin 14:749, 1987.

6. Oneal RM, Beil RJ, Schlesinger J: Surgical anatomy of the nose. Clin Plast Surg 23:195, 1996.

7. Firmin F: Discussion on Letourneau A, Daniel RK: The superficial musculoaponeurotic system of the nose. Plast Reconstr Surg 82:56, 1988.

8. Griesman BL: Muscles and cartilages of the nose from the standpoint of typical rhinoplasty. Arch Otolaryngol Head Neck Surg 39:334, 1994.

9. Letourneau A, Daniel RK: The superficial musculoaponeurotic system of the nose. Plast Reconstr Surg 82:48, 1988.

10. Daniel RK, Letourneau A: Rhinoplasty: Nasal anatomy. Ann Plast Surg 20:5, 1988.

11. Wright WK: Surgery of the bony and cartilaginous dorsum. Otolaryngol Clin North Am 8:575, 1975.

12. Burget GC, Menick FJ: Nasal support and lining: The marriage of beauty and blood supply. Plast Reconstr Surg 84:189, 1989.

3

Preparation of the Patient

Sam Naficy

Surgical restoration of the nose is, with few exceptions, a multistage procedure with a potentially protracted healing period before the final aesthetic outcome is evident. The initial reconstructive procedure is usually the most influential in predicting the aesthetic and functional result. Mucosa, cartilage, and facial skin are limited commodities. If the initial reconstructive effort squanders these resources through poor planning or execution, subsequent options for surgical restoration become more limited. The surgeon must carefully analyze the nasal defect and develop a cohesive surgical plan.

For many patients, the diagnosis of facial skin cancer and the perceived potential for unsightly scarring and distortion of facial features are traumatizing and create a great deal of anxiety. The patient must be prepared, emotionally and medically, through detailed explanation of the surgical plan. A thorough discussion of the required reconstructive stages is helpful in creating a trusting relationship between patient and surgeon.

Preoperative Consultation

Most of our patients undergo Mohs' surgery for a cutaneous malignancy. We work with the referring surgeon to provide an efficient and convenient coordination of care. Every attempt is made to schedule reconstruction on the day following surgery. To enable a smooth transition between the two procedures, all patients are seen preoperatively by the Mohs surgeon and the facial plastic surgeon. The consultation provides the opportunity to anticipate the extent of the defect to be repaired, assess the aesthetic demands of the patient, and discuss the reconstructive options. Depending on the location and anticipated size of the defect, patients may be provided with several reconstructive options.

Consideration is given to patient age, occupation, and aesthetic demands. As a general rule, younger patients have the highest aesthetic concerns and are more willing to tolerate a complex, multistage operation in order to obtain an optimal aesthetic result. While many older patients also have high aesthetic standards, some are willing to compromise the outcome in return for a single-stage operation with a more rapid recovery. The occupation of the patient may influence the choice of reconstructive procedures. Patients whose occupations require much public interaction are unable to perform their duties during the initial stage of reconstruction in which an interpolated forehead flap is used. The interpolated cheek flap, however, may be covered with a surgical bandage and allow the patient an earlier return to his or her occupation. Occupational use of corrective or protective eyewear or protective headwear should be considered when an interpolated paramedian forehead flap is required, as these items will be issues for the patient.

Factors are considered that may influence the extent of the nasal defect. These include tumor size, histology, and depth and whether the tumor represents a recurrence. Recurrent tumors or those with aggressive histologic features often require significantly larger excisions of nasal tissue than may be anticipated.

Most patients have a difficult time visualizing flaps

used in nasal reconstruction. This is especially true in the cases of interpolated cheek and paramedian forehead flaps. In order to prepare patients, they are shown a photograph album displaying representative preoperative and postoperative photographs of their anticipated operation. For staged repairs such as with interpolated flaps, photographs are shown that display an individual at each stage of the reconstruction. We have found this to be especially useful for younger patients for whom the shock of the initial deformity caused by an interpolated flap, without prior visual preparation, can be devastating and may create in the patient a feeling of hostility or resentment toward the surgeon. Photographs also allow patients to view the outcome of representative examples of different reconstructive techniques. The forehead or cheek scar and differences in skin color and texture are pointed out, particularly to those patients with the greatest aesthetic concerns. In order to develop realistic expectations of the outcome, patients with fair to average surgical results are included in the photograph album. A realistic estimate of when the patient may return to work and social activities is discussed, aided by photographs of representative reconstructive sequences.

The average number of surgical procedures and length of time required to complete all stages of the reconstruction are discussed with the patient (Table 3–1). In cases where an interpolated covering flap is planned, the reconstructive sequence includes initial flap transfer, pedicle division 3 weeks later, a contouring procedure 2 or 3 months following pedicle division, and possibly dermabrasion in the office 2 months after contouring the flap. We therefore advise patients that up to 6 months may be necessary to complete the restoration.

Preoperative consultation with the patient is ideally scheduled 4 to 6 weeks before surgery, allowing adequate time for the patient to stop anticoagulant agents. Medications to be avoided beginning up to 3 weeks before surgery include all nonsteroidal anti-inflammatory drugs and vitamin E supplements (Table 3–2). Coumadin should be discontinued 3 to 5 days before surgery. A number of herbal supplements also possess anticoagulant properties and should be avoided.

A medical history is obtained from the patient, and a

■ **Table 3–1. Estimated Number of Surgical Procedures and Recovery Periods**

TYPE OF PROCEDURE	NUMBER OF PROCEDURES	INITIAL RECOVERY
Local flap	1–2	1–2 weeks
Skin graft	2	1–2 weeks
Interpolated flap	2–4	4 weeks

■ **Table 3–2. List of Medications to Avoid Before Surgery**

NSAIDs (STOP 2–3 WEEKS PRIOR TO SURGERY)

Aspirin
Celecoxib
Diclofenac
Diflunisal
Etodolac
Fenoprofen
Flurbiprofen
Ibuprofen
Ketoprofen
Naproxen
Ketorolac
Rofecoxib
Sulindac
Tolmetin
Indomethacin

COUMADIN (STOP 3–5 DAYS PRIOR TO SURGERY)
NATURAL SUPPLEMENTS (STOP 2–3 WEEKS PRIOR TO SURGERY)

Asian ginseng
Bromelain
Cayenne fruit
Chinese skullcap root
Dan Shen root
Feverfew
Garlic
Ginger rhizome
Ginko biloba
Horse chestnut bark
Papain
Sweet clover plant
Sweet-scented bedstraw plant
Sweet vernal grass
Tonka bean seeds
Vanilla leaf leaves
Woodruff plant

VITAMIN E (STOP 3 WEEKS PRIOR TO SURGERY)

physical examination is performed as part of the consultation. The general health of the patient is noted, with special attention given to hypertension, symptomatic coronary artery disease, and smoking history. Smokers are strongly encouraged to quit and are instructed on the higher risk of complications for users of tobacco products. An electrocardiogram is obtained from all males older than 40 years and females older than 50 years. All patients older than 60 years are tested for hematocrit and blood levels of urea nitrogen, creatinine, and glucose (Table 3–3). During the physical examination, note is made of prior nasal or septal surgery, septal perforation, or ear surgery involving the cartilage. The patient is examined for scars on the forehead or cheeks that may potentially influence the design of flaps. The position of the anterior hairline is noted when a paramedian forehead flap is anticipated. Patients with low hairlines are informed about the possibility of the flap extending to hair-bearing scalp and the need for subsequent depilation procedures on the nose.

We provide patients with prescriptions for medica-

Table 3-3. Preoperative Requirements

AGE	MEN	WOMEN
<40	None	None
>40	ECG	None
>50	ECG	ECG and HCT
>60	ECG, HCT, BUN/Cr, Glu	ECG, HCT, BUN/Cr, Glu

Special Circumstances

1. Childbearing potential—puberty through menopause (1 year without a period). Obtain a pregnancy test if the patient:
   a. Has missed or late period or irregular periods.
   b. Is having unprotected intercourse.
   c. Has any of the symptoms of pregnancy—breast tenderness, nausea, bloating, etc.
   d. Believes there is a chance she might be pregnant.
2. Diabetics—fasting glucose on day of surgery
3. Patients on digitalis (Lanoxin) or diuretics—potassium level is required
4. Bleeding problems
   a. Patient is on anticoagulants—obtain PT.
   b. Patient complains of bleeding disorder—obtain PT/PTT, complete blood cell with platelet count, and a bleeding time.
5. Kidney disease—for patients with known renal insufficiency or on dialysis, obtain electrolytes, BUN, creatinine, and HCT
6. Chest radiograph or radiograph report—required if the patient has been hospitalized for treatment of CHF, pneumonia, or other lung disease (chronic obstructive pulmonary disease, asthma) within the last 6 months

BUN, blood urea nitrogen; CHF, congestive heart failure; Cr, creatinine; ECG, electrocardiogram; Glu, glucose; HCT, hematocrit; PT, prothrombin time; PTT, partial thromboplastin time.

tions at the time of the preoperative consultation (Table 3–4). Oral diazepam (5 to 10 mg) is prescribed, with instructions to take the evening before and 1 hour prior to the operation. Benzodiazepines help reduce preoperative anxiety and counteract the toxic effects of local anesthetics used during the procedure. In instances when skin or composite grafting is planned or when cartilage and bone grafting is anticipated, patients are given a postoperative course of an oral antistaphylococcal antibiotic for 5 to 7 days. A tapering dose pack of prednisone is prescribed for those patients undergoing composite grafting. An analgesic of choice is prescribed in appropriate quantity. In addition to the standard medications, those patients requiring a forehead flap are prescribed a 2-day supply of antiemetic suppositories.

Patients are encouraged to visit the office on the day of their Mohs surgery following completion of tumor resection. This visit enables the surgeon to examine and photograph the defect and to confirm or modify the surgical plan. This visit is often reassuring to the patient and allows the surgeon sufficient time to make adjust-

ments and alterations of the surgical plan and the operative schedule.

Photography

My technique for photography has been consistent over the past 12 years. Most photographs in this book were obtained using the following setup. My system utilizes two 35-mm SLR camera bodies, each outfitted with a 90-mm macro lens. One camera is used for slide photography, using 100 ASA, E-8 processed color slide film. The other camera uses 100 ASA color print film. Two ceiling-mounted strobe flashes are aimed at an angle of 25 to 30 degrees, 6 feet from the subject. The strobe flashes are hard-wired to the camera bodies for synchronization. A backlight illuminates a blue background to eliminate shadow. Blue is chosen as the background color as it provides an excellent contrast to the color of flesh and hair.

Photography in the operating room utilizes a 35-mm SLR camera with a macro lens. I use a 55-mm lens or a 60-mm lens. The cameras are equipped with a mounted ring flash for close-up photography. The operating room

Table 3-4. Recommended Medications

LOCAL FLAP OR INTERPOLATED CHEEK FLAP

Diazepam (preoperative)
Narcotic analgesic with acetaminophen

LOCAL FLAP OR INTERPOLATED CHEEK FLAP AND CARTILAGE GRAFT

Diazepam (preoperative)
Cephalexin (5–7 days)
Narcotic analgesic with acetaminophen

SKIN GRAFT

Diazepam (preoperative)
Cephalexin (5–7 days)
Narcotic analgesic with acetaminophen

COMPOSITE GRAFT

Diazepam (preoperative)
Cephalexin (5–7 days)
Prednisone dose pack
Narcotic analgesic with acetaminophen

INTERPOLATED FOREHEAD FLAP

Diazepam (preoperative)
Phenergan suppositories (postoperative)
Narcotic analgesic with acetaminophen

INTERPOLATED FOREHEAD FLAP AND CARTILAGE OR BONE GRAFTS

Diazepam (preoperative)
Cephalexin (5–7 days)
Phenergan suppositories (postoperative)
Narcotic analgesic with acetaminophen

lights are turned away from the subject because they give an undesirable yellow color to the photograph. In the operating room, a blue or green surgical towel often serves as an adequate substitute for the photographic background.

Photographic documentation is similar to that for rhinoplasty and includes those views that illustrate the nasal defect. These typically consist of a full-face frontal view, with oblique and lateral views on the side of the defect. If the defect extends to the infratip lobule or alar margin, a base view is also obtained. Close-up views of the defect may be obtained when appropriate. For nasal cutaneous malignancy, we have found it helpful to obtain photographs of the lesion at the time of initial consultation, prior to surgery. Photographs of the defect are obtained in the office photography suite if the patient is seen on the day before repair. Otherwise, photographs are obtained in the holding area or operating suite with proper regard for lighting and background.

Anesthesia

Monitored anesthesia care is appropriate for the majority of reconstructive nasal procedures, including all skin grafts, local or regional flaps, and cartilage grafts. The patient is placed on the operating table, with the head turned 90 to 120 degrees from the anesthetist but near enough to the anesthetist to allow manipulation of the airway if necessary (Fig. 3–1). The patient is positioned supine without a special headrest. A doughnut-shaped

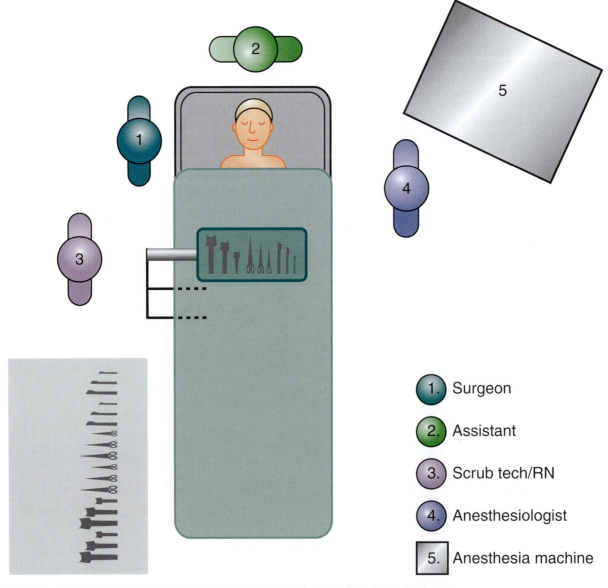

1. Surgeon
2. Assistant
3. Scrub tech/RN
4. Anesthesiologist
5. Anesthesia machine

Figure 3–1. Operating room setup for nasal reconstruction using monitored anesthesia care.

foam pillow is placed under the patient's head, and a towel roll supports the shoulder. A standard-sized pillow is placed under the knees to provide flexion and reduce back strain. The bed is placed in an appropriate degree of reverse Trendelenburg's position to reduce venous pooling in the face. Oxygen is administered at the rate of 2 to 4 L/min via nasal canula tubing either nasally or orally. Preoxygenation reduces the toxic effects of local anesthetics and accommodates for brief periods of apnea caused by intravenous sedation. It is important to reduce or stop the flow of oxygen during cautery to prevent the risk of fire.

After adequate oxygenation, the patient is given a bolus of intravenous sedatives and narcotics, achieving an adequate depth of anesthesia to enable the surgeon to infiltrate the local anesthetic. It is not uncommon for the patient to require a chin thrust at this point to prevent transient apnea. Following infiltration of the local anesthetic, the patient is maintained at an appropriate level of intravenous sedation for the duration of the procedure.

General anesthesia is used when cranial bone grafting is performed or when large septal mucoperichondrial flaps are required to repair full-thickness defects. An oral RAE tube taped in the midline to only the lower lip and chin offers the least amount of obstruction and distortion of the surgical field. An alternative is the use of laryngeal mask ventilation. The nose and face are painted with iodine, and a surgical drape is wrapped around the head in a turban fashion, exposing the entire face and donor sites if applicable. Moistened eye pads are place over the eyes to protect them from the intense overhead light and accidental injury. A preoperative intravenous dose of an antistaphylococcal antibiotic is administered when grafting is performed.

Local Anesthesia

The four methods of local anesthesia applicable to nasal surgery are topical, local infiltration, field block (ring block), and peripheral nerve block. Topical anesthesia and vasoconstriction of nasal mucosa are performed for all procedures where the inside of the nose is manipulated. Inside the nose are placed half- × 3-inch surgical cottonoids treated with an equal mixture of topical lidocaine 4% and oxymetazoline hydrochloride. The topical medicine is left in contact with the nasal mucosa for a few minutes prior to injecting the mucosa with local anesthetic. The septum is injected in the subperichondrial plane with a 27-gauge needle and a 3-mL syringe for adequate hydraulic force.

It may be useful to perform nerve blocks before injection of the external nasal tissue. An anesthetic block of the lateral nose can be obtained by infiltrating the infraorbital (V2) nerve as it exits the maxilla. The nerve exits the infraorbital foramen 1 cm below the level of the inferior orbital rim, vertically aligned with the pupil (Fig. 3–2). The nerve is blocked by injecting 1 mL of lidocaine (1% with 1:100,000 concentration of epinephrine) just above the periosteum around the site of exit of the nerve from the foramen. The injection may be performed percutaneously with a 30-gauge needle or through the gingivobuccal sulcus using a 27-gauge needle. The external nasal branch of the anterior ethmoidal nerve supplies the skin of the caudal half of the nasal dorsum and most of the tip. This nerve is blocked by injection of anesthetic in the subfascial plane of the nasal sidewall at the junction of nasal bone and upper lateral cartilage approximately 1 cm lateral to the midline. The infratrochlear nerve supplies the skin of the upper nasal vault. This nerve is blocked by infiltration of anesthetic under the thin skin of the lateral nasal sidewall, medial to the medial canthus and root of the nose. Bilateral blocks of these nerves will result in anesthesia of the majority of the skin and soft tissue of the nose, medial cheek, and upper lip.

Local anesthetic solution is injected in the desired plane of dissection and more superficially to the level of the subdermis using multiple punctures with a 30-gauge needle. A longer, 27-gauge needle is used for injection of the septum and turbinates and for infraorbital nerve blocks.

Choice of local anesthetic depends on the length of the procedure and the desired amount of postoperative analgesia. Procedures lasting less than 1.5 hours are performed using lidocaine (1% with 1:100,000 concentration of epinephrine). Longer anesthesia of up to 2.5 hours may be obtained by using lidocaine (2% with 1:100,000 concentration of epinephrine). One of our preferred local anesthetic formulations prepared just prior to injection is an equal (1:1) mixture of lidocaine (1% with 1:100,000 concentration of epinephrine) and bupivacaine (0.25% to 0.5% plain). The lidocaine provides immediate anesthesia and vasoconstriction while the longer acting bupivacaine provides an additional 3 to 6 hours of anesthesia. The lidocaine compensates for the longer onset of action of bupivacaine. The diluted epinephrine in the mixture is just as effective for hemostasis because there is no additional vasoconstrictive benefit with concentrations of epinephrine greater than 1:200,000.

Postoperative Care and Supplies

Written postoperative instructions that cover general wound care (Table 3–5) are provided. Patients are provided with an adequate supply of cotton tip applicators,

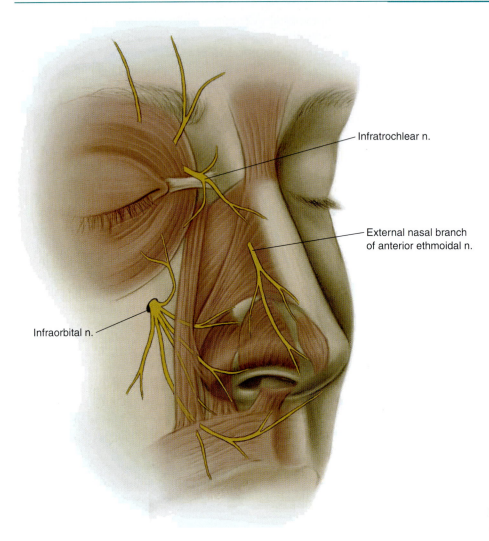

Infratrochlear n.

External nasal branch
of anterior ethmoidal n.

Infraorbital n.

Figure 3–2. Nerve blocks for nasal surgery.

hydrogen peroxide, and antibiotic ointment. Patients are instructed to avoid heavy lifting, bending, straining, and nose blowing. There are other postoperative instructions specific to each procedure.

Table 3–5. General Wound Care Instructions

1. Remove compression dressing the day following the procedure.

2. Clean sutures with cotton-tip applicators and peroxide or soap and water 3 times a day.

3. Apply bacitracin ointment 3 times a day for 3 days.

4. Patient may shower the day following the operation using lukewarm water on the face and avoiding a direct forceful spray to the operative site. Patient should apply ointment to the sutures after showering.

Hospitalization

The majority of cases of nasal reconstruction are performed on an outpatient basis. There are three categories of patients who are admitted overnight following the procedure. Patients requiring interpolated paramedian forehead flaps are admitted for control of pain and nausea. Nausea and vomiting are common following use of forehead flaps and are presumably due to tension on the galea aponeurotica. Patients requiring hinged septal mucoperichondrial flaps are admitted for observation and to decrease risk of early postoperative bleeding. Patients requiring cranial bone or rib grafting are admitted for pain control and because of the prolonged duration of such operations.

4

Internal Lining

Shan R. Baker

When a portion of the nose is missing, the ideal surgical approach is to repair it with an equal quantity of similar tissue. This is particularly important when dealing with the lining of the nasal passages.

The nine aesthetic units of the nose are identified by topographically distinct convex or concave surfaces. These units are the nasal tip "lobule," dorsum, paired sidewalls, paired alae, paired nasal facets (soft triangles), and columella. The lining tissue for each of the nine units is distinctive.[1, 2] Thin, non–hair-bearing skin lines the nasal tip, whereas the nasal facets and alae are lined by thicker skin, the caudal aspect of which is hair-bearing. The columella is backed by the membranous septum, which is skin-lined. At the piriform aperture, the skin lining the tip and alae transition to mucosa that lines the dorsum and sidewall units. Whenever possible, epithelial lining similar to these lining tissues should be used to resurface the interior of the nose.

In the past, full-thickness skin grafts were commonly used for nasal lining. However, skin grafts not only contract and possibly compromise the airway but also do not provide vascular support to cartilage and bone grafts. Turn-in hinge flaps harvested from the nasal skin adjacent to the wound margins have also been used for lining. These flaps, which are tenuously based on scar tissue formed at the edge of the wound, also lack sufficient vascularity to nourish cartilage and bone grafts necessary for the nasal framework. Partial or complete necrosis frequently leads to exposure and subsequent extrusion of the grafts, in turn leading to constriction of the airway as the wound contracts.

Because skin grafts function poorly as nasal lining, folding the covering flap internally was advocated so that the distal portion of the flap would line the defect and the more proximal portion would serve as external cover. When used at the nostril margin, however, this technique causes an abnormally thick alar margin and obstructs the aperture. Flap bulkiness also prevents the manifestation of the contour of structural framework grafts. This technique of folding a flap on itself should not be used in the region of the internal nasal valve, because tissue bulk will invariably obstruct the airway.

Cutaneous flaps from the cheek were used by Millard and others[3, 4] to line the caudal nose. These flaps usually take the form of superiorly based melolabial flaps that are positioned as closely as possible to the site of an alar defect. The flap is hinged on a subcutaneous or cutaneous base and turned medially to line lateral alar defects or the entire nasal vestibule. Millard delayed flaps such as these prior to their transfer to the nose. Although cheek flaps are more vascular than the distal portion of a covering flap folded on itself, they have the disadvantage of providing a lining with excessive bulk that will crowd the airway and overwhelm the cartilaginous grafts that are used for the nasal framework.

The evolution of the central forehead flap from midline to paramedian has allowed the development of dual flaps that are able to be harvested simultaneously. One flap may be used for lining the internal nasal defect while the other serves as a covering flap. The paramedian forehead flap used for lining provides vascular tissue that readily supports framework grafts. As the thick skin of the forehead presents the same problems of bulkiness and inflexibility as the nasal turn-in and hinged cutaneous cheek flaps, its use should be restricted to total and near-total nasal defects where there is inadequate tissue for lining flaps consisting of mucoperichondrium.

Fortunately, the lining for the majority of full-thickness nasal defects can be provided from intranasal donor sites. These sites include skin of the vestibule, mucosa of the middle vault, turbinate mucosa, and mucoperichondrium of both sides of the septum. Flaps from these sites are sufficiently flexible to conform to overlying cartilage and bone grafts used for the nasal framework; most critically, they are vascular enough to nourish the grafts. Except for limited situations, intranasal flaps are the preferred source of lining when available.

Primary Closure

Primary closure may be accomplished with certain internal lining defects of the nasal vestibule that are limited in size to less than 0.5 cm without compromising the results of the repair. This situation arises most commonly with alar defects where the surgeon is confronted with a small hole in the vestibular skin. The use of hydrodissection facilitates undermining the adjacent skin to enable primary repair and prevents inadvertent perforation of the mobilized skin. Defects that cannot be closed in this manner may require a releasing incision that consists of an intercartilaginous incision between the lower and upper lateral cartilages. The wound created by the releasing incision is left to heal by secondary intention only if the gap in skin continuity is less than 4 mm. Larger gaps should be covered with a thin full-thickness skin graft to prevent contraction of the lateral aspect of the internal nasal valve.

Full-thickness Skin Grafts

Although intranasal flaps are preferred for lining full-thickness nasal defects, there are occasions when full-thickness skin grafts may be appropriate for repair of limited lining defects. An example of this is the repair of the donor site for a bipedicle vestibular skin advancement flap used to resurface nostril margin and caudal alar lining deficits. In this case, the donor site for the advancement flap is located on the undersurface of the remaining lateral crus and caudal aspect of the upper lateral cartilage. The soft tissue on the underside of these cartilages is left intact and, thus, the donor site may be repaired with a thin full-thickness skin graft. The graft is most frequently harvested from the standing cutaneous deformity of the cheek that results from clo-

sure of the donor site of a cheek flap used externally for covering the nasal defect. The graft should be slightly oversized to accommodate wound contraction.

Skin grafts have no intrinsic blood supply and must be placed in a highly vascular recipient site to ensure their survival. Primary cartilage grafts should not be interposed between the graft and its recipient bed because they will prevent neovascularization of the graft and result in the loss of skin and cartilage. Small skin grafts (less than 1 cm in diameter) are occasionally capable of surviving by a bridging effect of peripheral tissue and may not compromise an underlying cartilage graft. To overcome this difficulty of graft survival, surgeons have placed skin grafts under delayed covering flaps prior to transfer to the nose. Similarly, composite nasal septal grafts have been buried beneath covering flaps in a delayed fashion; although these grafts survive, they undergo considerable tissue shrinkage from wound contraction. The process inevitably creates a thick rigid flap that cannot readily be contoured. Burget and Menick[5] have, to a degree, circumvented this problem by performing a staged sequential approach that combines primary and delayed cartilage grafts placed between the skin and frontalis muscle of a forehead flap and a skin graft on the undersurface of the frontalis muscle. This technique is possible because the skin and subcutaneous tissue of a paramedian forehead flap have an axial blood supply that is independent of the axial supply to the underlying galeofrontalis muscle and fascia. Both components are supplied by the supratrochlear artery and their anastomoses with adjacent vessels. At the initial operation, the paramedian forehead flap is transferred to a full-thickness nasal defect, and contour cartilage grafts are placed within tunnels developed between the skin and muscle of the flap. A full-thickness skin graft is simultaneously applied to the undersurface of the muscle to line the defect completely. The second stage is performed 3 weeks later. Excessive subcutaneous tissue and scar are excised from the flap, and additional cartilage or bone is inserted cephalic to the original grafts to restore a complete nasal framework. The forehead flap is then detached from the brow or is subsequently divided at a third stage. This approach addresses the three requirements of aesthetic nasal reconstruction: a thin epithelial lining that is backed by the frontalis muscle; support provided by a contouring framework of cartilage and bone; and the coverage of a contouring skin flap.[5] However, this approach requires a two- or three-stage procedure and offers few advantages over the use of intranasal lining flaps. This method should be limited to situations where the nasal septum is not available as a donor site for a mucoperichondrial lining flap. The vestibule, septum, and inferior and middle turbinates are the preferred donor sites for lining flaps. Only tissue from these areas provide thin, well-vascularized flaps that conform readily to a fabricated framework.

Bipedicle Vestibular Skin Advancement Flap

Full-thickness defects of the ala and hemitip that have a vertical height of 1.0 cm or less can be lined by a bipedicle vestibular skin advancement flap. This skin-only flap is based on the floor of the vestibule laterally and nasal septum medially. An intercartilaginous incision is made between the upper and lower lateral cartilages from the nasal septum to the lateral floor of the vestibule (Fig. 4–1). For a wider flap, the incision may be placed more cephalically under the ventral aspect of the upper lateral cartilage. Attachment of the skin to the overlying upper lateral and remaining lower lateral cartilages is released by careful dissection to prevent perforating the thin but vascular flap. Hydrodissection using a local anesthetic solution is helpful. The solution is injected between the vestibular skin and overlying alar cartilage to increase the thickness of the tissue plane between these two structures. The remaining lower and upper lateral cartilages with their intact perichondrium are left attached to the septum. The flap is mobilized sufficiently to allow easy caudal advancement to the level of the alar margin in cases of full-thickness alar margin defects. The donor site for the flap is resurfaced with a thinned full-thickness skin graft. This is usually harvested from the standing cutaneous deformity that forms at the donor site for the cheek flap that is used to provide external cover for the reconstructed ala. The skin graft is supported by the overlying perichondrium of the lower lateral cartilage and does not constrict the internal nasal valve. It is not necessary to include portions of the upper lateral cartilage or lateral crus in the bipedicle vestibular skin advancement flap. This maneuver has been recom-

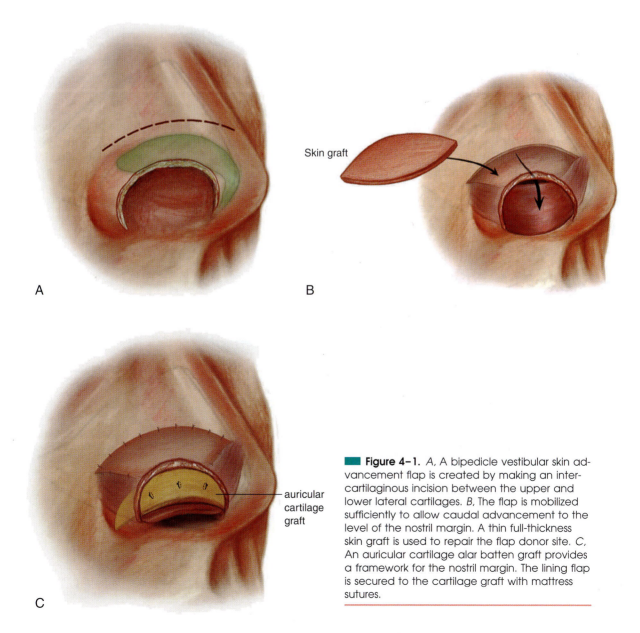

Skin graft

A

B

C

auricular cartilage graft

■ **Figure 4–1.** *A,* A bipedicle vestibular advancement flap is created by making an intercartilaginous incision between the upper and lower lateral cartilages. *B,* The flap is mobilized sufficiently to allow caudal advancement to the level of the nostril margin. A thin full-thickness skin graft is used to repair the flap donor site. *C,* An auricular cartilage alar batten graft provides a framework for the nostril margin. The lining flap is secured to the cartilage graft with mattress sutures.

mended by Burget and Menick[5] presumably because it provides a composite flap that simultaneously provides lining and a framework of cartilage for structural support of the nostril margin. An auricular cartilage alar batten graft will serve the same purpose of providing contour and support to the nostril while avoiding the need to disturb intact alar cartilage. Including the alar cartilage in the flap enlarges the defect cephalically, and if the overlying nasal skin is absent in the area of the alar cartilage, it creates a larger full-thickness defect. This, in turn, mandates a septal mucoperichondrial flap to close the donor site of the advance flap.

Septal Mucoperichondrial Hinge Flap

The posterior arterial supply to the mucosa of the nasal septum flows from the septal branches of the sphenopalatine arteries, and the anterosuperior arterial supply is derived from the ethmoid arteries (Fig. 4–2). The anteroinferior blood supply of the septum is derived principally from bilateral septal branches of the superior labial arteries. The labial arteries arise from the facial arteries to form a vascular arcade with each other across the upper lip, with the arteries positioned just deep to the mucosa and adjacent to the wet line of the vermilion. The septal branches of the superior labial arteries arise lateral to the philtrum columns passing vertically to the septum at the level of the anterior nasal spine. Blood supplied from this source is sufficient to nourish a flap of either unilateral or bilateral septal mucoperichondrium with or without intervening septal cartilage.[2] Based on this blood supply, Burget and Menick have shown that large flaps of septal mucoperichondrium will survive. The mucoperichondrium covering the entire height of the septum and extending posteriorly well beyond the anterior border of the perpendicular plate of the ethmoid bone may be developed as a flap based on a single septal branch of the superior labial artery. This flap has been shown to survive if based on a pedicle 1.3 cm wide located in the zone between the anterior plane of the upper lip and the inferior medial border of the piriform aperture.[2] The narrow pedicle is created by extending a back-cut inferiorly toward the anterior nasal spine from a dorsal incision near the anterior septal angle. The author prefers to base ipsilateral septal flaps on the entire height of the caudal septum and then turn the flap laterally as a hinged flap in contrast to the greater pivotal movement advocated by Burget and Menick.[1] The author's design may enhance the survival of longer flaps and has allowed the successful use of extended septal mucoperichondrial hinge flaps even when the ipsilateral septal branch of the labial artery may have been resected (Fig. 4–3). An alternative in these situations is to raise a unilateral hinge flap based on the contralateral septal branch of the superior labial artery. The flap is

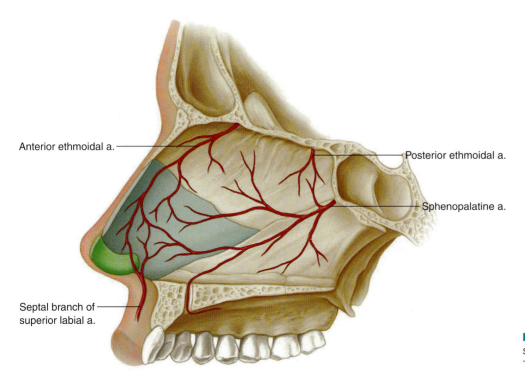

Anterior ethmoidal a.

Posterior ethmoidal a.

Sphenopalatine a.

Septal branch of superior labial a.

Figure 4–2. The arterial supply to the nasal septum.

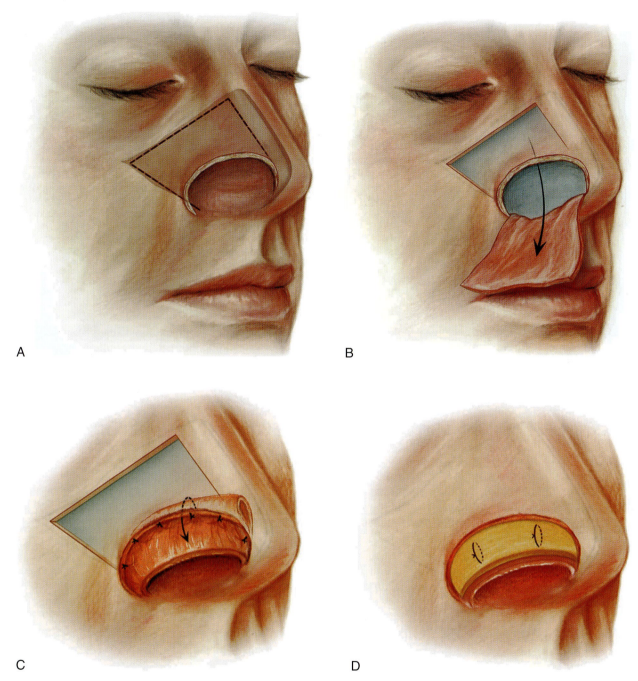

A

B

C

D

■ **Figure 4–3.** *A,* A unilateral septal mucoperichondrial hinge flap is developed by incising through the mucosa and perichondrium along the floor of the nose and 1.5 cm below and parallel to the cartilaginous dorsum. Incisions extend posteriorly beyond the septal bony cartilaginous junction. *B,* The flap is dissected from superior to inferior and from posterior to anterior. The anterior dissection remains 1 cm posterior to the caudal border of the septum and 1.5 cm posterior to the nasal spine. The flap is based on the intact mucoperiochondrium of the caudal septum and the region of the nasal spine. *C,* Hinged on the caudal septum, the flap is reflected laterally to line the lower nasal vault. *D,* A cartilage graft provides the nasal framework. The lining flap is secured to the framework with mattress sutures.

used to line a contralateral hemitip or alar lining defect. It is delivered through a fenestrum that is created 1 cm posterior to the caudal aspect of the septum (Fig. 4–4) (see Chapter 11).

The anterior ethmoid artery is the predominant source of vascular supply to the anterosuperior septum. This vessel supplies a mucoperichondrial flap hinged on the dorsal septum. Originally described as a composite flap,

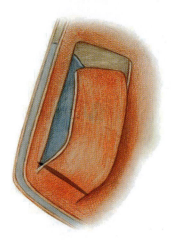
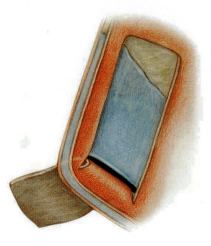

Figure 4-4. When the ipsilateral septal branch of the labial artery is absent, a contralateral septal mucoperichondrial flap may be delivered through a septal fenestrum to line the lower nasal vault.

the mucoperichondrial flap has been used for nearly a century by many surgeons. Its dimensions may equal the height and length of the septum, and it is transferred laterally toward the contralateral side as a hinge flap, with the raw surface facing exteriorly. Although it may be transferred with septal cartilage attached, movement is facilitated by removing the cartilage and using it as a free graft. The dorsal septal mucoperichondrial hinge flap is most frequently used to provide lining to the contralateral nasal sidewall and roof of the middle vault. The flap may be delivered through a superiorly located fenestrum of the contralateral mucoperichondrium in situations where the more caudal nose is intact and lining is necessary only for the more cephalically located middle vault.

Unilateral septal mucoperichondrial hinge flaps based on the septal branch of the superior labial artery may be used to line the nasal tip and ala and are often used in combination with a contralateral dorsal septal mucoperichondrial hinge flap. The hinge flap based on the caudal septum is used to line the lower nasal vault; the contralateral dorsal septal flap is used to line the middle vault. Thus, the lining for an entire full-thickness heminasal defect can be provided by septal mucoperichondrium (Fig. 4–5).

Although the septal mucoperichondrial hinge flap based on the caudal septum has a sufficient vascular supply in the majority of patients, it is slightly less dependable in patients who use tobacco products. It has the disadvantage of extending across the nasal airway in order to reach the lateral aspects of the nasal vestibule and almost completely obstructs the involved nasal passage. Three weeks following the initial transfer, the flap is detached from the septum simultaneously with the detachment of the interpolated cheek or paramedian forehead flap used for external lining of the nasal defect. In contrast, the dorsal septal hinge flap usually does not require detachment as it is draped across the roof and sidewall of the middle vault to reline these areas and does not constrict the airway. Detachment may be required in instances where the roof of the middle vault is intact and the flap extends across the nasal passage below the roof to reach a lateral wall defect. In this case, the flap is detached 3 weeks following transfer.

Composite Septal Chondromucosal Pivotal Flap

The entire septum may be utilized as a composite chondromucosal flap lined by two mucous membranes. The composite flap may be pivoted 90 degrees anteriorly to provide lining and structural support for bilateral full-thickness nasal tip and columellar defects. To achieve tissue movement, it is necessary to remove a small amount of bone and cartilage in the region of the nasal spine to facilitate tilting of the composite flap outward in an anterocaudal direction. Thus, after a submucosal tunnel is created at the anterior nasal spine by elevating the mucoperichondrium away from the midline bilaterally, a rongeur is used to remove sufficient bone and cartilage to enable the flap to pivot with minimal resistance.

Composite flaps used to reconstruct full-thickness defects of the nasal tip and columella are designed to be 1.5 to 2.0 cm wide and are pivoted 90 to 110 degrees anterocaudally. If present, a dorsal cartilaginous strut 1.0 cm wide is preserved to maintain structural support of the middle vault (Fig. 4–6). As the flap pivots antero-

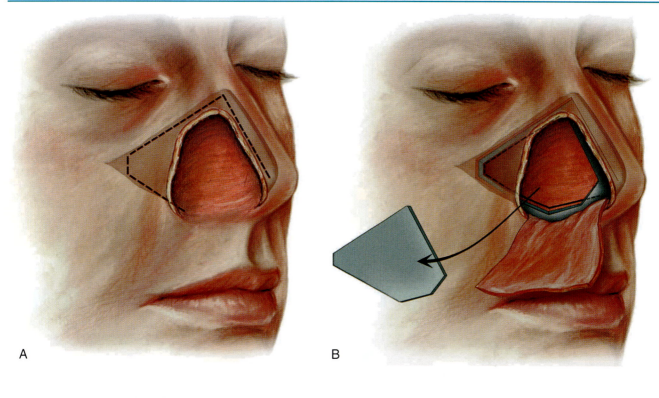

A

B

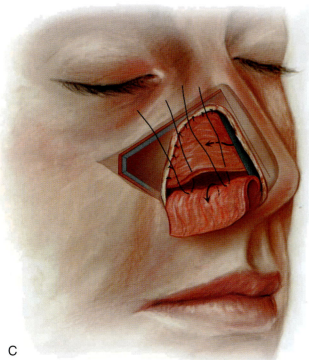

C

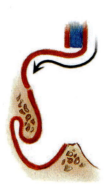

Figure 4–5. *A,* The broken line indicates the incision for an ipsilateral septal mucoperichondrial hinge flap. *B,* The ipsilateral flap is reflected outward, and exposed septal cartilage is removed. The *broken* and *solid lines* indicate the incisions for a contralateral dorsal septal mucoperichondrial hinge flap. *C,* A dorsally based flap is reflected laterally and sutured to the borders of the middle vault lining defect. The caudal border of the flap is sutured to the raw surface of the ipsilateral flap to seal the nasal passage from the exterior.

Illustration continued on following page

caudally, the cephalic aspect of the flap is locked in place by abutting it against the remaining dorsal cartilaginous septum. The flap is then secured to the remaining dorsal septum with a figure-of-eight suture.

The caudal aspect of the pivoted flap becomes the structural support and lining for the missing columella. Cartilage and bone are trimmed to prevent excessive visibility of the columella on profile. The mucosal

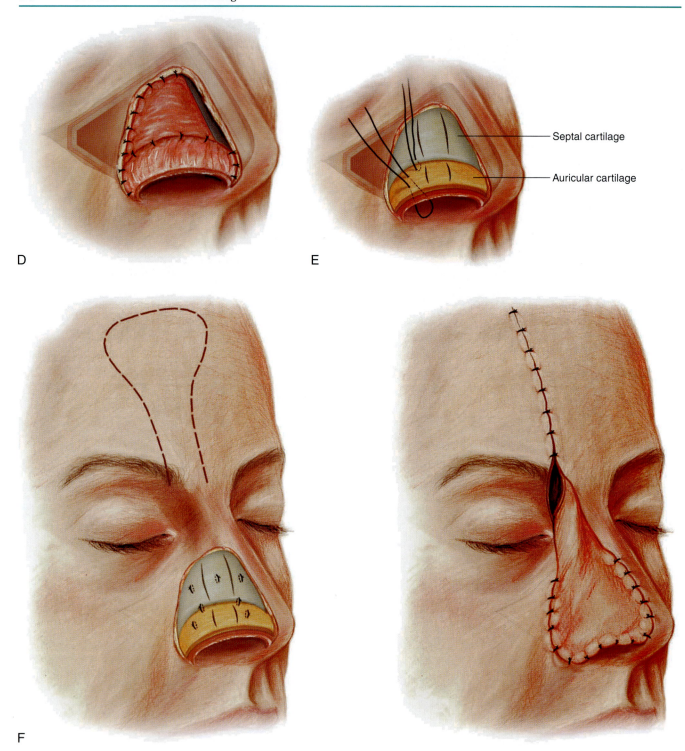

D

E

Septal cartilage

Auricular cartilage

F

Figure 4–5 *Continued. D,* The caudally based hinge flap provides the lining for the lower nasal vault; the contralateral dorsally based hinge flap provides the lining for the middle and upper nasal vaults. *E,* The septal cartilage (blue) provides a framework for the middle nasal vault; the auricular cartilage (yellow) provides a framework for the lower nasal vault. Cartilage grafts are scored to create the desired convex contour. The lining flaps are attached to the framework with mattress sutures. *F,* The nasal framework is covered by a paramedian forehead flap.

leaves of the anterior aspect of the positioned composite flap are peeled downward and reflected laterally to provide lining to the tip and vestibules. The greater the loss of nasal vestibular lining, the longer the composite flap must be in order to give sufficient length to the reflected mucoperichondrial flaps to adequately span the arc of the domes and line the lateral vestibules.

In instances where the nasal tip is present but the

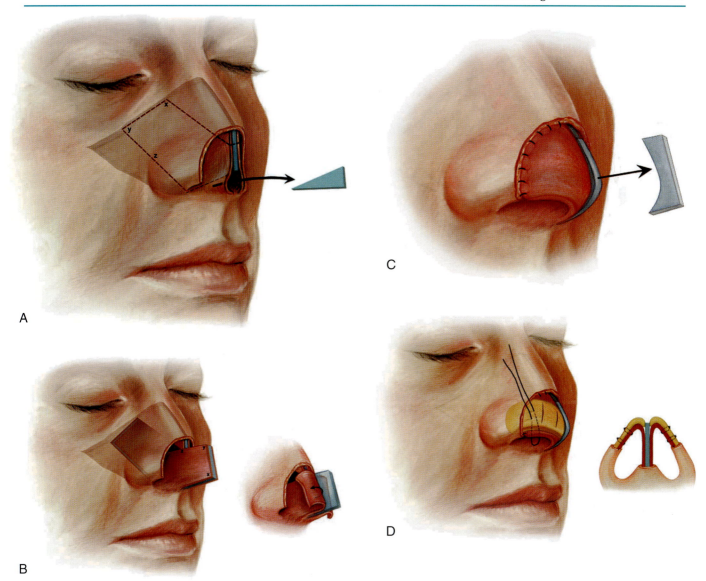

A

B

C

D

■ **Figure 4–6.** *A,* The *bold broken line* indicates a full-thickness incision through the septal cartilage, bone, and bilateral mucosa to create a composite septal chondromucosal pivotal flap. The *faint broken line* indicates an incision made only through the septal cartilage, preserving the overlying mucoperichondrium. A wedge of cartilage is removed to enable the flap to pivot anterocaudally. *B,* The cephalic aspect of the pivotal flap is locked into place by abutting it against the remaining cartilaginous dorsum. Bilateral mucoperichondrial flaps are reflected laterally to provide a lining for the nasal tip. *C,* Excess septal cartilage is trimmed. The reflected mucoperichondrial flaps are sutured to the borders of the lining defect. *D,* An auricular cartilage graft (yellow) provides a bilateral framework for the nasal tip, replacing the missing lateral crura. The septal cartilage (blue) of the composite flap serves as the medial crura for reconstruction. Mucoperichondrial flaps are attached to the framework with mattress sutures.

nasal bridge is missing, lining may be supplied with a composite pivotal flap 2.0 to 2.5 cm wide, often incorporating portions of the ethmoid perpendicular bony plate within the flap (Fig. 4–7). The flap typically has a pivotal arc of 45 to 90 degrees and is made to abut the remaining nasal bones or the nasal process of the frontal bone. In cases where both the nasal dorsum and tip are absent, a composite flap that encompasses the entire remaining septum is pivoted 90 to 110 degrees in an anterocaudal direction, buttressing the flap against the nasal process of the frontal bone.

In subtotal and total absence of the nose, the remaining septum may be adequate to provide sufficient mucoperichondrium to line both nasal vestibules but only if the composite flap is adequately mobilized caudally in a staged procedure. The entire remaining septum is delivered from the nasal passage as a composite septal chondromucosal pivotal flap (Fig. 4–8). The base of the flap should be 1.5 to 2.0 cm wide, and the pedicle is centered over the anterior nasal spine. In these cases, the nasal dorsum is absent, and the mobilized flap is delivered from the nasal passage and braced against

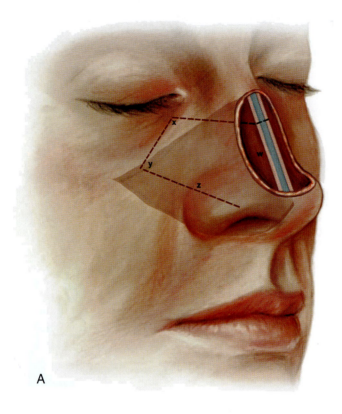

A

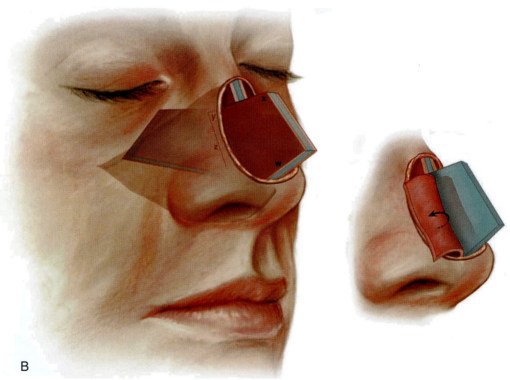

B

■ **Figure 4–7.** *A*, The *broken line* indicates a full-thickness incision through septal cartilage, bone, and bilateral mucosa to create the composite septal chondromucosal pivotal flap. *B*, The cephalic aspect of the pivoted flap is locked into place by abutting it against the remaining nasal bony septum. Bilateral mucoperichondrial flaps are reflected laterally to provide a lining to the nasal passage.

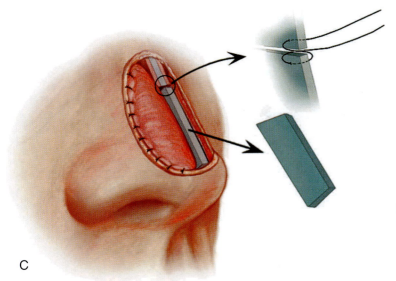

C

■ **Figure 4-7** *Continued. C,* Excess septal cartilage and bone are trimmed, and mucoperichondrial flaps are sutured to the borders of the lining defect. A figure-of-eight suture stabilizes the composite flap's connection to the remaining nasal bony septum.

the remaining nasal bones if present, or the nasal process of the frontal bone, and secured to the bone with sutures. The edges of the cartilage exposed along the borders of the flap are trimmed back sufficiently to allow the leaves of the mucoperichondrium to be approximated with 5-0 chromic sutures. The flap is secured in its new location for 4 to 6 weeks. This serves as a delay of the flap and has the effect of enhancing the vascularity of the mucoperichondrium. At a second stage, nasal reconstruction is completed by reflecting the mucoperichondrium and mucoperiosteum off of the more anterior portion of the flap. Exposed cartilage and bone are excised to a level that creates the ideal dorsal line. The reflected mucoperichondrial flaps are turned laterally to restore internal lining to the nasal passage. The flaps are well vascularized but flaccid and require support supplied by cartilage grafts from the septum and auricle, which are used to restore the nasal framework. The flaps are suspended to the overlying cartilage grafts with three or four mattress sutures that pass from the dorsal aspect of the exposed grafts through the flaps and then back again. When the entire inferior portion of the nose is absent, the septal composite pivotal flap must be designed so that it includes the entire length of the remaining cartilaginous and bony septum. The flap extends nearly to the choanae in order to maximize the tissue available for lining. In these situations, the composite flap must be pivoted as far as possible so that the reflected flaps will be positioned sufficiently anteriorly and caudally to reach the desired restoration areas of the tip and alae. Burget and Menick[1] described a technique in which the lining of the middle vault sidewalls is included in the composite pivotal flap to add an additional source of mucosa for lining the more caudal aspect of the nose. Figure 4-9 summarizes the variations in configuration of composite septal chondromucosal pivotal flaps, which differ according to the requirements for lining and extent of the nasal defect.

Septal mucoperichondrial hinge flaps and composite pivotal flaps should be designed for maximum length and sufficient width. Flaps that are insufficient in size will compromise the quantity of internal lining tissue available to the surgeon and will result in a reconstructed nose of inadequate length and height. The longest axis of the cartilaginous septum in an anteroposterior vector extends along a line that bisects the septum at the junction of the bony perpendicular plate of the ethmoid and the volmer. All composite septal chondromucosal pivotal flaps should be designed so that the axis of the flap is centered at this junction. The width of the flap depends on the required height of the mucosal lining. Because the caudal aspect of the septum is always included in the flap, it may require submucosal trimming to prevent inferior displacement of the columella. This depends on the arc of pivotal movement and whether the columella is present. It is far more important to line the caudal nasal passage with mucosa than the cephalic portion. Therefore, in circumstances where the length of the remaining septum is limited, the flap should be mobilized as far anterocaudally as possible so that it may reach the area of the reconstructed tip and alae. Then, if necessary, the upper nasal vault may be lined by turbinate flaps, adjacent turnover flaps, or a paramedian forehead flap.

Turbinate Flaps

The inferior turbinate may be used as an intranasal source of mucosa for lining small full-thickness alar defects.[6] A flap is created by incising the inferior turbinate so as to develop a mucoperiosteal flap based on

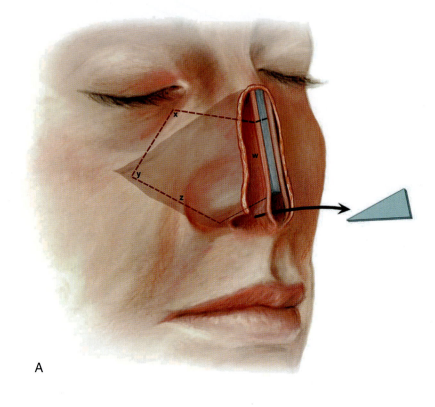

A

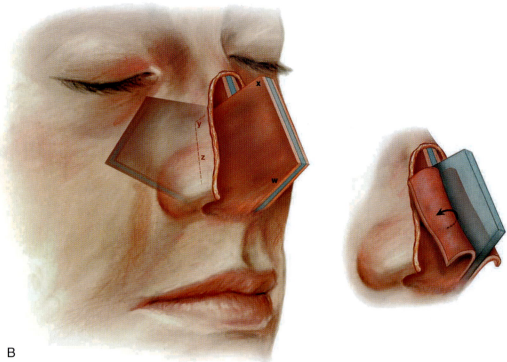

B

■ Figure 4–8. *A*, The *bold broken line* indicates a full-thickness incision through septal cartilage, bone, and bilateral mucosa. The *faint broken line* indicates an incision made only through the septal cartilage, preserving the mucoperichondrium. A wedge of cartilage is removed to enable the flap to pivot anterocaudally. *B*, The cephalic aspect of the pivoted flap is locked into place by abutting it against the nasal process of the frontal bone. Bilateral mucoperichondrial flaps are reflected laterally to provide a lining to the nasal passages.

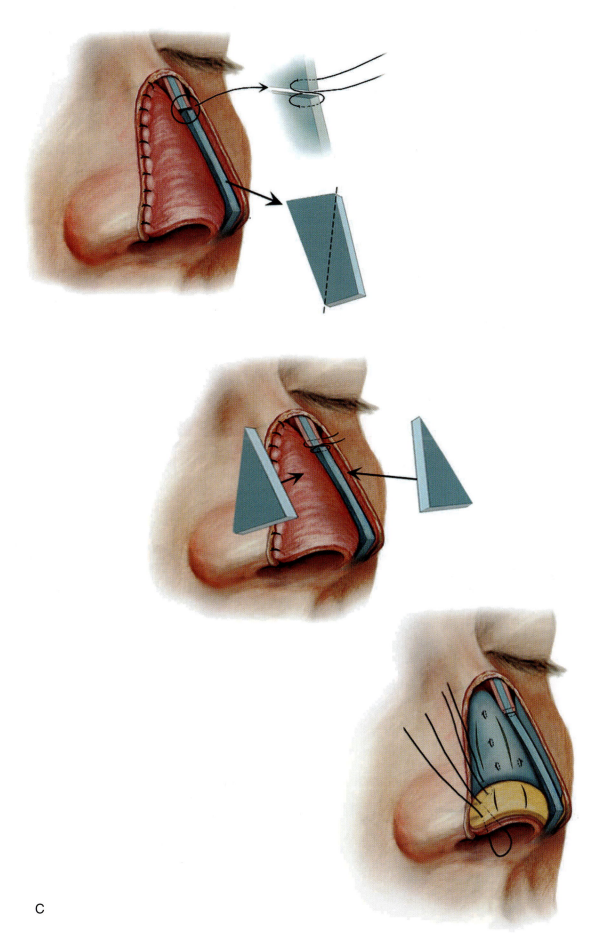

C

■ **Figure 4–8** *Continued. C,* Excess septal cartilage and bone are trimmed, and mucoperichondrial flaps are sutured to the borders of the lining defect. A figure-of-eight suture stabilizes the composite flap to the nasal process. Septal cartilage (blue) and auricular cartilage (yellow) provide the nasal framework. Cartilage grafts are scored to create the desired convex contour. Mucoperichondrial flaps are attached to the framework with mattress sutures.

Illustration continued on following page

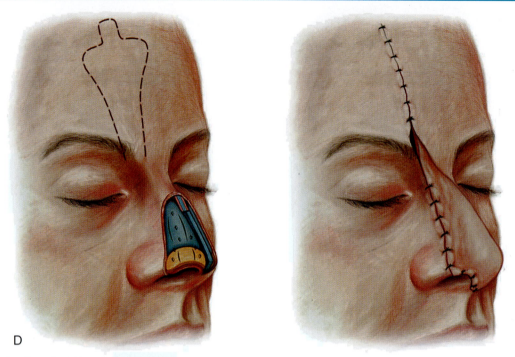

■ **Figure 4–8** *Continued. D,* The nasal framework is covered by a paramedian forehead flap.

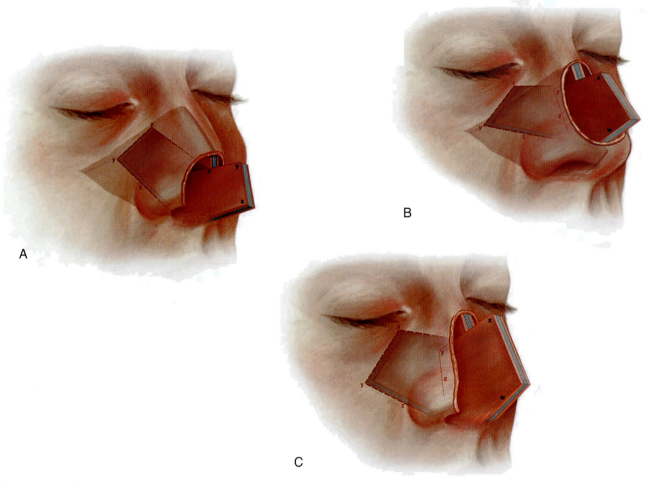

■ **Figure 4–9.** Variations in the configurations of composite septal chondromucosal pivotal flaps.

the anterior attachment of the turbinate. A sickle knife is used to release the posterior and central attachments of the turbinate from the nasal sidewall. The turbinate is delivered out of the nasal passage by pivoting it 180 degrees. Turbinate bone is carefully removed to create a filet of thin mucoperiosteum that may be used to line the lateral vestibule. Similar to all lining flaps, the inferior turbinate flap is suspended to overlying contour cartilage grafts with a limited number of mattress sutures. Nasal packing is recommended for 3 to 5 days to control hemorrhage, but precise cautery of the donor site borders may reduce the need for packing. The size of the flap is limited by the size of the inferior turbinate and also limits the usefulness of the flap. In addition, by pivoting the flap 180 degrees, a standing cone of mucosa that may obstruct the airway is created, requiring a second procedure to debulk or remove the redundant tissue.

Comparable to the inferior turbinate, the middle turbinate may provide a limited source of lining for full-thickness nasal defects. Similar to its inferior counterpart, the flap is created by making an incision starting posteriorly and extending forward, leaving a 1-cm pedicle at the anterior attachment of the turbinate. Compared with the inferior turbinate, the smaller size and superior position of the middle turbinate flap prevents it from reaching the nasal vestibule. Nonetheless, it is still able to provide sufficient mucoperiosteum to reline the roof of the middle vault or cephalic portions of the nasal sidewall.

Forehead Flap

The cross-sectional dimensions of the nose at the internal valve are the narrowest of the nasal airway. Whenever possible, the nasal passage caudal to the area of the internal nasal valve should be lined with mucosa because it provides the thinnest, most vascular lining available to support primary framework grafts without crowding the airway. Thin skin flaps have less risk of significantly compromising the airway if placed cephalic to the valve. The absence of the septum in the area of the internal valve in cases that call for composite septal pivotal flaps for lining the caudal nose is a benefit to the airway. The lack of the septum provides a greater cross-sectional area to accommodate a turn-in or paramedian forehead flap to line the more cephalic portion of the nose. Thus, in instances where the nasal septum is not available as a source for lining flaps or can provide lining only to the caudal aspect of the nose, a paramedian flap may serve as a source for lining. The flap is raised in a fashion similar to that used for covering flaps. The frontalis muscle and galea are removed, and the flap is thinned of its subcutaneous tissue. The flap is then folded on itself and delivered to the nasal passage by tunneling it under the glabellar skin to reach the lining defect (Fig. 4–10). The flap is suspended to framework grafts of bone and cartilage with mattress sutures. A second paramedian

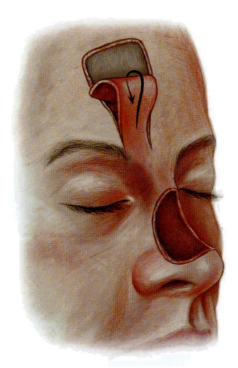
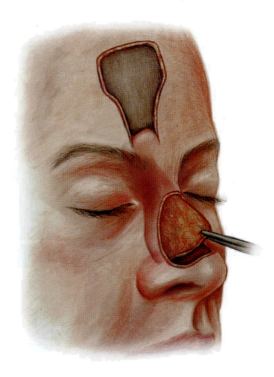

■ **Figure 4–10.** Paramedian forehead flaps may be used to line the nasal passage when nasal septum is not available as a source for intranasal lining flaps.

forehead flap is then used as a cover flap for the exterior of the nose. In cases where the upper nasal vault is intact, the lining flap may be delivered to the middle vault through the lateral aspect of the middle vault defect. In this case, to accommodate the flap, the necessary framework in the area of the fenestrum is delayed until the flap is detached. The forehead flap used for lining is detached from the brow after 3 weeks. Detachment of the external flap is delayed an additional 3 to 6 weeks to maximize revascularization of the framework grafts.

Microsurgical Flaps

Microsurgical flaps may be used to provide nasal lining in instances where there is total or near total loss of the nose and the remaining septum is insufficient for the development of adequate mucoperichondrial flaps for nasal lining. In these cases, the surgeon is often confronted with loss of portions of the adjoining lip or cheek. Reconstruction of the nose should be delayed until a foundation for the new nose is created by repairing adjacent soft-tissue deficits with local, regional, or microsurgical flaps. The next step is to create lining for the nose. In the event of massive loss of tissue of the midface, a microsurgical flap may be used in a staged procedure to provide soft-tissue replacement of the cheeks and upper lip. Subsequently, portions of the flap are developed as turnover flaps to provide a lining to the nose.

A number of donor sites exist from which to harvest a microsurgical flap suited for reconstruction of nasal lining defects. Although the radial forearm flap is the preferred source, two other potential sources are revascularized omentum and temporoparietal fascia.[7] The latter two flaps require skin grafting in order to provide an epithelial surface to the nasal passage. The forearm skin has a constant and reliable vascular supply that makes it suitable for free tissue transfer. This forearm flap has the advantages of ease of flap evaluation, large donor vessels, and a long pedicle, which greatly simplify the technical aspects of flap transfer. However, the greatest advantage of this flap is the thin, pliable tissue that is capable of being draped beneath a nasal framework. The vascular pedicle is tunneled laterally and inferiorly, usually deep to the melolabial crease, to recipient vessels in the upper neck. The flap is carefully designed so that the configuration and surface area of the skin are appropriate for the lining deficit. The flap is transferred concomitant with construction of the nasal framework, which is essential to prevent flap contraction. The flap is suspended to the overlying framework with mattress sutures, and the framework is then covered with a paramedian forehead flap. The radial forearm flap may survive independent of its vascular pedicle as early as 2 weeks following transfer. However, any thinning or sculpturing of the flap should be delayed a minimum of 6 weeks following microsurgical transfer.

References

1. Burget GC, Menick FJ: Aesthetic Reconstruction of the Nose. St. Louis, CV Mosby, 1994.

2. Burget GC, Menick FJ: Nasal support and lining: The marriage of beauty and blood supply. Plast Reconstr Surg 84:189, 1989.

3. Millard DR: Reconstructive rhinoplasty for the lower two-thirds of the nose. Plastic Reconstr Surg 57:722, 1976.

4. Spear SL, Kroll SS, Romm S: A new twist to the nasolabial flap for reconstruction of lateral alar defects. Plastic Reconstr Surg 79:915, 1987.

5. Burget GC, Menick FJ: Nasal reconstruction: Seeking a fourth dimension. Plast Reconstr Surg 78:145, 1986.

6. Murakami CS, Kriet D, Ierokomos AP: Nasal reconstruction using the inferior turbinate mucosal flap. Arch Facial Plastic Surg 13:97, 1999.

7. Soutar DS: Radial forearm flaps. In Baker SR (ed): Microsurgical Reconstruction of the Head and Neck. New York, Churchill Livingstone, 1989, p 139.

5

Structural Support

Sam Naficy

The goal of nasal reconstruction is to replace missing segments with autologous tissue of similar shape, size, and structural integrity. There are a number of available donor sites for obtaining grafts used to provide structural integrity to the nose (Table 5–1). Structural grafts must have sufficient intrinsic strength to maintain support of the constructed portion of the nose. Whenever possible, grafts are selected that have an intrinsic shape and contour similar to those of the missing portion of the nasal skeleton. This reduces the need for graft contouring and bending that could ultimately compromise structural integrity.

The three functions of grafts used in nasal reconstruction are restoration, support, and contour. Restorative grafts replace defects of the nasal skeleton and may be of bone or cartilage, depending on the missing framework. Support grafts provide reinforcement to the existing nasal skeleton. Contour grafts are used to enhance the shape of the nasal tip or to correct topographical irregularities. Support and contour grafts usually consist of septal or auricular cartilage.

Restorative grafts of bone and cartilage replace missing nasal framework. These grafts reestablish the structural continuity of the nasal framework and restore volume and contour to the nose. Cartilage grafts are secured to the native nasal cartilage with figure-of-eight sutures that maintain end-to-end contact between the two. This prevents shifting or overlapping.

The restorative graft is the only type of graft required for most cases of nasal reconstruction. There are a number of instances, however, where support grafts are necessary in addition to restorative grafts. Support grafts are not used to replace missing nasal cartilage or bone but rather to reinforce nasal structures that are not directly supported by the nasal skeleton or to enhance the strength of nasal cartilages. Examples of support grafts include alar batten grafts, spreader grafts, and columellar struts. These grafts are required when the constructed portion of the nose lacks sufficient support to withstand the distorting forces of scar contracture. It is critical with all support and restorative grafts that the cartilage or bone is in intimate contact with the nasal lining. This is ensured by using mattress sutures to secure the lining to the graft.

Contour grafts of septal or auricular cartilage are occasionally used in nasal reconstruction to enhance the shape and projection of the nasal tip or to correct contour irregularities. In the region of the nasal tip, enhancing contour with septal or auricular cartilage is achieved in the same manner as in open rhinoplasty. Cartilage tip grafts are used to gain additional definition, projection, or rotation to optimize the aesthetic proportions of the constructed nose. Onlay grafts of cartilage are used to improve areas of contour irregularity.

Restorative Grafts

■ Upper Nasal Vault

Structural support of the upper nasal vault is provided by the bony pyramid and its attachments to the frontal bone and the ascending processes of the maxillae. The bony pyramid is further supported by attachments to the bony septum. Defects of the bony pyramid are best

Table 5-1. Donor Sources of Structural Support for Nasal Reconstruction

CARTILAGE

Alar cartilage
Septum
Auricle
Rib
Composite chondrocutaneous auricular graft
Composite septal chondromucosal pivotal flap

BONE

Septum
Cranium
Rib

ALLOPLASTIC

Titanium mesh

reconstructed with autologous bone grafts sculpted to fit the defect. Bone grafts are contoured to the precise size and shape of the defect by using a drill or a bone cutter and are secured to the remaining framework by permanent suture or plate fixation (see Chapter 8). Most defects of the bony pyramid are repaired by using outer table cranial bone grafts (Fig. 5–1). Smaller defects may be repaired with septal bone harvested from vomer or ethmoid bone. Limited bony defects may also be repaired with septal cartilage (see Chapter 23). Suture fixation may be adequate as long as the structural integrity of the bony pyramid is intact. Larger defects of the bony pyramid require a three-dimensional reconstruction using cranial bone and fixation plate stabilization as discussed in Chapter 8. Rib grafts are an alternative method of restoring the bony pyramid. They are usually employed as a single composite graft of bone and cartilage to replace the entire structure of the nasal dorsum.

Middle Nasal Vault

The upper lateral cartilages and the dorsal cartilagenous septum compose the skeleton of the middle vault of the nose. The upper lateral cartilages are supported by connections to the bony pyramid and to the dorsal aspect of the cartilaginous septum and by fibrous attachments to the piriform aperture. At its caudal border, the upper lateral cartilage has a scroll-like fibrous connection to the cephalic border of alar cartilage. The caudal border of the upper lateral cartilage and the angle it forms with the dorsal septum define the internal nasal valve.

Defects of the upper lateral cartilage are best repaired with septal cartilage (Fig. 5–2). Septal cartilage has a flat contour and an appropriate thickness for replacement of middle vault skeletal defects. The graft

is cut to the size of the cartilage defect and is secured to remaining nasal cartilage and the periosteum of the nasal bone superiorly. Figure-of-eight suturing prevents displacement of the graft by scar contracture during wound healing. When replacing the lateral aspect of the upper lateral cartilage, the base of the graft is positioned so that a border lies just lateral to the piriform aperture to stabilize the graft and to prevent medial displacement into the nasal passage. The alar cartilage is positioned superficial to the caudal margin of the graft used to replace the upper lateral cartilage to recreate their natural relationship. The graft is secured to the underlying tissue or lining flap by using several mattress sutures of 5.0 polyglactin.

Large full-thickness defects of the central nose may result in loss of dorsal projection of the middle vault and disruption of mucosal continuity. Small mucosal defects may be repaired primarily. Onlay graft of layered septal cartilage or rib cartilage is the preferred grafting material for restoring dorsal support and projecting the middle vault. When there is loss of dorsal cartilage and a large deficit of mucosa lining, both lining and cartilaginous support for the middle vault may be restored with a composite septal chondromucosal pivotal flap (see Chapter 4). Dorsal support is restored by the septal cartilage in the center of the flap. This cartilage is secured to remaining stable elements of the nasal framework, such as the bony dorsum and tip cartilages, by using permanent sutures. Mucoperichondrial flaps are elevated from each side of the composite flap and approximated to the borders of the lining defect, restoring mucosal continuity of the middle vault.

When there is loss of the bony and cartilaginous dorsum, a cranial bone graft consisting of a single piece may be used to restore structure of the upper and middle vault. Likewise, when there is loss of the entire nasal sidewall, a cranial bone graft is usually utilized to provide structural support of the sidewall of both the

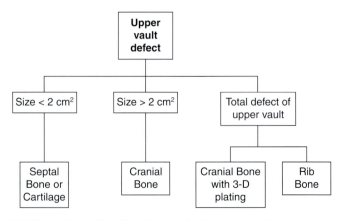

Figure 5-1. Algorithm for structural support of the upper vault.

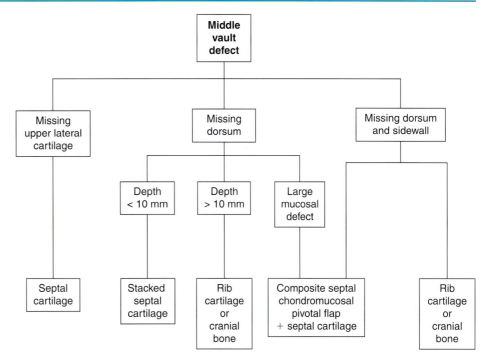

■ **Figure 5–2.** Algorithm for structural support of the middle vault.

1. Use spreader grafts for any defect with narrow middle vault.
2. Use lateral alar batten grafts for any defect with flaccid upper lateral cartilages.

upper and middle vaults. If the dorsum is also missing, two or more cranial bone grafts are combined with three-dimensional plating to restore structural support to both nasal vaults.

■ Lower Nasal Vault

The anterior septal angle forms a pedestal on which the paired alar cartilages are attached. The major support system of the lower nasal vault comprises the alar cartilages and their attachments to each other and to the upper lateral cartilages.

Missing segments of the alar cartilages are replaced with cartilage grafts of appropriate contour, size, and thickness to restore continuity of each structure (Fig. 5–3). Conchal cartilage has the ideal contour and thickness for this purpose. In addition to replacing missing alar cartilage, all full-thickness and partial-thickness defects of the ala are supported with cartilage grafts to avoid notching and retraction of the nostril margin (Fig. 5–4). Full-thickness defects of the nasal tip are often reconstructed with a composite septal chondromucosal pivotal flap. The flap has the advantage of providing structural support to the tip and internal lining to the nasal domes. Additional auricular or septal cartilage grafting is usually required to complete restoration of the arc of each alar cartilage.

■ Total Nasal Defect

Restoring the framework in cases of total and near total nasal defects is accomplished with multiple grafts of bone and cartilage (Fig. 5–5). If the septum and an adequate covering of mucoperichondrium remain, a composite septal chondromucosal pivotal flap is used to restore the structure of the columella and lower dorsum and provide internal lining to the lower nasal vault. Cranial bone is used to construct the framework of the cephalic half of the nose; bilateral auricular cartilage grafts are used to restore the framework of the caudal half. If the septum is missing or inadequate, the columella is restored with rib cartilage or cranial bone. The framework of the upper and middle nasal vaults is restored with cranial bone or a rib graft composed of bone and cartilage. Wafers of rib cartilage may be used to support the nasal sidewalls. The lower nasal vault framework is restored with bilateral auricular cartilage grafts.

Structural Grafts

■ Batten Grafts

Defects extending to the alar margin may result in retraction or partial collapse of the nostril if the ala is not properly supported with a batten in the form of a cartilage graft. Only superficial defects of the ala or defects situated 1.5 cm or more from the alar margin should be repaired without a cartilage graft to provide structural support to the soft tissue of the ala. A cartilage graft 2 to 3 cm in length and 0.75 to 1.5 cm in width is usually

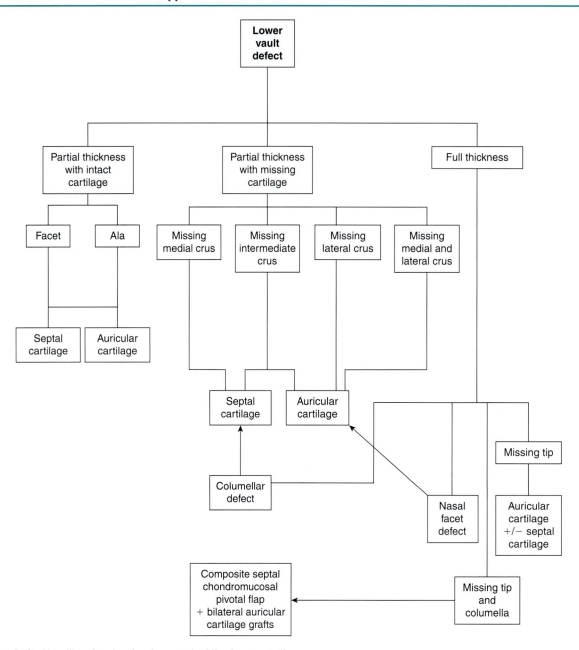

■ **Figure 5-3.** Algorithm for structural support of the lower vault.

obtained from the contralateral conchal cartilage (see Chapter 7). The graft is secured in a soft-tissue pocket created at the alar base with a 3.0 polyglactin suture tied inside the nasal cavity. Medially, the graft is secured to the caudal aspect of the alar cartilage just lateral to the dome with figure-of-eight 5.0 polyglactin sutures (see Fig. 5–4; Fig. 5–6). The entire alar aesthetic unit is resurfaced in the majority of cases. In these instances the batten graft is made to span the entire distance from alar base to nasal tip. After medial, lateral, and cephalic fixation, the graft is secured to the exposed raw surface of the internal nasal lining, with the inferior margin of the cartilage positioned 1 mm

above the alar margin. The defect is then resurfaced with a skin flap to provide external coverage over the graft.

Structural grafts may also be used to strengthen the region of the internal nasal valve to prevent nasal obstruction. Structural grafts in the form of alar batten grafts are more often utilized for this purpose for patients with weak alar cartilages or with narrow middle nasal vaults. In patients where two or more nasal aesthetic units (including the tip) of the nose are resurfaced with a covering flap, the mass of the flap with accompanying scar contracture may cause constriction of the valve. Batten grafts help prevent this constriction

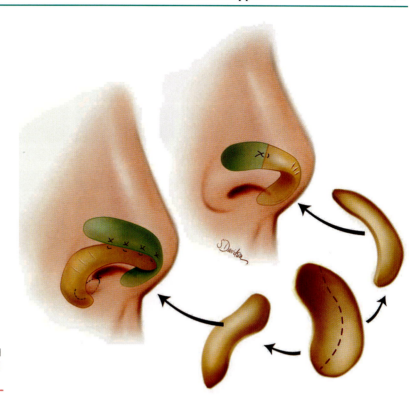

■ **Figure 5–4.** Auricular cartilage grafts are used to replace missing segments of alar cartilage and for support of the ala.

by reinforcing the upper lateral and alar cartilages. These grafts are positioned beneath the alar cartilages between the lateral crura and vestibular skin and are of sufficient length to extend from the crura to the alar bases (Fig. 5–7). The batten graft is sutured to the lateral crus in such a manner to cause the ala to flare slightly outward. This is accomplished by medial ad-vancement of the lateral crus on the batten and fixation with permanent mattress sutures.

■ Columellar Struts

Columellar struts are structural grafts often used during rhinoplasty to maintain or augment tip projection. Struts

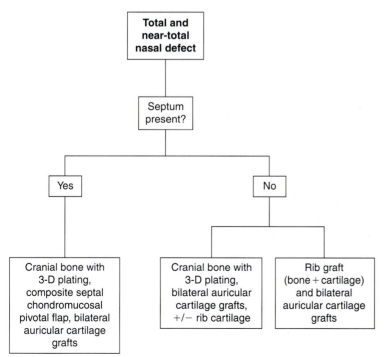

■ **Figure 5–5.** Algorithm for structural support of a total and near-total nasal defect.

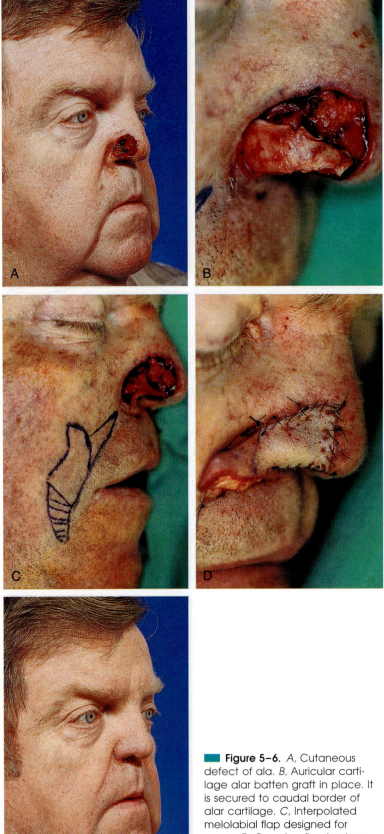

■ **Figure 5–6.** *A,* Cutaneous defect of ala. *B,* Auricular cartilage alar batten graft in place. It is secured to caudal border of alar cartilage. *C,* Interpolated melolabial flap designed for cover. *D,* Covering flap in place. *E,* Three months following detachment of pedicle of cheek flap.

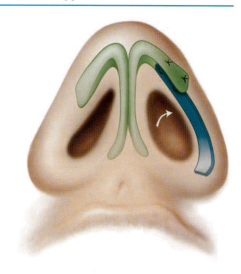

■ **Figure 5–7.** Lateral alar batten graft is fashioned from septal or auricular cartilage and produces slight lateral flaring of alar cartilage at region of the internal and external nasal valves, increasing nasal aperture.

also help reduce the risk of warping and deformity of the medial crura. A strut graft may also be used to increase columellar show and improve columellar retraction. Struts play a similar role in nasal reconstruction. Defects of the alar cartilage that involve the medial crura are repaired with auricular or septal cartilage grafts that restore continuity of the cartilage. Placement of an additional cartilage graft in the form of a columellar strut along the reconstituted medial crus reinforces and stabilizes the graft used to restore the crus (Fig. 5–8). Septal cartilage is the optimal graft material for a columellar strut. The strut is usually 1 to 2 mm in thickness, 3 to 5 mm in width, and 15 to 20 mm in height. A pocket is dissected bluntly between the medial crura, maintaining soft tissue over the nasal spine. The graft is placed inside the pocket, and the medial crura are secured to the graft with multiple mattress sutures of 5.0 polypropylene. Hydrodissection followed by sharp dissection of vestibular skin away from the medial crura facilitates placement of sutures.

Auricular cartilage may also be used as a columellar strut if septal cartilage is not available. Because of the cartilage's natural curvature, it is necessary to create a straight strut by creating a double layer graft. The graft is incised longitudinally through the full thickness of cartilage, but perichondrial continuity is maintained on the opposite side. The graft is then folded in half lengthwise, apposing the perichondrial surfaces together. Multiple mattress sutures of 6.0 polypropylene are placed through both layers to yield a stable and straight graft suitable for a strut (Fig. 5–9).

■ Spreader Grafts

Spreader grafts are structural grafts. They are constructed as long rectangular grafts of septal or auricular cartilage that are placed between the dorsal margin of the upper lateral cartilages and the dorsal margin of the septum. Spreader grafts strengthen the dorsal septum and widen the medial aspect of the internal nasal valve during reconstruction of the middle nasal vault. Sheen[1] described their placement with the endonasal approach, and Johnson and Toriumi[2] described it using the external approach. When required, spreader grafts are inserted through the external approach afforded by the reconstructive procedure. Septal mucoperichondrium is hydrodissected with lidocaine (1% with 1:100,000 concentration of epinephrine), and bilateral mucoperichondrial flaps are dissected. The dissection starts at the anterior septal angle and extends cephalically beneath the nasal bones. Using a Cottle elevator and a Freer septum knife, the upper lateral cartilages are detached from the cartilaginous septum along their entire length to the level of the rhinion. This provides wide exposure to the dorsal cartilaginous septum and prepares the middle vault for placement of the grafts. Preserving a dorsal and caudal strut of cartilage 1.5 cm wide, sufficient septal cartilage is harvested for grafting. The mucoperichondrial flaps are approximated using a continuous quilting stitch of 3.0 chromic suture. Grafts are cut with a no. 15 scalpel blade to a thickness of 1 to 2 mm, width of 3 to 4 mm, and length of 15 to 25 mm. Length depends on the vertical height of the upper lateral cartilages. Thickness depends on the septal

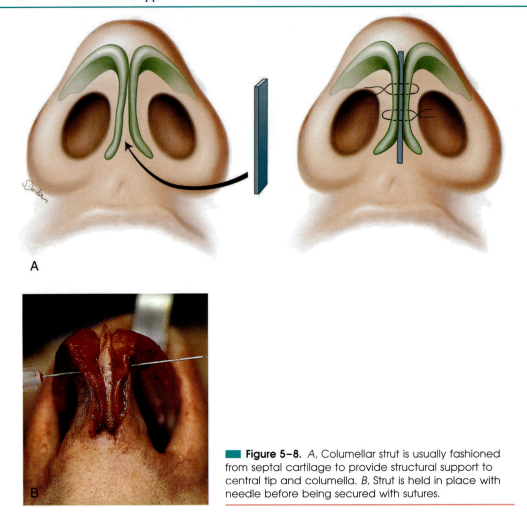

A

B

Figure 5–8. *A*, Columellar strut is usually fashioned from septal cartilage to provide structural support to central tip and columella. *B*, Strut is held in place with needle before being secured with sutures.

cartilage and the desired degree of lateral displacement of the upper lateral cartilages. Grafts are placed on each side and parallel to the dorsal septum (Fig. 5–10). Cephalically, the grafts extend to the junction of the upper lateral cartilages with the nasal bones. In aesthetic rhinoplasty, spreader grafts are frequently used when reducing a markedly overprojected dorsum to prevent constriction of the middle vault. A double-layer spreader graft is occasionally placed, either bilaterally or unilaterally, for particularly narrow noses or to correct a long-standing crooked nose deformity. Spreader grafts are held on either side of the septum with Brown-Adson forceps. The upper lateral cartilages are retracted laterally. Placement of a half-inch 30-gauge needle through all three structures is at times helpful in stabilizing the grafts prior to suture placement. Several horizontal mattress sutures of 5.0 polydioxanone or polypropylene are then passed through both grafts and the septum. The upper lateral cartilages are secured to the spreader grafts and septum with similar sutures.

Contour Grafts

■ Tip Grafts

Shield grafts, as described by Johnson and Toriumi,[2] are used to augment anterior projection of the tip and caudal projection of the columella (Fig. 5–11). The graft is usually fashioned from septal cartilage. The thicker portion of the graft is placed at the tip, and the graft is tapered toward the columella. The portion of the shield graft overlying the columella is made thicker if additional columellar show is required on lateral view. The projecting portion of the graft may be bidomal or unidomal, depending on the desired effect and on thickness of the external covering. The edges of the graft are tapered for a smooth transition. The graft is fixed to the tip complex using multiple simple interrupted 5.0 polypropylene sutures. Longer grafts are more stable and less likely to tilt or shift.

An alternative to the shield graft is the cap graft as

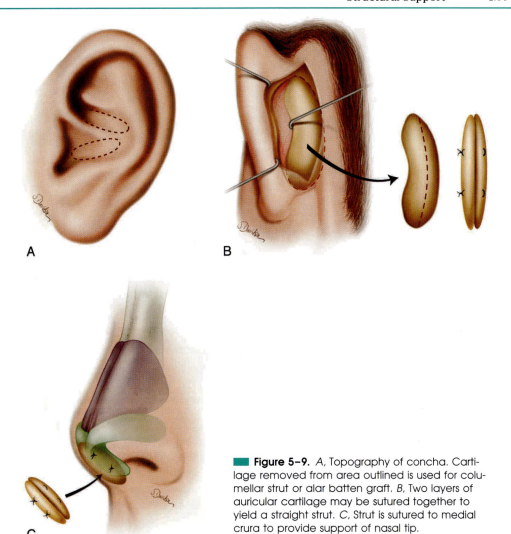

■ **Figure 5–9.** *A*, Topography of concha. Cartilage removed from area outlined is used for columellar strut or alar batten graft. *B*, Two layers of auricular cartilage may be sutured together to yield a straight strut. *C*, Strut is sutured to medial crura to provide support of nasal tip.

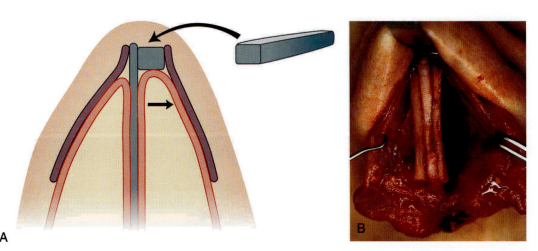

■ **Figure 5–10.** *A*, Spreader grafts are used to lateralize upper lateral cartilage and increase aperture of internal nasal valve. *B*, Grafts are secured with mattress sutures along both sides of dorsal margin of septum.

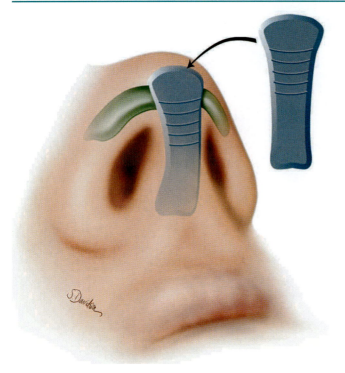

Figure 5-11. Shield graft of septal or auricular cartilage is used to enhance tip definition, projection, and rotation. Partial-thickness scoring of graft may be used to obtain desired curvature.

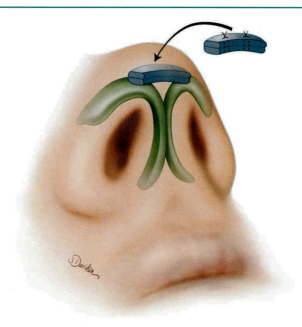

Figure 5-12. Cap graft of cartilage is used in single or double layers to enhance tip definition, projection, and rotation.

described by Peck[3] (Fig. 5-12). The cap graft may be used to enhance tip projection and cephalic rotation. The graft is fashioned from septal or auricular cartilage and is secured, using multiple 5.0 polydioxanone sutures, to the surface of the alar cartilages making up the domes. A single- or double-layer graft may be used to yield the optimal surface topography. By placing the

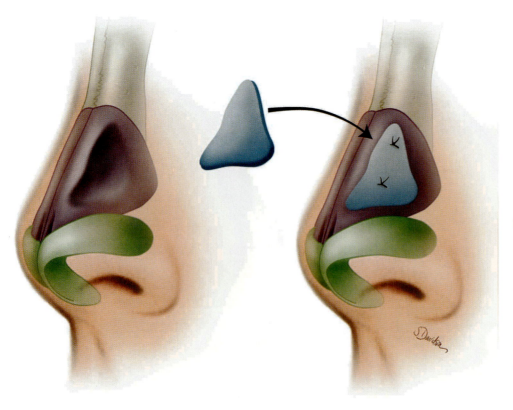

Figure 5-13. Septal or auricular cartilage is used to correct areas of contour depression on surface of nose. Edges of grafts are tapered or morselized, and grafts may be stacked to correct areas of deep contour depression. Whenever possible, graft is sutured to underlying nasal skeleton.

graft more cephalically on the tip complex, a greater degree of cephalic tip rotation is achieved. The edges of the graft are tapered or, alternatively, the graft may be covered by a second layer of morselized cartilage.

■ Onlay Grafts

Surface deformities on the nasal dorsum and sidewalls may be improved with contour grafts positioned over the nasal skeleton. Septal and auricular cartilage is used to augment areas of depression and smooth areas of irregularities. Edges of the grafts are carefully tapered or morselized to avoid a visible or palpable border (Fig. 5–13). Multiple layers of cartilage are stacked to correct deeper contour deformities. Onlay grafts may be placed primarily at the time of initial nasal reconstruction or secondarily as a revision procedure. When placed primarily, the grafts are fixed in place using multiple 5.0 polyglactin or polydioxanone sutures. Alternatively, the graft may be secured with 5.0 polyglactin mattress sutures placed through the recipient site and tied inside the nose. As a secondary procedure, the area of contour deformity is marked on the surface of the nose. The onlay graft is meticulously tailored before dissecting the nasal skin in the area of the deformity. This is accomplished by placing the graft on the surface of the skin overlying the depressed contour to determine the ideal size and configuration of the graft. As the graft is being sculpted, the thickness and shape are frequently assessed by replacing it on the nasal skin overlying the deformity. A soft-tissue pocket is then dissected over the recipient area, preferably through an endonasal incision. The pocket is made 15% to 20% larger than the graft. The graft is positioned in place and, when possible, secured to the underlying nasal skeleton with a suture. The access incision is repaired with 5.0 polyglactin or chromic gut suture.

Onlay grafts may also be placed in the infratip or columellar region to enhance the aesthetic proportions of the tip. These grafts are usually at least partially morselized and are inserted through a limited marginal incision.

References

1. Sheen JH, Sheen A: Aesthetic Rhinoplasty, 2nd ed. St. Louis, Quality Medical Publishing, 1987.

2. Johnson CJ, Toriumi DM: Open Structure Rhinoplasty, Philadelphia, WB Saunders, 1990.

3. Peck GC: The onlay graft for nasal tip projection. Plastic Reconstr Surg 79:27, 1983.

6

External Covering

Sam Naficy

Restoration of the external covering is required for repair of all defects of the nasal skin that result from removal of cutaneous malignancy. The majority of surgical defects involve only the skin and are repaired using a number of options. These include primary closure, healing by secondary intention, cutaneous flaps, skin and composite grafts, interpolated flaps, and microsurgical flaps.

Selection of the optimal reconstructive method is influenced by the defect's size, depth, and location. The defect is analyzed for missing muscle, cartilage, bone, or internal lining. Involved aesthetic units of the nose and adjacent facial regions are noted. Other important factors include the thickness, texture, and mobility of the remaining nasal skin and the relative size of the defect compared with the surface area of the nose. Medical, social, and psychological variables of each patient are also considered. This chapter provides a general overview of methods used to repair skin defects.

When planning facial reconstruction, it is helpful to divide the face into eight aesthetic regions: forehead, nose, right and left periorbita, right and left cheeks, and upper and lower lips. Each of these regions may be subdivided into various aesthetic units to assist in the design of cutaneous flaps. This is particularly applicable to the nose. A well-described principle of facial reconstruction is to repair defects that involve more than one aesthetic region with separate flaps for each region.[1, 2] This places scars along boundary lines separating aesthetic regions and maintains the natural contours between them. For instance, if a nasal defect extends to the upper lip or cheek, these portions of the defect are repaired with separate flaps or grafts. Adhering to this principle maintains a natural transition from the nose to the rest of the face, helping to hide scars in the boundaries between the nose, cheek, and upper lip (Fig. 6–1). Burget and Menick[1] recommend resurfacing an entire nasal aesthetic unit if more than half of the surface area of the unit has been removed. This is particularly important when repairing defects of the ala and tip. Removing the remaining skin of the nasal unit and covering the entire area with a flap places scars in the shadows along the borders between aesthetic units. This helps to maximize scar camouflage.

Preparation of the Defect

The aesthetic units of the nose are based on a recognizable pattern of contour elevations and depressions that result from subsurface anatomy.[1] Optimal repair of a nasal cutaneous defect often requires removal of additional skin and soft tissue from the involved unit. When interpolated cheek or forehead flaps are used as a covering, skin defects that involve half or more of the surface area of the unit are enlarged to encompass the entire aesthetic unit. When resurfacing the nasal tip aesthetic unit, the very thin skin of the alar rim and infratip lobule is not removed because it is difficult to match the thickness of this thin skin with skin of similar thickness from a flap. The same is true for skin of the nasal facet, which is considered its own aesthetic unit. Removal of the skin of the facet may predispose to retraction and notching of the nostril. When repairing

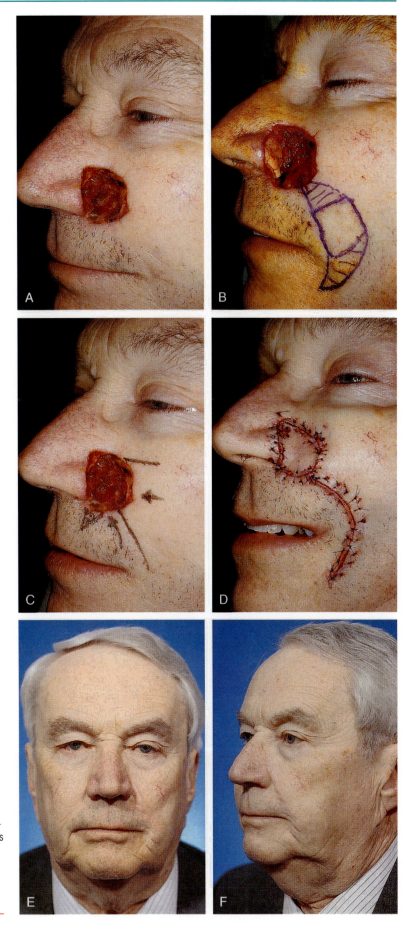

■ **Figure 6–1.** *A,* Cutaneous defect of nose, medial cheek, and very limited portion of upper lip. *B,* Auricular cartilage alar batten graft in place. Melolabial cheek flap based on subcutaneous pedicle is designed to cover ala and sidewall defect. *C,* Lip and cheek advancement flaps designed to repair their respective aesthetic region. *D,* Flaps in place. *E* and *F,* Eleven months postoperative. Contouring procedures (see Chapter 15) not required.

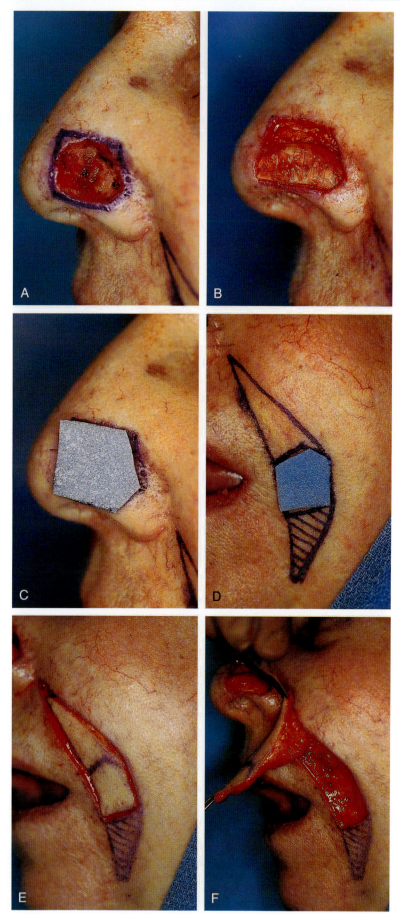

■ **Figure 6–2.** *A*, 2.0 × 2.0 cm superficial skin defect of medial ala and lateral tip. *B*, Defect converted from round to rectangular configuration. Auricular cartilage graft provides structural support to nostril margin. *C* and *D*, Template of defect used to design interpolated melolabial flap. *E*, Flap incised. Skin marked with blue hash marks below flap represents standing cutaneous deformity that is removed when donor wound is closed. *F*, Flap elevated on subcutaneous pedicle.

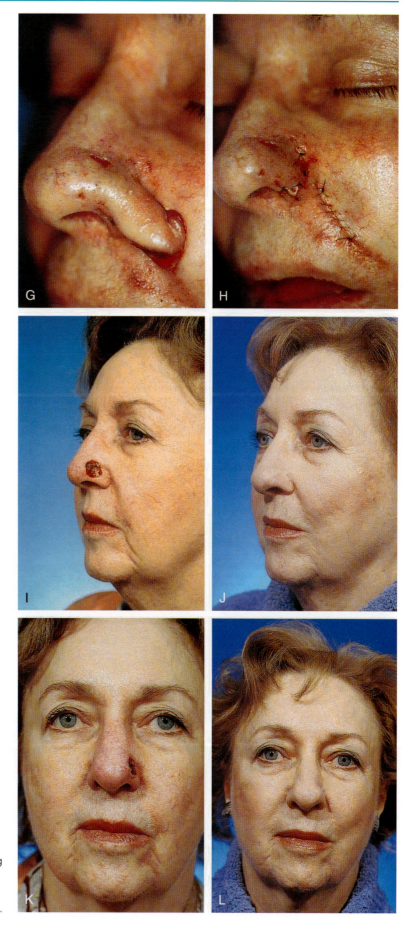

Figure 6–2 *Continued. G,* Three weeks following transfer of flap to nose. *H,* Immediately following detachment of pedicle. *I–L,* Preoperative and year postoperative.

the nasal dorsum with a forehead flap, the thin skin of the rhinion is generally not replaced with the flap if the cutaneous defect does not involve the rhinion. Likewise, the extreme cephalic portion of the sidewall skin in the area of the medial canthi is also preserved when using a flap to repair defects of the sidewall. When resurfacing the ala, the author preserves a 1-mm rim of the ala just beyond the alar-facial sulcus (see Chapter 13). However, there are a few exceptions to this rule.

In addition to enlarging a defect, occasionally it is beneficial to resect tissue in the depths of the wound to create a more uniform depth. Mohs' surgery for cutaneous tumors typically creates a 45-degree bevel at the margin of the defect. The specimen is excised in this manner in order to optimize it for histologic examination. Before repair of any defect resulting from Mohs' surgery, the beveled tissue at the borders of the wound is removed. The two circumstances in which this tissue is left intact are when the defect is left to heal by secondary intention or when a skin graft is planned for covering the wound and the graft is thinner than the skin surrounding the recipient site. Removing beveled tissue ensures that a covering flap of uniform thickness may be developed to resurface the defect with less risk of contour deformity. The skin adjacent to any nasal defect is undermined in the subfascial plane to minimize trap-door deformity. Another method of reducing this deformity is angulation of the peripheral margins of curvilinear defects. Compared with nasal skin defects that are angled or square, round defects are more likely to undergo concentric scar contraction and result in trap-door deformity. Modifying the periphery of a defect by creating 90-degree angles often reduces this risk (Fig. 6–2). For this reason, when enlarging a defect so it encompasses the entire nasal tip, the line of transition between the tip and sidewall or tip and lower dorsum should be straight with 90-degree angles at the cephalic borders of the defect.

A set of algorithms has been developed to guide the surgeon in selecting the optimal method of repairing nasal cutaneous defects (Fig. 6–3). They are based on a number of factors related to the defect and the patient. A separate algorithm has been developed for each aesthetic unit of the nose.

Primary Closure

Small defects of the nasal skin (less than 1.0 cm) may on occasion be repaired with primary closure. This is especially true when the defect has an oval or linear configuration (Fig. 6–4). The mobility of skin and soft tissue of the cephalic two-thirds of the nose may allow

closure of defects up to 1 cm in diameter after wide undermining in the subfascial plane. Larger skin defects may be repaired in this fashion if a concurrent reduction rhinoplasty (when indicated) is performed. Reducing the volume of the nasal skeleton creates a relatively greater amount of nasal skin, which facilitates nasal repair. Small cutaneous defects located near the glabella are often approximated in a horizontal orientation so that scars are parallel to the transverse creases caused by the procerus muscle. The wound is approximated in two layers with deep buried sutures of 4.0 or 5.0 polydioxanone placed through the fascia and dermis and by vertical mattress 5.0 or 6.0 nylon or polypropylene cutaneous sutures. Excision of standing cutaneous deformities and soft tissue is performed laterally on both sides of the wound closure. Defects of the middle and caudal third of the dorsum may be repaired in a transverse fashion if additional cephalic rotation of the tip is desired. If this is not desirable, the wound is approximated with a vertical orientation.

Healing by Secondary Intention

Small to medium cutaneous and superficial soft-tissue defects involving stable concave surfaces of the nose such as the upper bony sidewall and lateral alar groove may be allowed to granulate with a satisfactory aesthetic outcome. The force of wound contracture in these areas is countered by the rigid underlying bony and soft-tissue support, resulting in minimal distortion. Granulating wounds are kept moist by frequent application of topical petroleum-based ointments. Our regimen involves bacitracin ointment applied three times daily for 3 days to keep the granulating surface moist. After 3 days the antibiotic ointment is switched to petrolatum and continued until epithelialization is complete. Wounds are cleaned with soap and water, and debris may be removed with a wet washcloth. Based on the size of the defect, it may take 4 to 6 weeks for the wound to become epithelialized.

Delayed Skin Grafting

Some cutaneous nasal defects appropriate for skin grafting may be repaired on a delayed basis. In these instances, the defect is allowed to granulate for 2 to 4 weeks before the grafting procedure is performed. Granulation tissue fills the depth of the wound, reducing a step-down deformity along the borders of the skin graft. It also provides a rich vascular recipient site for the skin graft. During the delay, wound care is similar to

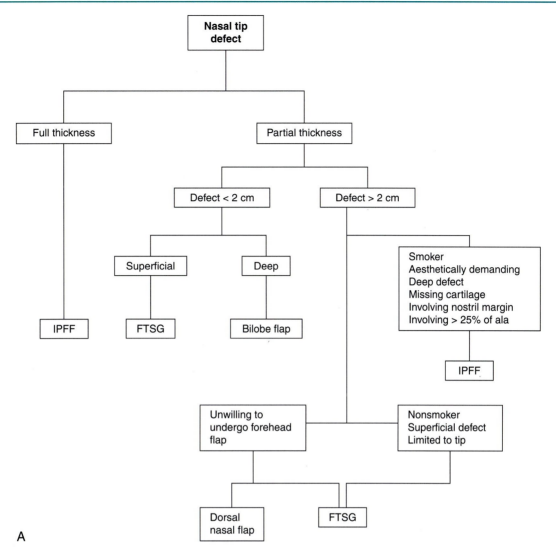

Figure 6–3. *A,* Algorithm for external covering of nasal tip defects. (FTSG: full-thickness skin graft; IPFF: interpolated parame-dian forehead flap).

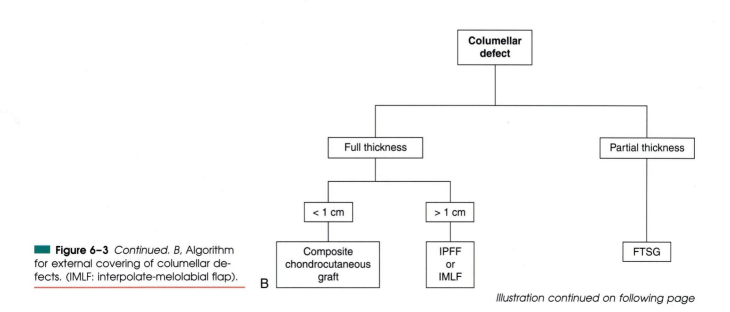

Figure 6–3 *Continued. B,* Algorithm for external covering of columellar de-fects. (IMLF: interpolate-melolabial flap).

Illustration continued on following page

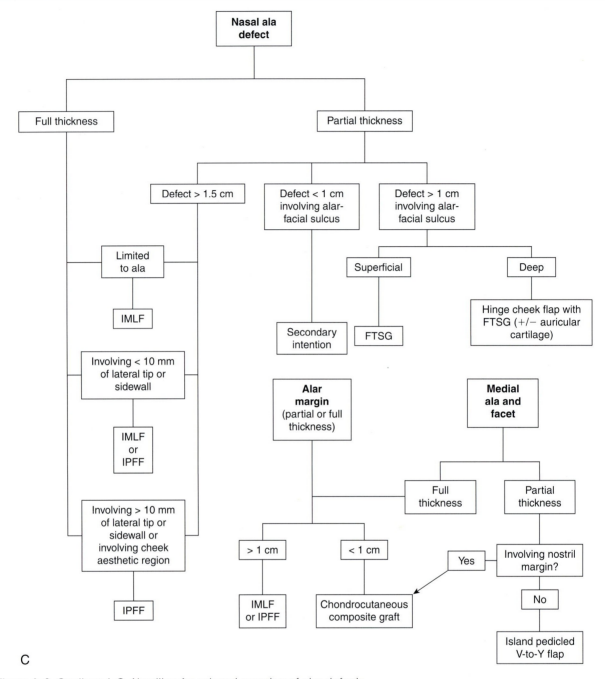

C

Figure 6–3 *Continued. C,* Algorithm for external covering of alar defects.

that for wounds healing by secondary intention. The wound is continually occluded with petrolatum. When sufficient granulation tissue has developed to nearly fill the depths of the wound, the area is covered with a full-thickness skin graft. Patients are started on a course of antistaphylococcal antibiotics 3 days before grafting to reduce bacterial colonization of the wound. The upper layer of the granulation tissue is bluntly débrided with a 4 × 4 gauze before the skin graft is transferred. In addition, the edges of the wound are débrided of the thin epithelial cover that forms over the granulation tissue. A full-thickness skin graft harvested from an appropriate donor site is sutured on top of the granulation tissue and bolstered in the standard fashion (see Chapter 9). A 7-day course of postoperative antistaphylococcal antibiotic is continued. Delayed grafting of a deep wound allows for restoration of the soft-tissue volume by granulating tissue and reduces the contour deformity that may result from primary grafting. Exposed cartilage and bone with missing perichondrium or periosteum

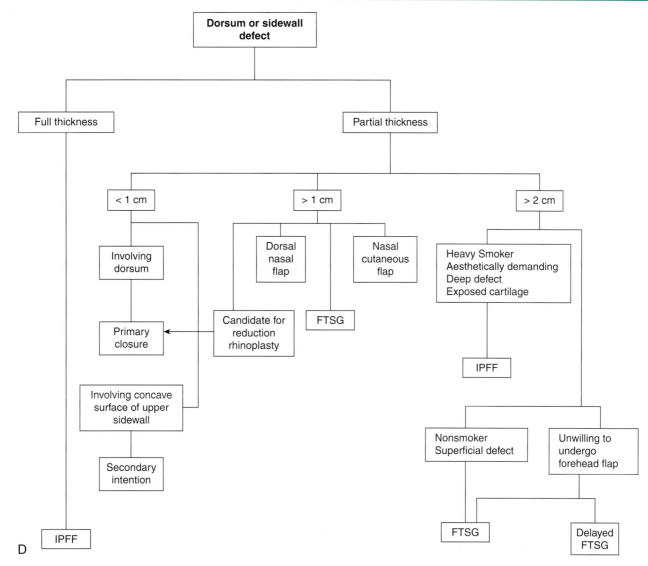

Figure 6–3 *Continued. D*, Algorithm for external covering of dorsum and sidewall defects.

Illustration continued on following page

are less likely to support a skin graft. With proper wound care, limited areas of exposed cartilage and bone will granulate and subsequently support a skin graft. This is often an acceptable alternative for repair of deep soft-tissue defects in patients unwilling to undergo reconstruction with a cutaneous flap.

Skin Graft

Cutaneous defects involving the nasal tip, columella, dorsum, or sidewalls may be repaired with a full-thickness skin graft in instances where the structural support is not disrupted and the wound depth is not excessive. Factors to consider in selecting a donor site for the skin graft include the match of color, texture, and thickness with that of the recipient site and the amount of skin required (see Chapter 9).

Perichondrocutaneous Graft

The perichondrium of the conchal bowl and its tightly adherent lateral conchal skin is a unique source of skin graft used for covering nasal cutaneous defects. The main disadvantage of this technique is that repair of the donor site requires another graft or flap. In our experience, the aesthetic outcome of perichondrocutaneous grafts is not superior to that obtained with a full-thickness skin graft.

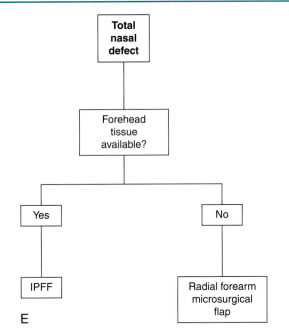

■ **Figure 6–3** *Continued. E,* Algorithm for external covering of total nasal defect.

Composite Graft

The composite chondrocutaneous graft has the advantage of providing a single-stage simultaneous repair of internal lining, structural support, and external cover of small full-thickness defects involving the nasal facet, alar margin, or columella (see Chapter 9). Its use is limited to nonsmokers and defects not exceeding 1 cm. The volume of the graft is slightly oversized to accommodate tissue contraction following transfer.

Nasal Cutaneous Flaps

Small cutaneous and soft-tissue defects of the nose can often be repaired with adjacent nasal tissue. Nasal skin clearly provides a color and texture match that is superior to that of any other source of skin. There is limited laxity of nasal skin, and the use of nasal cutaneous flaps is generally restricted to defects that do not exceed 2 cm.

The bilobe pivotal flap may be used to repair small cutaneous defects of the nasal tip with excellent results. It is ideal for repair of defects of the tip up to 1.5 cm in diameter. The zone of transition between the tip, ala, and sidewall is also an excellent location for repair using this technique. Defects involving the skin of the

infratip lobule, ala, or columella are not optimally suited for repair with a bilobe flap because it often results in deformity of the nostril margin, which may include retraction and distortion. Reconstruction of the ala with a bilobe flap requires the pedicle of the flap to cross the alar groove, thus distorting the topography of this important nasal contour.

Transposition flaps may be used to repair small skin defects of the cephalic third of the nose in the region of the radix, upper dorsum, and medial canthus. However, tension lines often create contour deformities that may take several months to improve.

The dorsal nasal flap (Rieger's flap) is an alternative for repair of small to medium defects involving the tip or caudal dorsum and sidewall. The technique has the disadvantage of causing juxtaposition of thick skin from the glabella and thin skin of the medial canthus. The dorsal heminasal flap (see Chapter 10) avoids this disadvantage by maintaining the thin skin of the cephalic nasal sidewall.

Like the dorsal nasal flap, the island pedicled V-to-Y nasal cutaneous flap has specific indications for its use. The flap is based on a soft-tissue pedicle in the depths of the alar groove and is used to repair skin defects positioned in the anterior portion of the alar groove (Fig. 6–5).

Interpolated Melolabial Flap

The interpolated melolabial flap is used to transfer skin and soft tissue of the cheek to the region of the ala, lateral tip, columella, and caudal nasal sidewall. The skin is similar in thickness and texture to the thicker, more sebaceous skin of the ala. This is the covering flap of choice for repair of subtotal or total cutaneous defects of the ala (see Figs. 6–1 and 6–2). The utility of the flap may be expanded to include cutaneous defects with limited (1.0 cm or less) involvement of the tip or caudal portion of the nasal sidewall.

Interpolated Paramedian Forehead Flap

This is the most common covering flap used for repair of medium (greater than 2.0 cm) to large (greater than 3.0 cm) defects of nasal skin and soft tissue (Fig. 6–6). The flap can be designed to provide sufficient forehead skin to resurface the entire nose. Forehead skin has an excellent color and texture match with that of the nose. There is minimal long-term morbidity at the donor site.

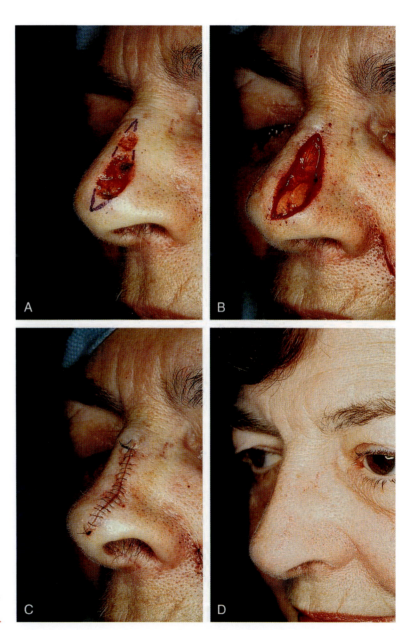

■ **Figure 6-4.** *A*, Superficial cutaneous defects of nasal dorsum and tip. Elliptical excision is planned to assist with primary closure of wound. *B*, Skin excised to level of cartilage. *C*, Wound closed primarily. *D*, Three months postoperative.

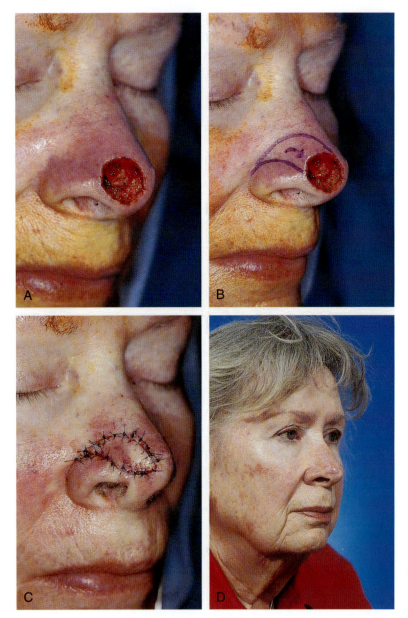

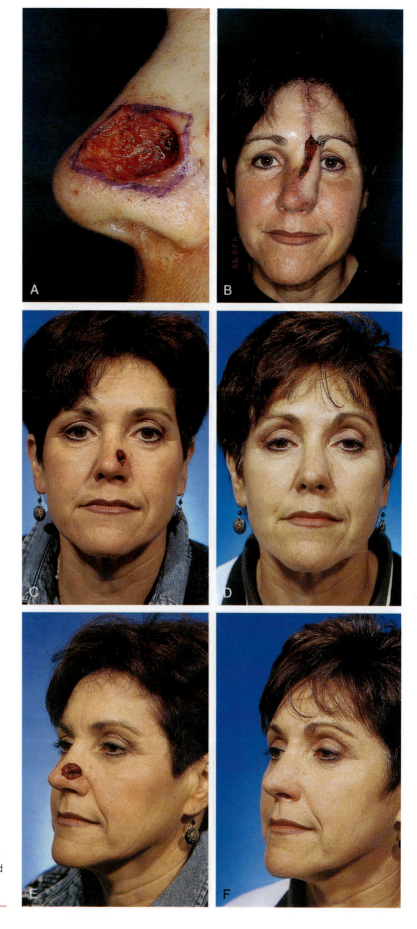

■ **Figure 6–6.** *A,* 2.0 × 2.0 cm cutaneous defect of lateral nasal tip and sidewall. Defect to be converted to rectangular configuration. *B,* Interpolated paramedian forehead flap used as covering flap. *C–F,* Preoperative and 17 months postoperative.

Complex cutaneous defects involving multiple aesthetic units, such as all or portions of the tip, facet, columella, dorsum, and sidewall, are most commonly repaired with this flap. This is also the flap of choice for repair of full-thickness nasal defects, with the exception of those limited to the ala.

Radial Forearm Microsurgical Flap

There may be instances of total or near-total nasal reconstruction in which forehead tissue is not available for resurfacing the entire nose. The glabella and central forehead may be missing because of tumor resection or trauma. In these instances, the thin skin of the volar aspect of the distal forearm is an acceptable substitute for forehead tissue. The radial forearm microsurgical flap has the advantages of ease of dissection, large donor vessels, and a long pedicle, all of which greatly simplify the technical aspects of flap transfer. The vascular pedicle is tunneled beneath the melolabial fold to recipient vessels in the upper neck. The flap is carefully designed so its configuration and surface area accurately replace the nasal skin deficit.

References

1. Burget GC, Menick FJ: The subunit principle in nasal reconstruction. Plastic Reconstr Surg 76:239, 1985.

2. Burget GC, Menick FJ: Aesthetic Reconstruction of the Nose. St. Louis, Mosby, 1994.

PART II

Technique

7

Cartilage Grafts

Sam Naficy

One of the most important steps in reconstruction of the nose is restoration of a structurally sound cartilaginous framework to provide a natural contour to the middle and lower nasal vaults. Grafting with cartilage is required in instances where the defect extends through the cartilage framework or when wound contracture during healing may result in collapse or distortion of the soft tissues of the nose. Therefore, in addition to replacing missing nasal cartilage, grafts may be used to reinforce portions of the nose that, in their natural form, lack cartilaginous support. Examples of the latter include the ala and nasal facet.

Three principal sources of autologous cartilage used for grafts in nasal reconstruction are the auricle, nasal septum, and rib. A limited amount of cartilage may also be obtained from the alar cartilages. Regardless of the source of cartilage, precise sculpting and fixation of grafts are required to achieve optimal contour. Cartilage grafts are covered with a cutaneous flap externally. Grafts used to repair full-thickness nasal defects are completely enveloped with a well-vascularized lining flap and cutaneous covering flap. These flaps ensure that cartilage grafts maintain their shape and volume indefinitely.

Auricular Cartilage Graft

Autologous conchal cartilage is ideal for providing a framework to reconstruct the entire lower nasal vault and portions of the middle vault. Auricular cartilage also serves as an excellent batten graft for supporting the ala. The auricle is easily included in the surgical field in preparation for nasal reconstruction, and there is minimal donor site morbidity and complication associated with harvesting the graft. The ear contralateral to the alar defect usually provides conchal cartilage that has the desirable contour.

The auricle consists of a single piece of highly convoluted elastic cartilage (Fig. 7–1). Auricular cartilage is nourished on both sides by a layer of perichondrium. Laterally, conchal perichondrium adheres tightly to the skin. Medially, there is a loose, relatively avascular plane between the skin and conchal perichondrium. The concha is bounded superiorly by the anterior crus of the antihelix and the crus of the helix, posteriorly by the antihelical fold, and inferiorly by the antitragus. Anteriorly, it funnels into the cartilaginous external auditory canal. The concha is made up of two concavities that are partially separated by the crus of the helix. The smaller, superiorly located concavity is the cymba; the larger, inferiorly located concavity is the cavum. The concha cymba typically has a contour that is remarkably similar to the size and contour of the contralateral intermediate and medial crura (Fig. 7–2). Likewise, the concha cavum often has dimensions and contour that closely replicate the configuration of the lateral crus and ala. Harvesting both segments of the concha in continuity provides sufficient cartilage to restore the entire intermediate and lateral crura of the alar cartilage. If the graft is sufficiently wide, it may be used to simultaneously provide a framework for the ala.

■ Technique

The procedure is performed with the patient under local anesthesia, usually with intravenous sedation. The

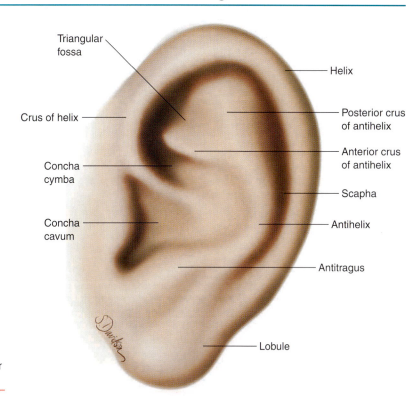

- Triangular fossa
- Helix
- Crus of helix
- Posterior crus of antihelix
- Anterior crus of antihelix
- Concha cymba
- Scapha
- Concha cavum
- Antihelix
- Antitragus
- Lobule

■ **Figure 7–1.** Topographic anatomy of auricular cartilage.

head is elevated on a foam cushion, and the surgical table is placed in 15 to 20 degrees of a reverse Trendelenburg position. Lidocaine (1% with 1:1,000,000 concentration of epinephrine) is used to anesthetize and hydrodissect the auricular skin and soft tissue. Laterally, injection is made in the subperichondrial plane and medially in the subcutaneous plane.

Two approaches are available to harvest conchal cartilage. Our preferred technique for harvesting auricular cartilage grafts is a medial approach. A postauricular incision is made halfway between the postauricular crease and the helix, spanning the entire vertical height

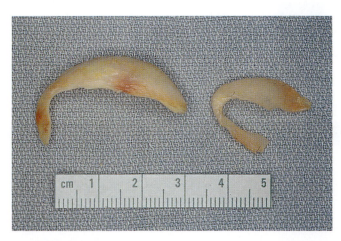

■ **Figure 7–2.** Lower lateral cartilage and conchal cartilage. Alar cartilage (right) has great similarity in contour to conchal cartilage (left) harvested from contralateral ear.

of the conchal cartilage. Dissection immediately superficial to perichondrium exposes the entire medial aspect of the conchal cartilage (Fig. 7–3). A full-thickness curvilinear incision is made through the conchal cartilage parallel and just medial to the crest of the antihelical fold. Subperichondrial dissection is performed using a no. 9 dental or Cottle elevator, exposing the entire lateral surface of the conchal cartilage. An appropriate-sized graft is harvested, taking care to preserve the helical crus, cartilage of the antihelix, and a rim of cartilage around the external auditory canal. The cartilage surrounding the external auditory meatus prevents collapse of the canal. Preserving the cartilage of the antihelix, including the anterior and posterior crura, supports the helical rim and prevents deformation of the auricle. The cartilage graft is placed in an isotonic solution containing an antistaphylococcal antibiotic. Following hemostasis of the wound, the postauricular incision is repaired in a single layer with a simple continuous 5.0 fast-absorbing gut suture. A bolster dressing consisting of two dental rolls, one placed inside the concha and one place behind the ear, is secured using three sutures of 4.0 nylon placed full-thickness through the ear and around the dental rolls (see Fig. 7–3). The bolster sutures are positioned to straddle the suture line of the postauricular access incision and are removed on the first postoperative day. The sutures are tied lightly to prevent excessive compression of the auricular skin. Advantages of the medial approach include a hidden scar, easier access to the plane of dissection for the lateral aspect of the conchal cartilage, and greater

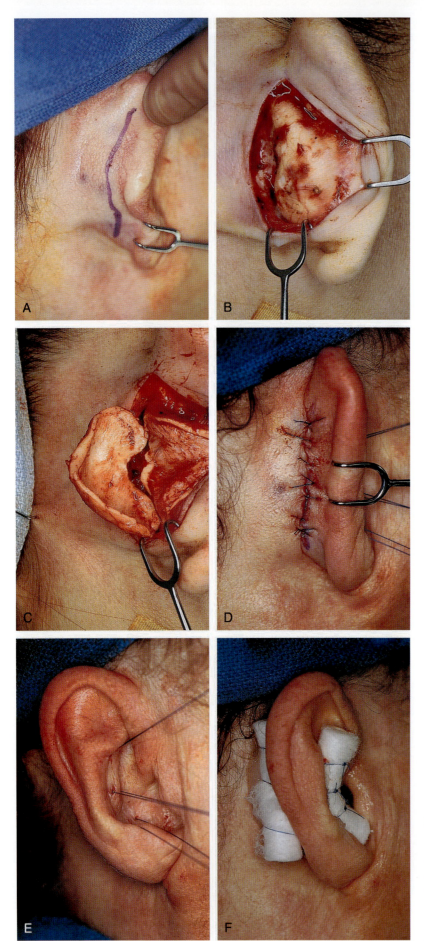

Figure 7–3. Technique for harvesting auricular cartilage through medial approach. *A* and *B*, Skin incision made and conchal cartilage exposed. *C*, Cartilage incised and lateral surface dissected in subperichondrial plane to deliver graft. *D*, Skin incision repaired. Three bolster sutures straddle incision. *E*, Bolster sutures evenly spaced along vertical axis of concha. *F*, Bolster dressing tied in place.

exposure of the entire conchal cartilage. This technique not only produces a superior aesthetic outcome but also reduces operative time.

Using the lateral approach, a perichondrocutaneous flap is elevated after making a curvilinear incision just anterior to the antihelical fold (Fig. 7–4). Careful subperichondrial dissection is performed, exposing the entire lateral surface of the conchal cartilage. A kidney bean–shaped piece of cartilage is incised full-thickness with a scalpel and elevated with scissors, maintaining the medial attachment of the perichondrium. Care is taken to preserve cartilage of the antihelix, a rim of cartilage around the external auditory canal, and the crus of the helix. Typically a 4.5 × 2 cm segment of curved conchal cartilage may be harvested without jeopardizing the shape of the auricle. Following hemo-

stasis, the access incision is closed in a single layer of simple continuous 5.0 fast-absorbing gut suture. A bolster dressing similar to that used for the medial approach is applied for 24 hours.

Perioperative care consists of a single dose of a preoperative intravenous antistaphylococcal antibiotic and 5 to 7 days of postoperative oral antistaphylococcal antibiotic therapy. Patients are instructed to clean the wound site with cotton tip applicators soaked in hydrogen peroxide two to three times each day and apply topical antibacterial ointment three times a day for 3 days. Then they are instructed to switch to a petroleum ointment for 3 additional days.

Complications of harvesting an auricular cartilage graft include hematoma and infection of the operative sites, both of which are quite rare. Hematoma in the

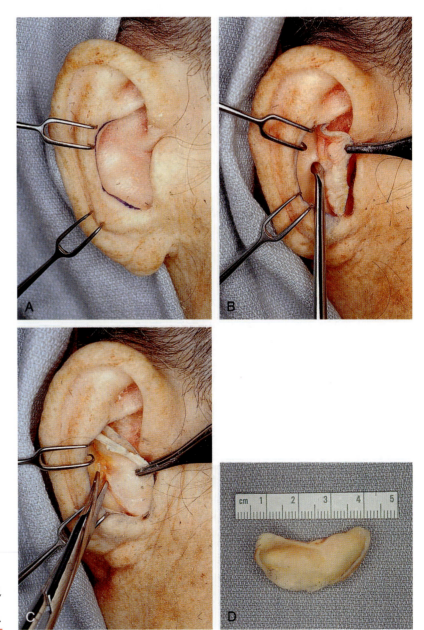

■ **Figure 7–4.** Technique for harvesting auricular cartilage through lateral approach. *A,* Skin incision made anterior to antihelix (blue marking). *B,* Auricular skin dissected from cartilage. *C,* Cartilage incised and medial surface dissected in supraperichondrial plane. *D,* Excised cartilage.

early stages may be aspirated with an 18-gauge needle in sterile conditions. Larger, more solidified hematomas may require wound exploration or performing a small incision to evacuate blood. Utilizing the bolster dressing previously described, we have not observed a single case of auricular hematoma in well over 200 cases. Wound infection, also a rare complication, should be treated with broad spectrum antibiotics that have effective coverage for staphylococcus and pseudomonas.

Septal Cartilage Graft

Septal cartilage is hyaline cartilage and provides an excellent source of grafting material for nasal reconstruction. It is particularly well suited for restoring the cartilaginous framework of the nasal dorsum, tip, columella, and caudal aspect of the nasal side walls. It is also extremely useful as a strut for support of the nasal tip or as a dorsal onlay graft. The septum is always in the surgical field, and septal cartilage grafts persist indefinitely if nourished by a covering flap. Septal cartilage is easily sculpted and maintains its shape over long periods. Septal cartilage lacks the natural curvature and flexibility of auricular cartilage and is not optimal for repair of alar defects where marked convexity of the framework is required. However, proper fixation and scoring of the cartilage will often allow a moderate degree of convexity. Septal cartilage is harvested through a standard septoplasty. In cases requiring septal mucoperichondrial hinge flaps, cartilage is removed through the exposure offered by flap dissection.

■ Technique

The nasal mucosa is vasoconstricted by placing inside the nasal cavity pledgets (0.5 × 3 in. surgical cottonoids) soaked with oxymetazoline hydrochloride. Lidocaine (1% with 1:100,000 concentration of epinephrine) is used to hydrodissect the mucoperichondrium from the septal cartilage on both sides. An incision 2 to 3 cm long is made through the nasal mucoperichondrium along the caudal margin of the septal cartilage. For a right-handed surgeon, the incision is usually made on the patient's left side. Sharp dissection is initially accomplished with a no. 15 scalpel blade or small dissecting scissors until the septal cartilage is visualized along the entire length of the incision. Careful scoring of the surface of the cartilage with the tip of a scalpel blade ensures penetration through the thin and tightly adherent inner perichondrial layer. Using a Cottle elevator, a mucoperichondrial flap is elevated from an anterior to a posterior direction. Wide exposure of the entire quadrangular cartilage is achieved, extending superiorly and posteriorly to expose the perpendicular plate of the

ethmoid and the vomer bone. A caudal and dorsal strut of cartilage 1 to 1.5 cm wide is preserved for nasal support, and the remainder of the quadrangular cartilage may be safely removed for grafting (Fig. 7–5). A no. 15 scalpel blade is used to incise the cartilage outlining the L-strut that will remain in situ. A Cottle elevator is then used to penetrate the cartilage and elevate the contralateral mucoperichondrium from the portion of cartilage to be removed. Using the blunt end of the Cottle elevator, the quadrangular cartilage is disarticulated from its posterior attachments to the vomer and perpendicular plate of the ethmoid bone. Inferiorly, the cartilage is separated from the fibrous attachments to the nasal crest and the vomer. The cartilage graft is removed and stored in an isotonic solution containing antistaphylococcal antibiotic. A composite graft of septal cartilage and bone may be harvested by maintaining the posterior attachments of the cartilage to the vomer and perpendicular plate of the ethmoid bone. Angled scissors are used to transect the bone horizontally 1 cm inferior to the level of the canthi. A 4 mm chisel is used to free the bony component of the graft from its inferior and posterior attachments.

The approach incision is repaired using multiple interrupted 5.0 chromic gut suture. The two mucoperichondrial flaps are approximated using a continuous horizontal mattress suture of 3.0 chromic gut. This "quilting stitch" eliminates the dead space and need for nasal packing and minimizes the potential for hematoma.

Postoperative care consists of cleansing the inside of

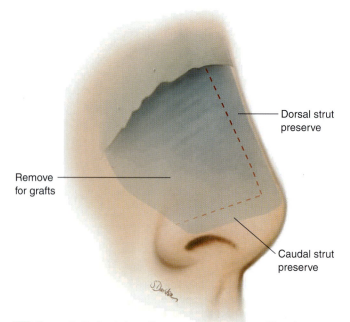

Dorsal strut preserve

Remove for grafts

Caudal strut preserve

■ **Figure 7–5.** Septal cartilage available for grafting. L-shaped dorsal and caudal strut (*dotted line*) preserved for nasal support.

the nose with cotton tip applicators soaked in hydrogen peroxide two to three times a day and applying a petroleum-based ointment to the sutures. Patients are prescribed a 5- to 7-day course of oral antistaphylococcal antibiotics to begin postoperatively.

In instances where a septal mucoperichondrial hinge flap is used for repair of an internal lining defect, septal cartilage is always exposed and readily accessible. A caudal and dorsal strut of cartilage 1 to 1.5 cm wide is preserved, and the remainder of the cartilage may be removed, preserving the contralateral mucoperichondrium. The exposed raw surface of the contralateral mucoperichondrium will heal by secondary intention and become resurfaced with epithelium. Crusting is minimized by periodic débridement and frequent use of isotonic saline nasal spray during the first few weeks after surgery.

Complications of harvesting septal cartilage grafts include hematoma, structural deformity of the nose, and infection. The risk of hematoma is minimized by elevation of the mocoperichondrial flaps in the proper anatomical plane and by coaptation of the flaps with a quilting horizontal mattress suture. Preserving an adequate strut of dorsal and caudal cartilaginous septum maintains support of the lower and middle nasal vaults, minimizing the risk of saddle deformity of the dorsum. Infections at the septal donor site are rare and, if seen, are usually subsequent to the development of a septal hematoma. Septal perforation may occur from bilateral overlapping injury to the mucoperichondrial flaps or from a septal hematoma.

Rib Cartilage Graft

Autologous rib cartilage provides an ample source of material for nasal framework grafts. A substantial amount of rib cartilage and bone may be harvested from one or several different ribs to provide material for reconstruction of large defects. Rib cartilage is hyaline and undergoes extensive ossification with advancing age. Ribs of older individuals may have only small amounts of nonossified hyaline cartilage.

Rib bones articulate with their corresponding thoracic vertebrae and curve anteriorly. Ribs bend at the costal angle, the lateral-most aspect of each rib, and continue medially, inferiorly, and anteriorly. The bony portion of the first ten ribs ends in a bar of hyaline cartilage at the costochondral synchondrosis. The cartilaginous segment of the second through seventh rib articulates with the sternum. The sternochondral joint of the sixth rib is at the level of the xiphisternal junction. The costal cartilages of the eighth, ninth, and tenth ribs extend medially and superiorly from the bone of their corresponding ribs to terminate on the costal arch, which connects superiorly to the costochondral syn-

chondrosis. The internal thoracic artery provides the blood supply to the anterior chest wall. Intercostal branches of this artery run along the pleural aspect of the ribs.

■ Technique

The straightest rib is palpated either at the inframammary line or along the costal margin. The fifth rib is usually the most suitable donor rib for nasal reconstruction. It has a long and fairly straight cartilaginous segment (Fig. 7–6). To expose the rib, a 3-cm incision is made through the skin, superficial fascia, anterior rectus sheath, and rectus abdominus muscle overlying the rib. This limited incision reduces postoperative pain but limits access for removing more than one or two ribs. The anterior perichondrium is incised in the shape of an H, with the central limb extending the full length of the exposed rib. Perichondrium is elevated circumferentially from above and below the rib with a no. 9 dental elevator, taking care to dissect all tissue from the underside of the cartilage. After circumferential dissection is accomplished, a rib stripper may be used to free the deep perichondrial attachments to the rib cartilage. After adequate release of the rib from its attachments, a section is freed by full-thickness incision. This is performed with a no. 10 scalpel blade after placing a malleable retractor on the deep side of the rib. If there is a bony nasal defect, the dissection may be extended laterally and posteriorly to include a portion of the bony rib along with the cartilage. An alternative to full-thickness resection is splitting the rib cartilage longitudinally, creating a split rib graft. The deeper portion of rib cartilage is left in situ. This lessens the risk of pneumothorax and postoperative chest pain. After harvesting the rib graft, the wound is tested for the presence of a pneumothorax by employing a sustained positive pressure breath while the depth of the wound is filled with saline. The escape of air bubbles suggests the presence of a tear in the pleura and warrants exploration and repair of the tear. The wound is irrigated with an antibiotic solution, and the anterior perichondrium is closed. The remaining layers of rectus muscle and sheath, superficial fascia, and skin are approximated following insertion of a suction drain in the depths of the wound. If the procedure has precipitated a tear in the pleura, a small red rubber catheter is inserted in the thoracic cavity. After wound closure, the catheter is placed on suction and withdrawn from beneath the skin. An upright chest radiograph is obtained postoperatively to ensure that a significant pneumothorax is not persistent. Injection of bupivacaine 0.5% in the subperichondrial space may provide relief of discomfort during the immediate postoperative period.

The main advantages of the rib cartilage graft are the ample supply and capability of harvesting a large segment of cartilage, or a composite of bone and cartilage, for repair of large nasal defects. The incision is reasona-

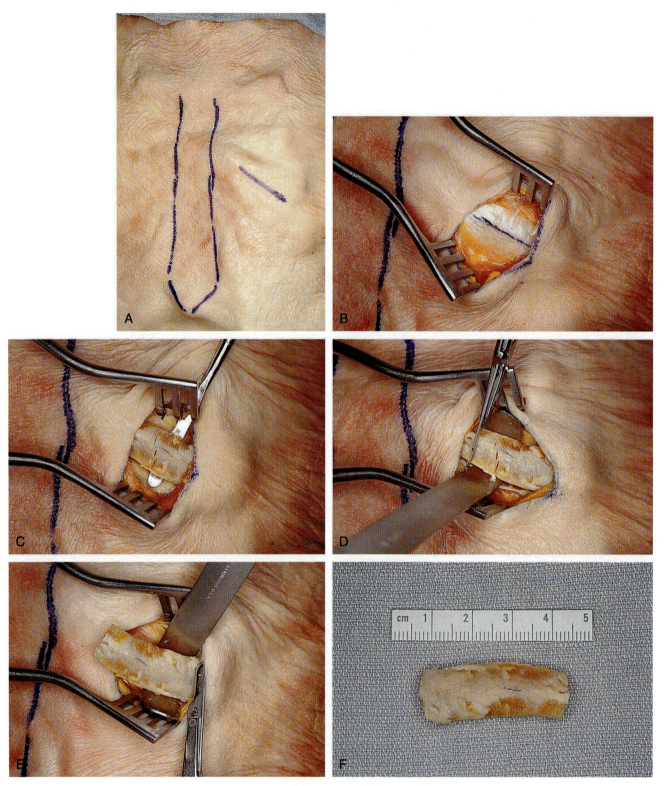

■ **Figure 7–6.** Technique for harvesting rib cartilage. *A*, Inframammary incision made (blue marking). *B*, Intercostal muscles bluntly separated to expose anterior perichondrium of rib. *B* and *C*, Perichondrium incised (blue marking) and dissected circumferentially. *D*, Rib incised full-thickness near sternocostal junction over malleable retractor. *E*, Deep side of rib is dissected laterally as necessary, and graft is excised. *F*, Rib graft demonstrating some degree of ossification.

bly well camouflaged, especially in women, where it may be placed in the inframammary fold. Disadvantages of using rib cartilage grafts are the painful donor site, potential for an unsightly donor scar, a tendency for long-term absorption, and warping and deformation of grafts over time. In elderly patients, rib cartilage may have a significant degree of calcification that may make it difficult to use in nasal reconstruction.

Alar Cartilage Graft

A limited amount of cartilage may be removed from the cephalic margin of the lateral crura of the alar cartilages when the defect provides exposure of these cartilages. This donor supply is limited because the alar cartilages are weakened and tip support is compromised if a large portion of the lateral crus is removed. The amount of cartilage that may be harvested safely depends on the size and intrinsic strength of the alar cartilages. Trimming the cephalic portion of the alar cartilages increases tip rotation; trimming should be limited to patients who desire this change. In most instances, a graft measuring 0.5 × 1.0 cm may be harvested without compromising structural support of the nasal tip. The cartilage has the ideal thickness and curvature for repair of small defects of cartilage in the nasal domes or columella. It is also an excellent graft for providing structural support to the nasal facets prior to coverage with a flap. Alar grafts may be used individually or sutured together as a double-layer graft for additional strength.

■ Technique

The alar cartilages are accessible through defects involving the nasal tip. Dissection is performed over the alar cartilages through the exposure offered by the defect. The line of excision is marked on the surface of both alar cartilages with a marker, or a partial-thickness incision is made with a no. 15 scalpel blade. In order to maintain tip symmetry, grafts are harvested bilaterally. The thin vestibular skin is hydrodissected away from the cephalic margin of the cartilages with a 30-gauge needle and a local anesthetic solution containing epinephrine. After a full-thickness incision is made through the alar cartilage, the leading edge of the cartilage is grasped with atraumatic forceps and dissected free with fine sharp scissors.

Contouring Grafts

Cartilage grafts are used to replace missing segments of nasal cartilage, thereby restoring the natural contour of the missing structures. Grafts are sculpted to provide a segment of cartilage that has the precise size, shape, and contour of the structure it is replacing. Grafts also serve as battens to maintain the shape and position of nasal structures that are vulnerable to deformation during the healing process (Fig. 7–7).

Grafts are contoured to the fullest extent possible prior to fixation. Further modifications may be accomplished in situ after the graft has been secured. We prefer a no. 15 scalpel blade for trimming cartilage grafts. The graft is held securely over a moist surgical towel with atraumatic tissue forceps, and the blade is used to plane away excess soft tissue or cartilaginous irregularities. The perichondrium of auricular cartilage is removed and, if necessary, the cartilage is shaved to a thickness of 1.5 mm. Structural integrity of a graft may be jeopardized by excessive thinning. After thinning, the graft is tailored to the precise shape of the corresponding nasal cartilage it is designed to replace by trimming redundant cartilage. The edges of the graft are sharply beveled. The graft may be further contoured by scoring, bending, and suture fixation to create the desired shape. When available for inspection, the contour of intact contralateral structures serve as an ideal template for fashioning the graft. Grafts and all excised soft tissue are stored in an antibiotic solution until the time of grafting. All patients having cartilage grafting to the nose are maintained on postoperative antistaphylococcal antibiotics for 5 to 7 days.

Depending on circumstances, septal cartilage usually requires minimal contouring except for trimming to the required size. Septal cartilage is inherently straight; creating convexity is more difficult than when dealing with auricular cartilage grafts. Convexity may be accomplished by thinning the cartilage and by partial-thickness scoring. Occasionally, horizontal mattress sutures of 5.0 polypropylene may be used to enhance convexity. If septal cartilage is used to restore the intermediate crus, it is helpful to attach the graft to the remnant of the medial crus using 5.0 polyglactin sutures placed in a mattress or figure-of-eight fashion. The graft is then bent laterally to restore the contour of the dome, using judicious scoring of the exposed outer surface of the cartilage.

Rib cartilage grafts may be used as a single onlay graft for reconstruction of major defects of the nasal dorsum. Defects with marked loss of projection of the nasal bridge are repaired using this technique. A platform is created to receive the graft by removing sufficient bone and cartilage to provide a stable foundation for the rib graft. If an internal lining defect is present, it must be repaired prior to placement of the graft. The rib is sharply sculpted with a no. 10 scalpel blade with appropriate tapering of the margins. Symmetric removal of perichondrium from all surfaces of the cartilage minimizes warping and graft deformation. A steel wire strut

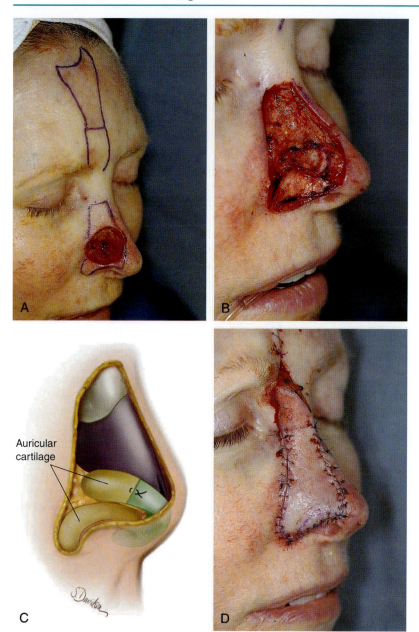

Auricular
cartilage

Figure 7–7. *A*, Cutaneous defect of ala and nasal sidewall. Portion of lateral crus was resected. Skin of aesthetic units marked for excision. Paramedian forehead flap designed as covering flap. *B*, Two auricular cartilage grafts outlined in blue used to replace missing portion of lateral crus and to serve as alar batten. *C*, Drawing showing structural grafts. *D*, Covering flap in place.

placed within the rib cartilage graft may reduce the risk of graft warping.[1]

Portions of the rib may be cut into cross-sectional wafers 2 mm thick and used as small independent grafts to correct contour irregularities.[2] These are most frequently used as grafts for reconstruction of the sidewall or tip.

■ Graft Fixation

Proper fixation of cartilage grafts to the native nasal skeleton creates a stable framework for the internal lining and external cover used to complete the reconstruction. The internal nasal lining is approximated to the underside of cartilage grafts with horizontal mattress sutures. This intimate contact between lining and graft helps nourish the graft. Multiple 5.0 polyglactin sutures are placed through the cartilage, the internal lining, back through both layers, and tied against the cartilage without excessive tension.

Fixation of cartilage to cartilage is accomplished by mattress suturing and figure-of-eight suturing. Mattress suturing of an overlapping segment of graft and native cartilage provides excellent mechanical stability. This technique is commonly used when restoring the medial or intermediate crus of the alar cartilage. To approximate the structures, horizontal mattress sutures of 5.0 polypropylene or polyglactin are passed through overlapping layers of cartilage and tied in place. In areas where end-to-end approximation is desired, figure-of-eight sutures of 5.0 polyglactin are used to fix cartilage grafts to native nasal cartilage (Fig. 7–8). The suture is passed full-thickness 2 to 3 mm from the free edge of

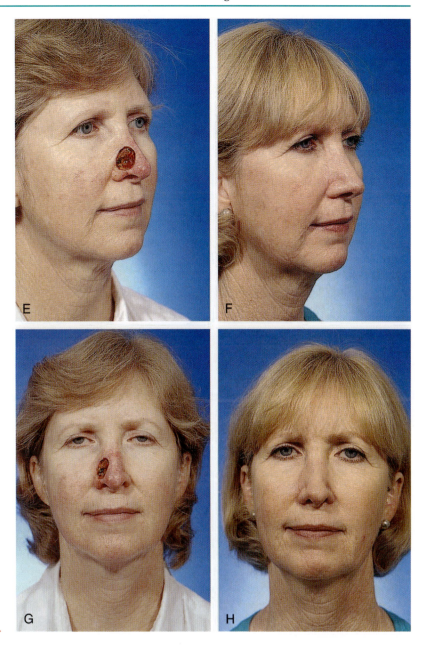

■ **Figure 7–7** *Continued. E–H*, Preoperative and 8 months postoperative.

each structure to be approximated. For a figure-of-eight suture, the same direction of travel is maintained through each pass of the needle. The knot is tied with minimal tension to avoid tearing the cartilage.

When reconstructing defects of the ala, an auricular cartilage batten graft (0.75 cm × 3.0 cm) is secured over the internal lining as a framework for the ala. Laterally, the batten graft is fixed to the periosteum and

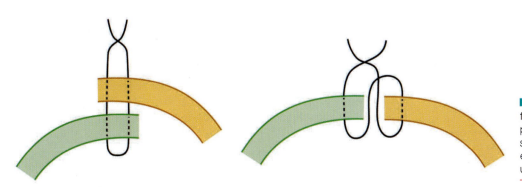

■ **Figure 7–8.** Graft fixation for structures that are overlapping are fixed with mattress suturing. Structures that are end-to-end are fixed with figure-of-eight sutures.

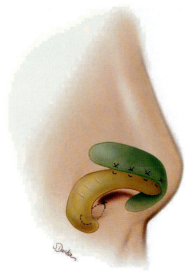

■ **Figure 7–9.** Cartilage batten graft spans entire surface of ala caudal to alar cartilage.

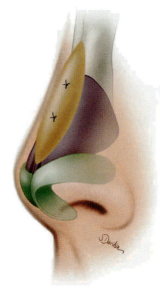

■ **Figure 7–11.** Auricular cartilage dorsal onlay graft fixed to septum with sutures.

soft tissue of the piriform aperture in a region corresponding to the alar facial sulcus. This is accomplished with a through-and-through mattress suture of 3.0 polyglactin that is tied inside the nasal vestibule. Medially, the graft is secured to the caudal aspect of the ipsilateral domal segment of the alar cartilage, creating a continuous arc of cartilage from the alar base to the nasal tip (Fig. 7–9). Greater curvature is achieved by using a longer graft. The cephalic border of the batten graft is stabilized against the caudal border of the alar cartilage with multiple figure-of-eight sutures of 5.0 polyglactin. If the lateral crus is missing, a wider (1.5 cm × 3.0 cm) segment of auricular cartilage is used to simultaneously replace the missing lateral crus of the alar

cartilage and batten the nasal ala (Fig. 7–10). If the entire domal segment of the alar cartilage is absent, the graft is extended from the alar base to the columella. Then, the concha cymba of the auricular cartilage graft is sutured to the ipsilateral medial crus. It is critical that during the reconstructive process the cartilaginous framework be viewed from all key positions (frontal, oblique, lateral, and basal) to ensure proper position and contour of the graft.

Grafts of the nasal tip and dorsum are placed in the same manner as in open rhinoplasty. Septal or auricular cartilage may be used to create cap grafts, shield grafts, infratip grafts, columellar struts, and dorsal onlay grafts (Fig. 7–11). The grafts are sutured to the underlying framework using 5.0 polypropylene or polydioxonone sutures. The borders of tip grafts are tapered or morselized to avoid a visible or palpable edge. In order to achieve an aesthetically desirable profile, the tip should project a minimum of 6 to 8 mm beyond the plane of the dorsum before repair of the external cutaneous defect.

Graft fixation to the nasal sidewall usually involves suture fixation to the periosteum of the piriform and nasal bones as well as to remnant upper lateral cartilage or dorsum. When the entire upper lateral cartilage is missing, the graft is secured to the nasal bone with sutures passed through multiple 1 mm holes drilled through the caudal margin of the bone.

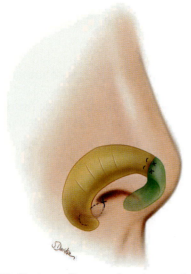

■ **Figure 7–10.** Single cartilage graft replaces missing lateral crus of alar cartilage and extends to caudal margin of nostril to batten alar region.

References

1. Gunter JP, Clark CP, Friedman RM: Internal stabilization of autogenous rib cartilage grafts in rhinoplasty: A barrier to cartilage warping. Plast Recontr Surg 100:161, 1997.

2. Burget GC, Menick FJ: Aesthetic Reconstruction of the Nose. St Louis, Mosby, 1994.

8

Bone Grafts

Sam Naficy

When a nasal defect involves all or part of the bony pyramid, the missing portion of nasal bone is usually replaced with autologous bone grafts. Bone grafts are sculpted to fit the defect and are secured to the remaining bony and cartilage framework. It is necessary for vascularized tissue to nourish both surfaces of bone grafts. The most common donor sites for autologous bone grafts used in nasal reconstruction are the cranium, rib, and septum.

Cranial Bone Graft

Extensive defects of the bony pyramid are best reconstructed with a three-dimensional structural framework of autologous bone. Outer table parietal bone, when properly sculpted, spatially oriented, and rigidly fixed, provides a stable replacement for defects of the bony pyramid. The donor site is adjacent to the operative field and, with the proper technique and precautions, morbidity and complications are rare.

■ Anatomy

Cranial bone is made up of three distinct layers (Fig. 8–1). The outer cortical layer is thicker than the inner cortical layer and is separated from it by a layer of cancellous bone called the diploic layer. A number of venous channels are present in the diploic layer. Both cortical layers are covered with periosteum on the nondiploic surface. The periosteum of the inner table is fused to the dura. Pensler and MacCarthy[1] found that

the adult parietal cranium ranges from 6.8 to 7.7 mm in thickness. There is regional variation, with thinner bone in the temporal region and thicker bone in the occipital region. Topographically, the coronal suture separates the frontal from the parietal bones. Anteriorly, the root of the nose marks the midline. The midline sagittal suture extends posteriorly from the coronal suture and separates the two parietal bones. It marks the midline of the vertex and the location of the superior sagittal dural sinus. The sinus measures as much as 1.5 cm in width and courses in the midline along the inner surface of the cranial vault. It is critical to identify the location of this vessel using anatomical landmarks to avoid harvesting bone within 2 cm of the midline.

■ Harvesting Technique

General anesthesia is used for cranial bone grafting. The patient is placed supine in approximately 15 to 20 degrees of a reverse Trendelenburg position to reduce venous pooling in the scalp and diploae. It is not necessary to use a special headrest. The patient is given an intravenous preoperative dose of an antistaphylococcal antibiotic. The technique for harvesting cranial bone has been modeled on descriptions by other authors.[2, 3]

The size of the graft will depend on the extent of the defect, but we have found that a graft measuring 4 × 3 cm will prove sufficient for reconstructing the dorsum and two sidewalls of the nose. A parasagittal scalp incision measuring 8 to 10 cm is marked halfway between the midline and the temporal line. The hair on either side of the planned incision is parted and rubber-banded to facilitate incisions and wound closure. Lidocaine (1% with 1:100,000 concentration of epinephrine)

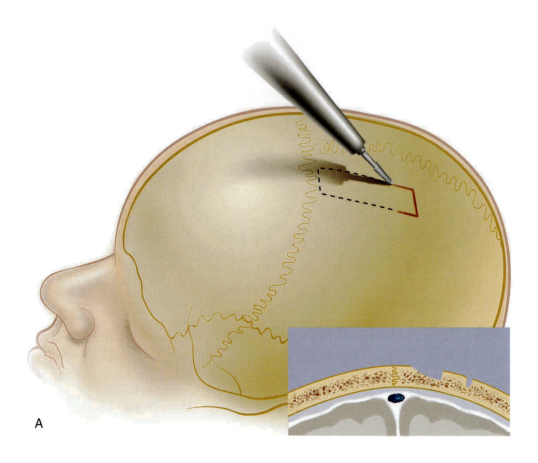

A

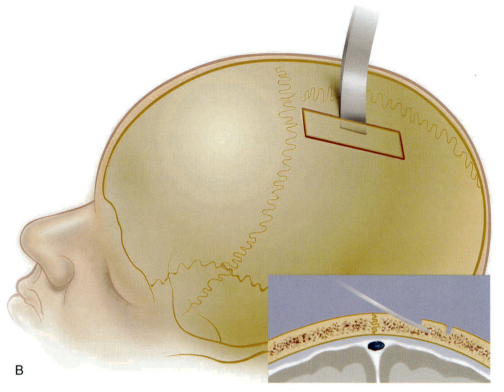

B

Figure 8–1. *A,* Side-cutting bur is used to drill trough at periphery of bone graft. *B,* Medial trough is beveled with cutting bur to allow placement of oscillating 90-degree saw blade, which traverses diploic space under the graft. Chisel is used to release bone graft.

is injected from the pericranium to the dermis along the entire length of the incision. After adequate time for vasoconstriction, the scalp incision is made to the level of the cranium, and wide subperiosteal elevation is performed. Self-retaining retractors are used for exposure (Fig. 8–2). The graft is harvested from the flattest portion of the exposed skull without extending laterally to the squama of the temporal bone. A template of the graft is used to create a pattern on the exposed bone in a parasagittal position with anterior to posterior orientation. The medial border of the template remains at least 2 cm lateral to the midline to avoid injury to the sagittal sinus. The template is traced with a surgical marker or drilled to score the bone lightly. Using a high-speed drill with a side-cutting bur (2 to 3 mm) and saline irrigation, a trough is drilled down to the diploic layer around the perimeter of the pattern (see Fig. 8–1). A large-bore cutting bur (6 mm) is used to bevel the trough outward around the circumference of the pattern. Beveling enables placement of a 90-degree angled oscillating saw blade within the diploic space of the cranial bone. The length of the oscillating portion of the saw blade should be at least half the width of the intended bone graft (Fig. 8–3). Using saline irrigation and protective eyewear, the diploic layer is traversed with the oscillating saw blade from the lateral and medial aspects of the bone graft. Great caution is exercised in orienting the blade of the saw parallel to the plane of the outer and inner cortical layer of the cranium to avoid penetrating the inner table. Wide bone chisels are used to free the remaining connections of the diploic layer to the outer table (see Fig. 8–1). The bone graft is wrapped in a sponge moistened with an isotonic solution. Bleeding from diploic veins is controlled with bone wax. After removal of the graft, the

edges of the skull defect are drilled down to avoid a palpable bony ridge. It is not necessary to repair the donor site. However, if a significant contour deformity of the skull is present, the depression may be filled with methylmethacrylate or hydroxyapatite cement. The wound is irrigated to remove bone debris and closed-in layers, using 2.0 polyglactin suture for the galeal layer. The skin is approximated with staples or 4.0 gut suture. A suction drain is usually not required. Local wound care consists of cleaning the staples or scalp sutures with hydrogen peroxide twice daily and applying a topical petroleum-based antibiotic ointment. The patient is maintained on a course of an oral antistaphylococcal antibiotic for 5 to 7 days. Staples are removed on the seventh to the tenth postoperative day.

■ Complications

The use of proper techniques and the awareness of cranial bone anatomy reduces complications when harvesting outer table parietal bone. Dural exposure is the most common complication and is usually of little consequence. Dural tear, cerebrospinal fluid leak, subdural hematoma, injury to the sagittal sinus, and intracerebral injury are rare and more serious complications requiring neurosurgical consultation.

Rib Bone Graft

The technique for harvesting rib cartilage is described in Chapter 7. The approach for harvesting rib bone is the same except that the dissection is extended laterally, in a subperiosteal plane, past the costochondral

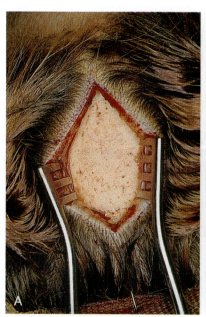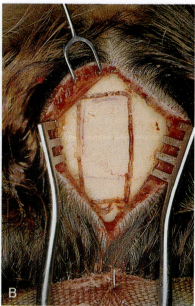

■ **Figure 8–2.** *A*, Parietal skull is exposed using parasagittal incision. *B*, Bone graft is outlined by a trough created with side-cutting bur.

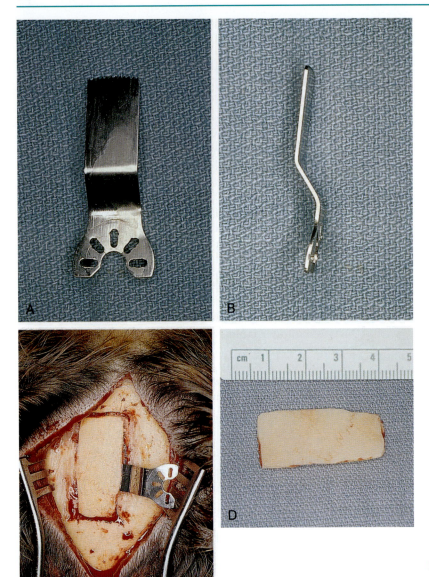

Figure 8–3. *A* and *B*, Oscillating 90-degree blade. *C*, Saw blade is used to transect diploic layer. Drill has been disconnected from saw blade to show placement. *D*, Outer table cranial bone graft.

junction to expose a segment of rib bone. The periosteum is dissected from the bone with a periosteal or no. 9 dental elevator. After adequate exposure, the rib bone is transected with a rib cutter. Wound closure is similar to that described for rib cartilage grafts.

Septal Bone Graft

Small bony defects of the nose are suitable for repair with ethmoid or vomer bone. This bone is generally thin and may require layering for optimal thickness and strength. Ethmoid and vomer bones are harvested using a septoplasty approach described in Chapter 7. Following elevation of a mucoperichondrial flap from the cartilaginous septum through a unilateral caudal incision, a mucoperiosteal flap is dissected exposing the bony septum. The bony cartilaginous junction is disarticulated with a Cottle or Freer elevator, and the contralateral mucoperiosteum is elevated. Angled scissors are used to transect the bone horizontally 1 cm inferior to the level of the canthi. A 4-mm chisel is used to free the graft from its inferior and posterior attachments.

Sculpting and Fixation of Bone Grafts

■ Cranial Bone Graft

When portions of the bony pyramid persist, the bone graft is tailored precisely to accommodate the remaining native bony vault. A template is made of the bony defect and used as a guide for precise sculpting of the bone graft. Beveled areas in the bony perimeter of the defect should be maintained to provide maximal surface contact with the graft. The graft is counterbeveled for a precise fit. A small (3-mm) bone-cutting bur is useful for contouring and shaping each graft so it fits the bony defect precisely.

When replacing the entire bony nasal vault, the cranial bone graft is usually divided into three segments with a 1-mm side-cutting bur. One rectangular graft is used for the dorsum, and two mirror-image grafts are used for the sidewalls (Fig. 8–4). A template is made of each component (dorsum and sidewalls) of the nasal skeletal defect and used to size the three segments before dividing the bone graft. After the planned cuts are marked, the graft is stabilized on each side of the marks with an Allis clamp. With copious saline irrigation, bone cuts are made with a 1-mm side-cutting bur. In preparation for rigid fixation, a 3-mm round cutting bur is used to smooth or bevel the edges of the grafts for maximal contact with the maxilla and with each other. Each graft is shaped to the appropriate size to replicate the missing nasal bone it is meant to replace. In the case of complete loss of the upper and middle nasal vault skeleton (nasal bones and upper lateral cartilages), bone grafts are designed sufficiently long to provide structural support for the entire length of the dorsum and sidewalls. Bone thus replaces the missing upper lateral cartilages and cartilaginous dorsum (see Chapters 25 and 27).

The grafts are thinned of the diploic layer, leaving a shell of cortical bone 2 mm thick. It may be necessary to lower the nasal process of the frontal bone with a drill in order to develop a flat surface for bone grafts used to replace the bony dorsum. This will maximize surface contact between graft and frontal bone, which in turn provides greater stability and integration of the graft. Drilling down the nasal process also accommodates for the added thickness of the cranial bone in the region of the nasion. Bone grafts to replace the dorsum are fixed to the frontal bone with fixation plates in the shape of a small rectangle. Fixation plates are used to position the grafts in the desired spatial configuration when more than one graft is necessary. The plates are bent and shaped in such a manner that when attached to the bone grafts a three-dimentional reproduction of the bony nasal vault is created.

Occasionally, the bony vault is restored with only two sidewall segments that meet in the midline to form a pyramid (Fig. 8–5). Each segment is precisely sculpted to fit the bony defect. The constructed bony framework is rigidly secured to the facial skeleton with additional fixation plates, positioned superiorly at the nasion and laterally at both medial maxillary buttresses (see Chapter 25). Titanium fixation plates (1.0 to 1.2 mm) in several geometric shapes are used for this purpose.

Several 1-mm drill holes are made through the bone grafts to allow passage of mattress sutures. The holes are drilled after the constructed framework is secured to the frontal bone and maxillae. Multiple 5.0 polyglactin sutures are passed through the holes and lining flaps to secure the flaps against the deep surface of the grafts. Drill holes are also placed through the caudal

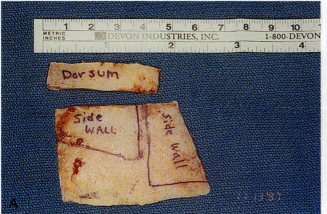
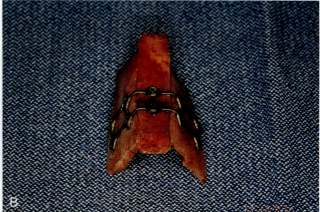

■ **Figure 8–4.** *A,* Bone graft is divided into three segments, a dorsum and two sidewalls. *B,* Segments are positioned to replicate shape of bony vault and are secured with fixation plates.

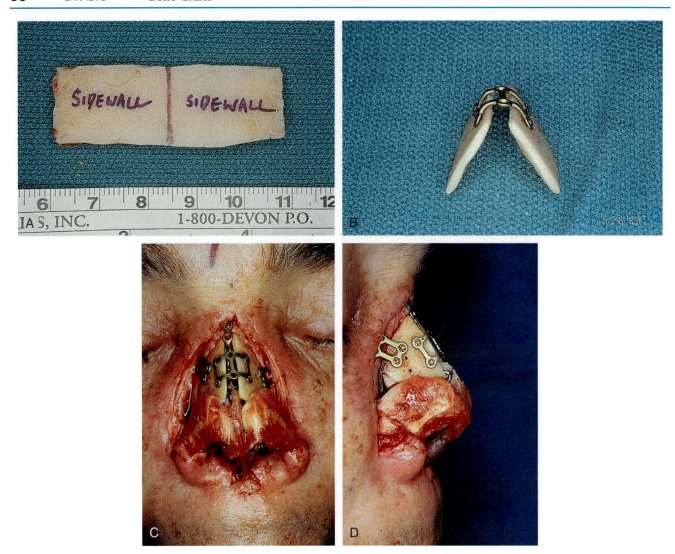

Figure 8–5. *A,* Bone graft is divided into two segments representing nasal sidewalls. *B,* Segments are positioned to form triangular pyramid and are secured with fixation plates. *C* and *D,* Constructed pyramid is secured to frontal bone and maxillae with fixation plates.

aspect of the bone grafts. These holes are for suture fixation to cartilage grafts for the lower framework of the nose.

■ Rib Bone Graft

Rib grafts are sculpted with a drill, using a 3-mm round cutting bur for the bony segment and no. 10 and no. 15 surgical blades for cartilage. The rib graft is stabilized with a bone clamp and contoured using copious irrigation. Remnant nasal bone may be drilled down to provide a stable platform for placement of the graft. The bony portion of the graft is secured to the frontal bone with an appropriately sized and angled fixation plate.

■ Septal Bone Grafts

Septal bone may be easily sculpted using a small bone rongeur. Several layers of septal bone may be stacked

together to produce the desired thickness. The grafts are secured to each other with 4.0 nylon mattress sutures placed through 1-mm holes drilled through each graft. The graft is secured to the bony recipient site with additional permanent sutures placed through 1-mm holes drilled in the perimeter of the bony defect.

References

1. Pensler J, MacCarthy JG: The calvarial donor site: An anatomic study in cadavers. Plast Reconstr Surg 75:648, 1985.

2. Frodel JL Jr, Marentette LJ, Quatela VC, et al: Calvarial bone graft harvest: Techniques, considerations, and morbidity. Arch Otolaryngol Head Neck Surg 119:17, 1993.

3. Kellman RM, Marentette LJ: Atlas of craniomaxillofacial fixation. New York, Raven Press, 1995.

9

Skin and Composite Grafts

Brian S. Jewett

The epidermis, the most superficial layer of skin, consists of keratinizing, stratified, squamous epithelium. The predominant cell type is the keratinocyte, which comprises 80% of the cells. Layers of the epidermis include the basal cell, prickle cell, granular cell, and keratin layers, with the overall thickness of human skin varying from 0.075 to 0.15 mm. The epidermis is thin at birth, becomes thicker during early adulthood, and thins during the fifth to sixth decades of life.

The epidermis is attached to the dermis by a basement membrane zone that extends from the epidermis to pilosebaceous units and sweat ducts in the dermis. Each pilosebaceous unit contains sebaceous glands, a hair shaft and follicle with associated arrector pili muscle, and a sensory end organ. Epithelialization of partial-thickness wounds occurs from wound edges and basement membrane zone around the hair follicles, sebaceous glands, and sweat ducts.[1]

The dermis consists of a fibrous connective tissue matrix made up of collagen, elastic tissue, and ground substance. Dispersed throughout the dermis are epidermal appendages, blood vessels, nerves, and cells. The most common cell in the dermis is the fibroblast. Fibroblasts have a synthetic role in wound healing, producing collagen, elastin, and ground substance. Fibroblasts behave like contractile cells during wound maturation.

The dermis is divided into a thin papillary and a thicker reticular dermis. The overall thickness of the dermis is variable, depending on its location. Eyelid skin has the thinnest dermis, measuring less than 1 mm. Dermal thickness measures 1.5 mm on the temple, 2.5 mm on the scalp, and more than 4 mm on the back. The dermis is thin at birth, increases in thickness until the fourth or fifth decade, and then decreases with further aging. On average, men have a thicker dermis than women.[1]

Cutaneous blood flow is directed toward the more metabolically active epidermis through dermal papillae, hair papillae, and adnexal structures. Two vascular plexuses connected by communicating vessels are present in the reticular dermis. A deep plexus lies at the junction of dermis and fat, and the superficial plexus gives rise to a rich capillary loop system in the superficial dermal papillae. This system provides nutrients to the epidermis through diffusion.[2]

Skin Grafts

Skin grafts can be harvested in several different forms, including full-thickness, split-thickness, and composite grafts. Regardless of the type of graft, graft viability depends on several factors: blood supply to the recipient site, microcirculation on the surface of the recipient site, vascularity of donor graft tissue, contact between graft and recipient site, and certain systemic illnesses. Contact between the skin graft and recipient site is essential. A bolster dressing is helpful to prevent fluid collection beneath the graft postoperatively. Bolsters also prevent shearing forces from disrupting fibrous connections between the graft and wound bed. Systemic illnesses that may compromise graft survival include rheumatoid arthritis, lupus, hematologic disorders, diabetes, nutritional deficiencies, and hypoxemia.[3] Use of tobacco products is also detrimental to the survival of skin grafts.

Recipient site conditions that are not favorable to graft survival include irradiated tissue; excessive fibrosis; exposed bone, cartilage, or tendon; and a bleeding wound. Grafts placed over avascular defects smaller than 1 cm² may survive through nutritional support via wound edges; however, grafting over avascular wounds larger than this is unlikely to succeed.[3]

For deeper wounds, skin grafting may be delayed until granulation tissue has filled the wound bed (2 to 3 weeks). Any epithelium on the surface of the granulation tissue is removed before grafting, and the tissue is cross-hatched so that myofibrils are released. Granulating wounds normally contain bacteria. Bacterial counts greater than 10⁵ organisms per gram of tissue often lead to graft loss.[4] When delayed grafting is planned, the patient is started on a 10-day course of an antistaphylococcal antibiotic 3 days before grafting. When necessary, wound cultures are obtained to direct antibiotic selection.

Split-thickness Skin Graft

The split-thickness skin graft consists of epidermis and a variable portion of underlying dermis. It has more capillaries exposed on its undersurface as compared with full-thickness grafts permitting greater absorption of nutrients from the wound bed. In addition, the graft consists of less tissue that requires revascularization.[3] As a result, the graft is often used for large wounds in which revascularization is a concern. However, the graft provides a relatively poor aesthetic result. Because of its poor color and texture match with normal skin and its tendency to contract, the split-thickness skin graft is not used in nasal reconstruction.

Full-thickness Skin Graft

The full-thickness skin graft consists of epidermis and full-thickness dermis. It resists contraction, has texture and pigmentation similar to those of normal skin, and requires a well-vascularized, uncontaminated wound site for survival. The graft survives initially by diffusion of nutrition from fluid in the recipient site, a process called plasma imbibition. Vascular inosculation may occur during the first 24 to 48 hours. After 48 to 72 hours, capillaries in the recipient site begin to grow into the graft to provide new circulation. By 3 to 5 days, a new blood supply has been established. Initially, the full-thickness skin graft appears blanched; over 3 to 7 days a pink color develops, signaling neovascularization. After 4 to 6 weeks, the pink color begins to fade, but the graft often remains lighter than the surrounding skin, especially in dark-skinned individuals.

Compared with the split-thickness graft, the full-thickness graft has the advantages of better color and texture match, less contour irregularities, no need for special equipment, and easier donor site wound care. The disadvantages include reduced survival rate for larger grafts and longer healing time.[3]

The ideal nasal defect to repair with a full-thickness skin graft is smaller than an aesthetic unit. Ideally, the defect should be superficial, with loss of skin but not

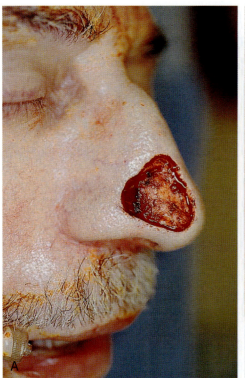

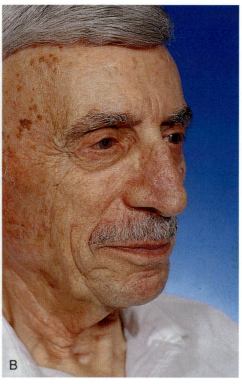

■ **Figure 9–1.** *A,* Superficial cutaneous defect of the tip of the nose. The patient requested the least complex repair possible. *B,* Four months after repair with a full-thickness skin graft obtained from a preauricular site. There are marked textural discrepancies between the graft and the nasal skin.

sal skin is an important preoperative consideration. For similar nasal defects, a skin graft may provide a perfect match in terms of thickness for one person and a poor match for another. There are individuals who have thin nasal skin covering the entire nose. These individuals are often fair-skinned females. Full-thickness skin grafts may be used in these cases for superficial cutaneous defects anywhere on the nose without significant contour or textural discrepancies between graft and nasal skin. The only exception is in the area of the nostril margin, where scar contraction following skin grafting will likely distort the border of the nostril.

A number of donor sites for skin grafts are available in most individuals, depending on the location and size of the nasal defect. Sites include the upper eyelid, forehead, melolabial fold, and preauricular, postauricular, and supraclavicular areas (Fig. 9–2). When selecting a donor site, the thickness of the skin surrounding the recipient site is assessed, and donor skin is matched accordingly. Defects of the nasal tip may be repaired with thicker skin from the forehead by means of a trichophytic incision for patients with a stable hairline. The melolabial fold also provides sebaceous skin with thickness and texture similar to those of the nasal tip. Skin defects of the cephalic two-thirds of the nose require thinner grafts, which are usually obtained from the preauricular or postauricular areas (Fig. 9–3). Skin

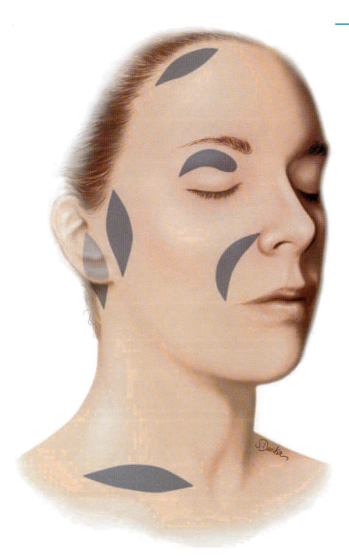

Figure 9–2. Common donor sites for full-thickness skin grafts used for nasal reconstruction.

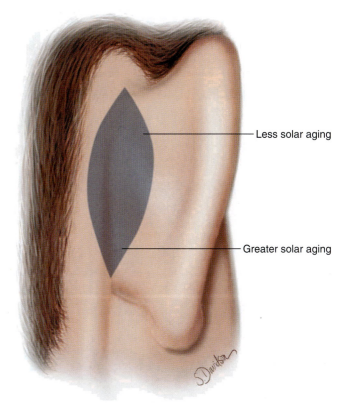

Less solar aging

Greater solar aging

Figure 9–3. The skin posterior to the auricle is an ideal source for full-thickness grafts to cover cutaneous defects of the cephalic nose. Skin from the inferior aspect of the region has greater solar aging and provides a better color match with nasal skin.

underlying muscle. The vascularity of shallow wounds is greater than that for defects extending through the muscle to the underlying cartilage or bone. The ideal defect is separated from the free margin of the nostril by 5 mm and is located in thin-skinned areas of the nose. These areas include the cephalic sidewalls, dorsum, and infratip lobule. Shallow wounds in these areas are typically completely filled by a full-thickness skin graft, leaving no step-down contour deformity.

The areas of the nose covered with thicker skin include the tip, ala, and caudal aspect of the sidewalls and dorsum. Although the nasal skin is thin in the area of the rhinion, it becomes thicker as it transitions toward the nasion. Full-thickness skin grafts used to repair defects of the nose in regions of thicker nasal skin tend to heal with a contour depression and noticeable textural discrepancies between graft and adjacent nasal skin (Fig. 9–1). This is because the nasal skin in these areas tends to have a more sebaceous nature than the graft.

There is a wide variation of nasal skin thickness among individuals, and the overall thickness of the na-

from the postauricular area is preferred for men whose skin defects are of limited size because it is hairless and tends to have a similar thickness to the skin covering the infratip lobule and cephalic sidewalls (Fig. 9–4). Because men tend to have shorter hair than women, the postauricular skin is likely to have solar aging, which provides an improved skin color match with the nasal skin. In contrast, preauricular skin is used as a source for grafts for females. Preauricular skin in females is hairless and has more solar aging compared with postauricular skin, which is often covered by hair. The supraclavicular region is an excellent source for skin grafts, especially if a large graft is required. The thickness of supraclavicular skin approximates that of the cephalic portion of the nasal dorsum.

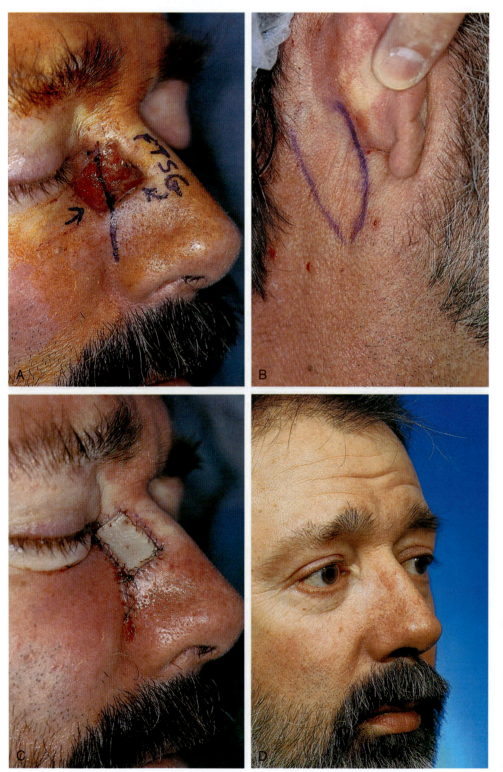

■ **Figure 9–4.** *A,* A skin defect of the cephalic nasal sidewall and medial cheek. The cheek skin is advanced to the nasal-facial sulcus. *B,* A full-thickness skin graft is obtained from the inferior aspect of the posterior auricular skin. *C,* The graft in place. *D,* Three years after surgery. The graft was dermabraded 6 weeks after grafting.

There are occasions when skin grafts are used to repair shallow skin defects of the nose even when it is anticipated that the graft will result in a contour depression or noticeable mismatch in skin texture or color. These situations often arise when caring for elderly debilitated patients who have life-threatening illnesses. At other times, patients comment that they are not in the least concerned about the appearance of their nose and request the simplest type of repair (see Fig. 9–1). For patients who have malignancies showing aggressive growth patterns and for whom tumor persistence or recurrence is a primary concern, skin grafts may be used as a temporary covering for 2 or 3 years while the patient is at greatest risk for recurrence.

In general, cutaneous flaps from the nose, forehead, or cheek are the preferred method of resurfacing cutaneous defects of the nose. However, the infratip lobule is one site where a full-thickness skin graft is preferred to a cutaneous flap. Provided the defect does not involve the margin of the nostril and there is no loss of the intermediate crura, cutaneous defects of the infratip lobule are best covered with a full-thickness skin graft harvested from the pre- or postauricular skin. The match in thickness and color between the skin from these sources and the skin of the infratip lobule is nearly perfect. Six weeks following grafting, the area may be lightly dermabraded to blend the graft with the nasal skin (Fig. 9–5).

■ Technique

All patients undergoing skin grafting receive preoperative intravenous antibiotics, usually consisting of 1 g of Kefzol or 600 mg of clindamycin if allergic to penicillin. Oral antibiotics are administered during the first week postoperatively. The procedure is performed with the patient receiving intravenous sedation and local anesthesia (1% lidocaine with 1:100,000 concentration of epinephrine). The wound and donor sites are cleansed with betadine solution. The 45-degree bevel of the defect after Mohs' excision is often maintained to help the transition between the graft and native skin. This creates an incline from the base of the wound to the surface of the surrounding skin and lessens the step-

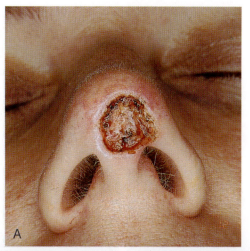

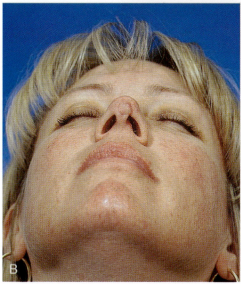
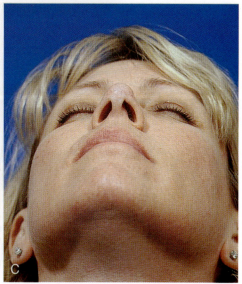

■ **Figure 9–5.** *A,* A superficial cutaneous defect of the infratip lobule. *B,* Four months after full-thickness skin graft and before dermabrasion. *C,* Sixteen months after dermabrasion of graft.

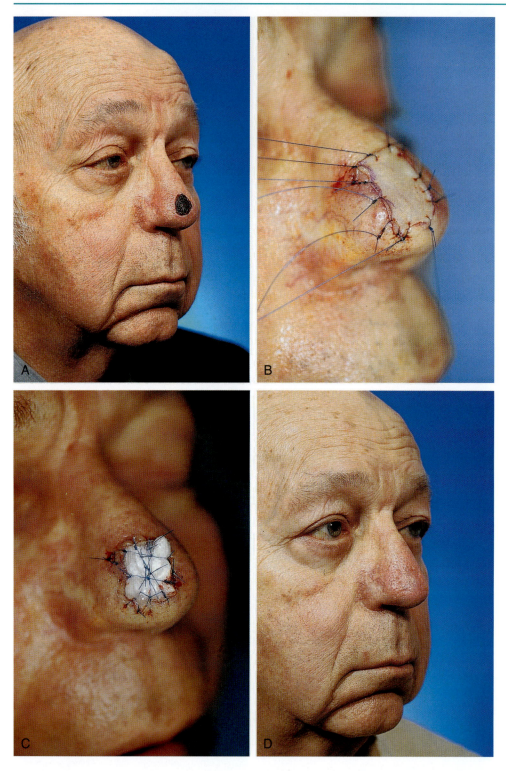

■ **Figure 9-6.** *A,* A superficial cutaneous defect of the tip of the nose. *B,* The circular defect converted to a rectangular configuration and covered with a full-thickness skin graft using preauricular skin. *C,* The graft is compressed with a bolster dressing made of nonadherent bandage. *D,* Six months after grafting. Graft and adjacent skin were dermabraded on two occasions.

down contour deformity that may develop. Additional beveling of the defect may be performed if the skin graft is substantially thinner than the depth of the recipient site. In other instances, the wound may be prepared by freshening the margins with a scalpel.

A template is made of the recipient site by outlining the periphery of the wound with a surgical marker and pressing a nonadherent dressing pad over the marking.

If the defect is round, the shape is often modified by excising skin to create "corners." This causes the defect and covering graft to have angulated borders, which lessens the likelihood of developing a trapdoor deformity (see Fig. 9–4). The template is fashioned and used to design the size and configuration of the graft. Because most full-thickness skin grafts contract 10% to 15% after excision from the donor site,[5] the graft is designed slightly larger than the defect to accommodate for this contraction. The donor skin is incised with a 45-degree bevel to match the bevel of the Mohs defect. The dermal tissue remaining at the periphery of the donor defect is trimmed prior to repair of the donor site. The graft is excised, and all subcutaneous tissue is removed with tenotomy scissors. This is best accomplished by placing the graft over the index finger, epidermal side down, and trimming off excess fat until shiny dermis is visible.

The graft is transferred to the recipient site and oriented in a manner to maximize contact between wound and graft. Excess graft is trimmed. The graft is secured with simple interrupted 5.0 polypropylene sutures. One end of each suture is left long enough to be tied with another suture at the opposing aspect of the graft. A bolster dressing is made from nonadherent bandage (Telfa) and secured with opposing sutures (Fig. 9–6). Placement of petroleum-based antibiotic ointment between the dressing layers helps to stabilize the bolster during suture fixation. The bolster is left in place for 5 days. Upon removal, any fluid collection beneath the graft is gently wicked away by a rolling motion with a cotton-tip applicator. Any type of sheering motion is avoided as it may disrupt vascularization of the graft. The patient is instructed to keep the graft dry and to return in 1 week to reassess the graft's condition. If the graft has survived and has adhered well to the recipient site, the patient is allowed to bathe the area.

The graft may appear cyanotic during the first few days following transfer. It then transitions to a hyperemic stage, which fades over weeks to months. Occasionally, a cyanotic graft may not survive. If the entire graft dies, it will suppurate and separate from the recipient site within 2 weeks. More commonly, the deeper portion of the graft survives while the more superficial portion forms an eschar, which remains fixed to the wound bed. When this occurs, the graft is left in place as a biologic dressing, allowing healing by secondary intention. Re-epitheliazation will occur from the wound edges and from the viable deeper dermal component of the graft. Often, sufficient dermis survives to prevent the development of a depressed scar following complete healing; however, pigmentary and textural differences between nasal skin and the graft are usually more apparent than when the graft survives completely.

When defects of the nasal sidewall that extend to the medial cheek are repaired with a skin graft, the cheek component of the defect is reconstructed with a cutaneous advancement flap developed from the remaining medial cheek skin. The flap is advanced to the level of the nasal facial sulcus and anchored in place with deep sutures that pass from the medial border of the flap to the periosteum of the nasal sidewall. A full-thickness skin graft is used to resurface the sidewall. The cheek advancement flap facilitates positioning

scars along the junctional zone between the aesthetic regions of the cheek and nose. If the cheek defect is of considerable size, the standing cutaneous deformities that occur from advancement of the cheek flap are excised and used as full-thickness grafts for covering the sidewall defect (Fig. 9–7).

Adjunctive procedures to optimize aesthetic appearance may be performed 6 weeks after grafting. Trapdoor deformities usually resolve over time, especially if steroids are injected beneath the graft. Grafts rarely require a surgical contouring procedure, but occasionally Z-plasties are performed at the border of the graft to enhance the appearance of the transition between graft and native nasal skin. The author recommends dermabrasion of all full-thickness skin grafts used to resurface nasal cutaneous defects. In addition to the graft, we dermabrade the nasal skin within the aesthetic units surrounding the graft (Fig. 9–8). Dermabrasion is accomplished in the office using local anesthesia and is usually performed 6 weeks following successful grafting. Skin flaps may occasionally become hypopigmented following dermabrasion. In contrast, the color and textural match of skin grafts nearly always improve after dermabrasion. Grafts are occasionally dermabraded a second time if the first treatment fails to yield acceptable results.

Composite Chondrocutaneous Grafts

Composite grafts contain two or more tissue layers and are often unsuccessful secondary to high metabolic demands.[6] They obtain their nourishment through plasma imbibition during the first 24 hours after transfer. This is followed by vascular inosculation. Ingrowth of capillaries from the edges of the graft begins by the third day.[7, 8]

Composite grafts were first described by Konig,[9] who used composite auricular grafts to repair alar defects and noted a 53% graft survival rate. Composite grafts have been used to repair columellar defects[10, 11] and deficiencies in nasal lining.[12] During the first half of the 20th century, Limberg[13] advocated the cavum and cymba of the concha as the preferred donor site for repair of the nose, and Gillies[14] described the transfer of composite grafts to the undersurface of forehead flaps for nasal reconstruction. Symonds and Crikelair[15] also used composite auricular grafts for nasal reconstruction, reporting an 89% graft survival rate.

The auricle is an excellent source for composite grafts for nasal reconstruction because it provides a contoured graft of skin and cartilage. Certain segments of the auricle loosely replicate the delicate topography of the columella, facet, and nostril margin where com-

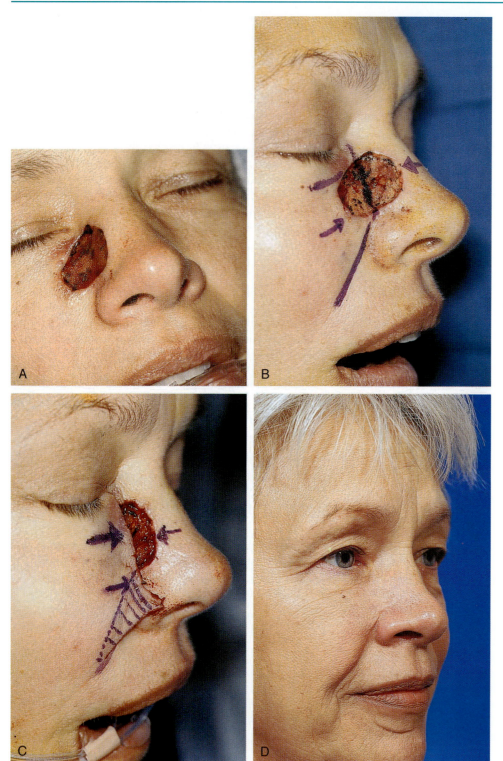

Figure 9–7. *A,* A superficial cutaneous defect of the sidewall, with extension to the medial cheek. *B,* A cheek advancement flap is designed to repair the cheek component of the defect. A vertical line through the defect indicates the level of the nasal-facial sulcus. *C,* The cheek skin is advanced and secured to the nasal-facial sulcus. A standing cutaneous deformity in the melolabial sulcus is marked with vertical lines, excised, and used as a full-thickness skin graft to cover the nasal component of the defect. *D,* Three years after surgery. The graft was dermabraded 2 months after the transfer.

posites grafts are commonly employed. The skin is tightly adherent to the underlying cartilage at the columella and to the fibrofatty tissue of the alae and facets. Likewise, the skin covering the lateral aspect of the auricle is firmly attached to the underlying cartilage. Common auricular donor sites are the helical crus, helical rim, antihelix, tragus, antitragus, and fossa triangu-

laris (Fig. 9–9). The helical crus provides a good contour match for small alar rim defects and provides the option of incorporating a segment of preauricular skin in the graft. This design of the composite graft may be used to resurface larger nasal defects requiring considerable skin but minimal framework replacement.

The traditional recommendation is to limit the size of

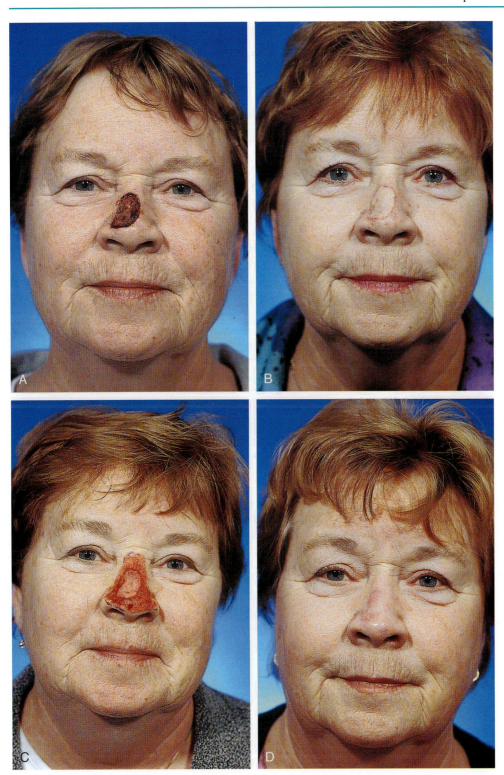

■ **Figure 9–8.** *A,* A superficial cutaneous defect of the dorsum and tip. *B,* Six weeks after a full-thickness skin graft. Note the discrepancy in the color match between the nasal skin and the graft. *C,* Immediately after dermabrasion of the graft and the adjacent aesthetic units occupied by the graft. *D,* One year after dermabrasion. Note the improvement in the color match between the graft and the nasal skin.

composite grafts to 1 cm or less.[16] Considerably larger grafts may be successful if they are placed in a vascular recipient site and the graft is designed so that no portion is more than 1 cm from a wound edge.[17–19] Skouge[4] advocated a tongue-and-groove technique when using composite grafts. This technique involves insetting the border of the graft between two layers of tissue at the recipient site. This method of graft attachment has the effect of increasing surface contact between the graft and the recipient site by 50%.[20] A hinge flap developed at the recipient site also increases the surface area for attaching a composite graft.[21]

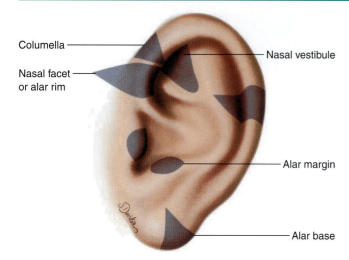

Columella

Nasal facet or alar rim

Nasal vestibule

Alar margin

Alar base

Figure 9–9. Common donor sites for the composite grafts used in nasal reconstruction.

The use of perioperative corticosteroids is beneficial in enhancing survival of composite grafts in animals. Rabbits treated with preoperative and postoperative methylprednisolone demonstrated improved graft survival compared with animals receiving no steroids or postoperative doses only. Attempts to salvage compromised grafts with delayed administration of steroids were not successful.[22, 23] Cooling of composite grafts has also been demonstrated to improve survival. Cooling reduces biologic requirements and improves graft survival in irradiated, atrophic, or scarred recipient sites. Conley and Van Fraenkel[24] demonstrated that constant application of ice and ice compresses for 14 days effected a fall in skin temperature from 38°F to 17°F. Grafts ranged in size from 1×1 cm to 2×2 cm. Of 12 composite grafts transferred to the nose and treated with ice compresses, 10 survived completely. Five of the grafts had been placed in recipient sites with scarring or postirradiation fibrosis.[24]

The ideal defect for a composite auricular graft is a small (1.0 cm or less) full-thickness defect of the facet or columella. The nasal skin in these areas is extremely thin, lacking subcutaneous fat, and is tightly adherent to the alar cartilage in the columella and to the fibrous connective tissue in the facet. Skin flaps used to repair the facet or columella convey skin with subcutaneous fat and are thicker than the native nasal skin. In contrast, composite auricular grafts obtained from the helical crus provide a graft with thin skin attached to a delicate segment of cartilage (see Fig. 9–9). The cartilage provides structural support, and the skin closely resembles the adjacent nasal skin of the columella and facet (Fig. 9–10).

■ Technique

Patient selection is an important consideration. We restrict the use of composite grafts to small alar margin or columellar defects (less than 2 cm) in patients who are younger than 65 years of age, do not use tobacco, and have no systemic illnesses that would compromise graft revascularization. Patients receive antibiotics, wound preparation, and anesthesia similar to those for skin grafts. In addition, 60 mg of prednisone is administered on the day of surgery. The steroids are tapered by 10 mg each day, eventually to 5 mg on postoperative day 7.

We have found an improved survival rate if grafting is delayed until the nasal defect has healed by secondary intention. The nasal defect is prepared by removing the epithelium and subepithelial scar tissue, and a template is created that measures 2 mm larger than the defect in all dimensions. Harvesting a graft that is slightly larger than the defect accommodates for the inevitable contraction of the graft. Whenever possible, a flap of soft tissue hinged on a border of the defect is developed to enhance surface contact with the graft (Fig. 9–11). A composite graft containing skin and cartilage that most closely matches the contour and thickness of the nose at the defect site is harvested from the auricle. The graft is placed in cold saline, and the donor site is closed primarily with 5-0 polydioxanone sutures to approximate the edges of the auricular cartilage and 5-0 polypropylene vertical mattress sutures for the skin. The graft is transferred to the recipient site and secured with 5-0 polypropylene simple cutaneous sutures while limiting the degree of manipulation of the graft. Subdermal or subcutaneous sutures are not used. Using as few sutures as possible, precise approximation of skin edges is accomplished. If the graft is small, no sutures are placed through the cartilage. Limiting the number of sutures used to fix the graft in place is thought to be beneficial in enabling earlier and more abundant vessel ingrowth.

An intranasal bolster in the form of a dental roll is occasionally used to limit motion of the graft and prevent fluid accumulation between graft and recipient site. Ice-saline compresses are applied for the first three days. Successful grafts transition in color during the first week: blanched at initial transfer, pink color at 6 hours, cyanotic by 24 hours, and gradual development of a pink color in 3 to 7 days. Dermabrasion may be performed after 6 to 8 weeks. Complications include partial or complete graft loss, contracture, pigmentary changes, and contour abnormalities.

Other Composite Grafts

Other types of composite grafts have been described for nasal reconstruction. Composite grafts consisting of skin and subcutaneous fat from the earlobe or contralateral alar base may be used to repair defects of the alar base

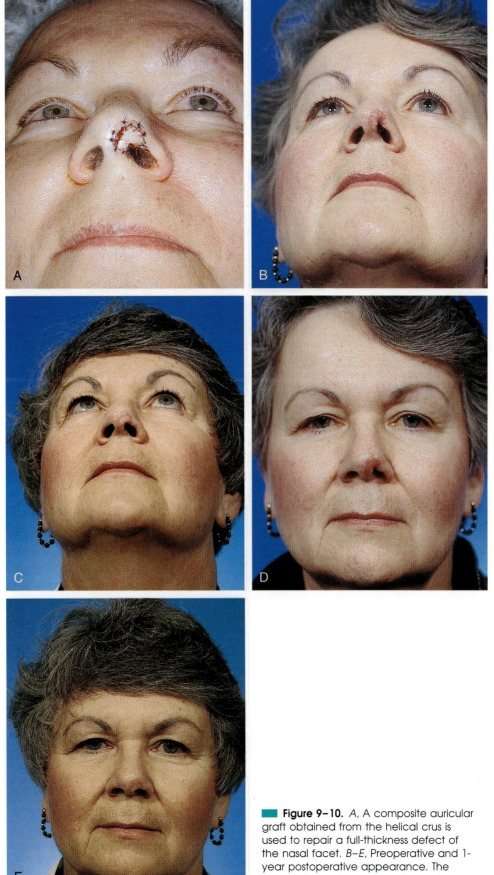

Figure 9–10. *A,* A composite auricular graft obtained from the helical crus is used to repair a full-thickness defect of the nasal facet. *B–E,* Preoperative and 1-year postoperative appearance. The composite graft was dermabraded.

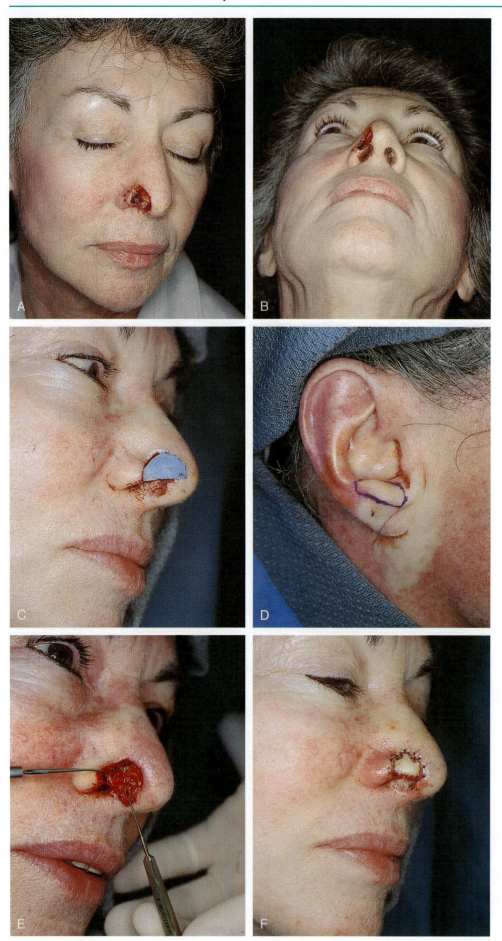

Figure 9–11. *A* and *B*, A full-thickness defect of the nostril margin that was allowed to heal by secondary intention before being repaired with a composite graft. *C* and *D*, A template 0.2 cm larger than the defect is used to design a composite graft of the right antitragus. *E*, A flap of soft tissue hinged on the border of the defect is developed to enhance surface contact with the graft. *F*, The composite graft is secured to the recipient site with a limited number of cutaneous sutures.

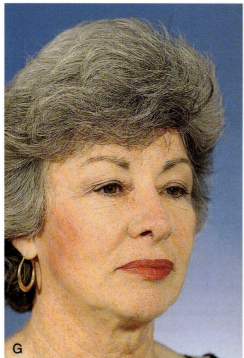 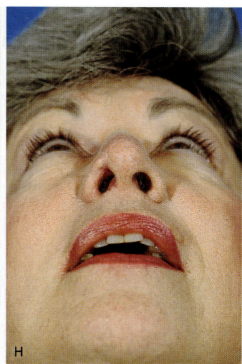

■ **Figure 9–11** *Continued. G and H,* Six months after grafting.

or nostril margin.[9] Stucker and Shaw reported on the use of perichondrocutaneous grafts that consist of epidermis, dermis, scant subcutaneous tissue, and a perichondrial layer.[25] The grafts are harvested from the cavum concha and an island pedicled skin flap from the postauricular sulcus is used to repair the donor site. These authors report excellent aesthetic results, with no contraction of the graft.[26] In our experience, the aesthetic outcome of this graft is not superior to that obtained with a full-thickness skin graft.

References

1. Johnson TM, Nelson BR: Anatomy of skin. In Baker SR, Swanson NA (eds): Local Flaps in Facial Reconstruction. St. Louis, Mosby, 1995, p 3.

2. Goding GS, Hom DB: Skin flap physiology. In Baker SR, Swanson NA (eds): Local Flaps in Facial Reconstruction. St. Louis, Mosby, 1995, p 15.

3. Glogau RG, Haas AF: Skin grafts. In Baker SR, Swanson NA (eds): Local Flaps in Facial Reconstruction. St. Louis, Mosby, 1995, p 247.

4. Skouge JW: Skin grafting, New York, Churchill Livingstone, 1991.

5. Hill TG: Reconstruction of nasal defects using full-thickness grafts: A personal reappraisal. J Dermatol Surg Oncol 12:995, 1983.

6. Konior RJ: Free composite grafts. Otolaryngol Clin North Am 27:81, 1994.

7. Clairmont AA, Conley JJ: The uses and limitations of auricular composite grafts. J Otolaryngol 7:249, 1978.

8. McLaughlin CR: Composite ear grafts and their blood supply. Br J Plast Surg 7:274, 1954.

9. Konig F: Über nasenplastik. Beitr Klin Chir 94:515, 1914.

10. Converse JM: Reconstruction of nasolabial area by composite graft from the concha. Plast Reconstr Surg 5:247, 1950.

11. Meade RJ: Composite ear grafts for construction of columella. Plast Reconstr Surg 23:134, 1959.

12. Dingman RO, Walter C: Use of composite grafts in correction of the short nose. Plast Reconstr Surg 43:117, 1969.

13. Limberg A: Rhinoplasty using free transplant from concha. Sovet Khir 9:70, 1935.

14. Gillies HD: A new free graft applied to the reconstruction of the nostril. Br J Surg 30:305, 1943.

15. Symonds FC, Crikelair GF: Auricular composite grafts in nasal reconstruction. Plast Reconstr Surg 37:433, 1956.

16. Ballantyne DI, Converse JM: Vascularization of composite auricular grafts transplanted to the chorio-allantois of the chick embryo. Plast Reconstr Surg 42:51, 1968.

17. Ruch M: Utilization of composite free grafts. J Int Coll Surg 30:274, 1958.

18. Becker OJ: Extended application of free composite grafts. Trans Am Acad Ophthalmal Otolaryngol 64:649, 1960.

19. Avelar JM, Psillakis JM, Viterbo F: Use of large composite grafts in the reconstruction of deformities of the nose and ear. Br J Plast Surg 37:55, 1984.

20. Davenport G, Bernard FD: Improving the take of composite grafts. Plast Reconstr Surg 24:175, 1959.

21. Converse JM: Reconstructive Plastic Surgery, vol 2. Philadelphia, W.B. Saunders, 1964.

22. Aden KK, Biel MA: The evaluation of pharmacologic agents on composite survival. Arch Otolaryngol Head Neck Surg 118:175, 1992.

23. Hartman DF, Good RL: Pharmacologic enhancement of composite graft survival. Arch Otolaryngol Head Neck Surg 113:720, 1987.

24. Conley JJ, Van Fraenkel P: The principle of cooling applied to the composite graft in the nose. Plast Reconstr Surg 17:444, 1956.

25. Stucker FJ, Shaw GY: The perichondrial cutaneous graft. Arch Otolaryngol Head Neck Surg 118:287, 1992.

26. Portuese W: Perichondrial cutaneous graft: An alternative in composite skin grafting. Arch Otolaryngol Head Neck Surg 115:705, 1989.

10

Nasal Cutaneous Flaps

Shan R. Baker

Primary wound closure is possible for smaller skin defects of the nose, especially in the elderly patient where nasal skin tends to be redundant. Defects that are 1.0 cm or smaller in size and located on the dorsum or sidewall are repaired most easily. This is accomplished by advancement of opposing wound margins after wide undermining of the skin adjacent to the defect. Standing cutaneous deformities (SCD) form at the margins of the repair and may require excision, although most of the skin cone dissipates without treatment over 4 to 6 weeks. Primary wound closure of defects of the tip and supratip area frequently distorts the free margins of the nostril. Fortunately, alar cartilages typically have sufficient intrinsic strength to counteract this distortion; over time, the nostril margin returns to its natural position (Fig. 10–1).

Primary repair of skin defects of the dorsum may be facilitated by concomitant reduction rhinoplasty if the patient has overprojection of the dorsal profile line and desires reduction. Occasionally, reduction rhinoplasty enables primary closure of a skin defect, which would otherwise not be possible (Fig. 10–2). This may spare the patient from a full-thickness skin graft or paramedian forehead flap. With reduction rhinoplasty, a more desirable profile line is created, and the dorsal skeletal reduction creates a relatively greater amount of skin redundancy, which in turn reduces wound closure tension. Most often, wound approximation is oriented vertically because the greatest amount of skin advancement is derived from the skin of the sidewalls rather than of the dorsum. Reduction of the dorsal nasal skeleton is accomplished directly through the skin defect. Likewise,

if the defect is sufficiently large, a concomitant septoplasty may be performed. When a medializing osteotomy is necessary, it is performed endonasally. After the skin defect is repaired, the nose is taped, and a cast is applied, typical of any standard rhinoplasty. The author has also successfully performed reduction rhinoplasty and septoplasty directly through dorsal skin defects of the nose in cases where the defect was repaired with local nasal cutaneous flaps.

When primary wound closure is not possible, cutaneous flaps harvested from the nasal skin may be an alternative for repair of centrally located nasal skin defects that measure up to 2.5 cm in greatest dimension. Nasal cutaneous flaps are particularly useful for elderly patients because their skin is lax and mobile. When designed properly, flaps harvested from nasal skin have the advantage of color, texture, and thickness similar to those of the missing skin of the defect. Nasal cutaneous flaps are not sufficient to resurface an entire aesthetic unit of the nose, and the scars resulting from flap transfer do not always fall in the borders between aesthetic units. However, the ultimate contour of the nasal repair is far more important aesthetically than the location or number of scars. Local flaps may take the form of pivotal, advancement, or V-to-Y island pedicle advancement. In general, pivotal flaps such as single lobe transposition and rotation flaps are confined to repair of skin defects of the central and upper nasal vault where the nasal skin is thin, mobile, and more redundant. V-to-Y island pedicle advancement flaps are limited to small defects of the anterior alar groove. For the caudal nose, the bilobe flap is the most versatile and useful of the nasal cutaneous flaps.

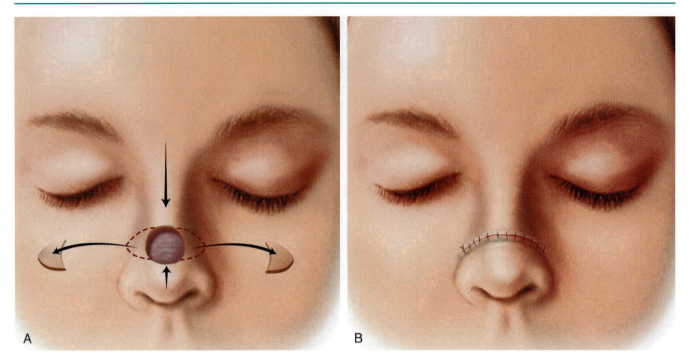

■ **Figure 10–1.** *A,* Skin defects of the nasal dorsum may be closed primarily if sufficient skin redundancy exists and nasal cartilages have sufficient intrinsic strength to resist marked displacement of the tip. Standing cutaneous deformities (SCDs) result from the advancement of wound margins. *B,* SCDs are removed laterally in alar grooves to create transverse nasal scars.

Technique

Nasal cutaneous flaps are dissected using local anesthesia containing epinephrine. Flaps should be designed to minimize thickness discrepancies between flap and skin surrounding the defect. This often necessitates converting a superficial skin defect into one that extends through the underlying muscle and fascia. The margins of the skin defect are freshened with a scalpel, and the flap is incised full-thickness to the level of the periosteum or perichondrium. The flap consisting of skin, subcutaneous tissue, and muscle is elevated just superficial to the periosteum and perichondrium of the nose in the loose areolar tissue between these structures and the overlying muscles of the nose. Flaps are not to be elevated in the subcutaneous plane because of risk of skin necrosis and the limited mobility achieved in this plane of dissection. The skin surrounding the flap and nasal defect are undermined in the same plane of dissection as the flap. For larger defects, this usually means complete undermining and mobilization of the entire remaining nasal skin. Wide undermining reduces trapdoor deformity and wound closure tension. Often, the alar branch of the angular artery located in the vicinity of the extreme lateral aspect of the alar groove is exposed and transected in order to fully mobilize the skin of the nasal sidewall.

The donor site of the flap is usually approximated by placement of 5-0 polydioxanone deep dermal sutures. The flap is then transferred to the recipient site and sutured in place. Skin incisions are closed with 5-0 polypropylene vertical mattress sutures. A compression dressing is applied overnight. Cutaneous sutures are removed in 5 to 7 days.

Although it may take 3 to 4 months for all the swelling of the nose to subside and 12 months for the scars to mature, we routinely perform dermabrasion of the nose in 6 to 8 weeks following flap transfer. This is accomplished in the office under local anesthesia with a diamond fraise and a Bell hand engine that provides an operating range from 1500 to 33,000 rpm. The donor site scar and entire aesthetic unit in which the flap is located are treated. The skin immediately adjacent to the reconstructed area is lightly dermabraded to transition the resulting skin changes. Bleeding is controlled with hydrogen peroxide, and the wound is covered with petroleum ointment. The wound is cleaned daily, kept moist with ointment, and covered with a nonadherent (Telfa) dressing for 5 to 7 days.

Starting on the first postoperative day, the patient is instructed to soak the treated area in warm water with moistened washcloths several times a day. After each 20-minute soak, petroleum ointment is applied. Reapplication is intermittently necessary to avoid drying. At bedtime, a heavy coat of petroleum ointment is placed

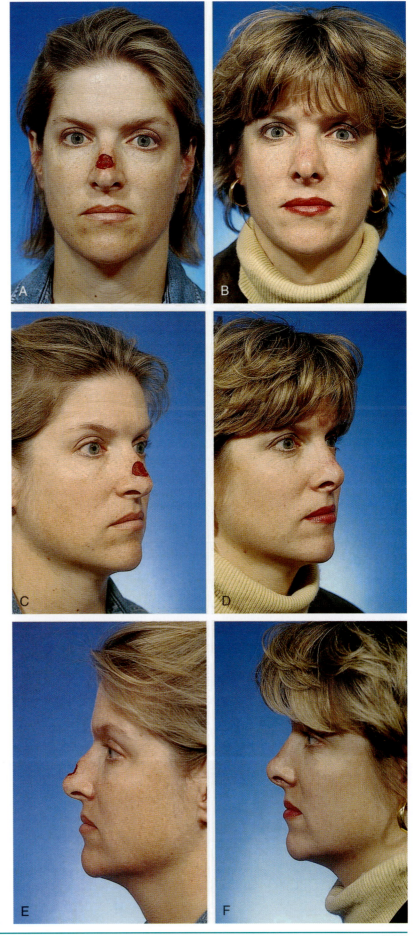

■ **Figure 10–2.** *A–F*, A skin defect at the junction of the dorsum and tip. Primary wound closure was achieved by reduction of the dorsal convexity, complete undermining of the nasal skin, and advancement of the skin margins. SCDs were excised in alar grooves. Preoperative and 1½-year postoperative views. Stiff lower lateral cartilages have prevented excessive cephalic rotation of the nasal tip. Some tip elevation has occurred; in this case it enhances the appearance of the nose.

over the wound, and the site is covered with a non-adherent dressing. Soaks are continued for approximately a week four to six times a day until the area has re-epithelialized. The patient is allowed to wear makeup in 10 days to camouflage the pinkness that results from the dermabrasion, provided the area has completely re-epithelialized. One to two weeks after complete re-epithelialization, 1% hydrocortisone cream is applied to the treated area once or twice a day to reduce erythema. This is continued for 4 to 8 weeks. The patient is instructed to avoid sun exposure to the treated area until all erythema has regressed and to use sunblocks daily.

Single Lobe Transposition Flap

Transposition flaps are pivotal flaps with a linear axis. The base of the flap is positioned adjacent to the defect, and the donor site is repaired primarily by advancement of surrounding nasal skin. The use of single pedicle transposition flaps is restricted to small defects 1.0 cm or smaller in size in the thin skin zones of the nose. Flaps confined within thick skin zones work poorly unless the defect is small (0.5 cm or smaller in maximum dimension). The thicker skin of the caudal nose is stiff and inelastic; transposition flaps created from this skin produce large standing cutaneous deformities and excessive wound closure tension. Transposition flaps are most useful for repair of defects located on the upper nasal sidewall and dorsum in the vicinity of the rhinion. In these areas, the mobility of nasal skin allows ease of transposition and enables dissipation of most of the standing cutaneous deformity that forms from transferring the flap. Any remaining cone of tissue may be safely removed without influencing the vascularity of the flap, thus making the repair one-stage. Confining transposition flaps to thin skin zones of the nose reduces contour irregularities by maintaining similar tissue thickness of the flap and recipient site. In contrast, transposition flaps transferred from thin to thick skin zones inevitably result in a mismatch of tissue thickness and create a permanent unnatural topography in the region of reconstruction.

Transposition flaps are designed with angulated rather than curved borders, thus giving a "corner" to the flap. To facilitate this design, it may be necessary to modify the configuration of the skin defect from a more common round shape to one that has an angulated configuration. The angulated borders of the repair retard concentric scar formation and reduce the problem of trapdoor deformity commonly observed with curvilinear scars. Wide undermining of adjacent nasal skin is also helpful in preventing this problem.

Rotation Flap

Rotation flaps are pivotal flaps that have a curvilinear configuration. They have limited usefulness in repairing skin defects of the nose. The flap may be used anywhere on the nose except the ala but should be restricted to defects that are 1.0 cm or smaller in size. Rotation flaps are best for repair of triangular defects because portions of the standing cutaneous deformity that naturally form as the flap is pivoted are used to fill the triangle, reducing the need for its excision. Rotation flaps are designed immediately adjacent to the defect, with the advancing border of the flap representing one border of the defect. The flap is designed so the length of its curvilinear border is four times the width of the defect. With a 4:1 ratio, excision of a Burrow triangle is usually not necessary, and wound closure tension is minimized. A Z-plasty at the pivotal point of the flap facilitates transfer and may also eliminate the need to excise a Burrow triangle, which is sometimes necessary to equalize the length of the wound borders (Fig. 10–3).

V-to-Y Island Pedicle Advancement Flap

Small skin defects located in the region of the anterior alar groove between the ala and tip can be effectively repaired with a V-to-Y advancement flap transferred as a cutaneous island and based on a subcutaneous tissue pedicle consisting of nasalis muscle and subcutaneous fat. This flap was described by Herbert and DeGeus[1, 2] and later by Staahl.[3] Millman and Klingensmith[4] modified the flap design to include only a subcutaneous pedicle containing no axial vessels. It is useful for skin defects up to 1.5 cm in maximum dimension located in the junctional zone between the nasal tip and ala, including the nasal facet (Fig. 10–4). A triangular flap, with its base making up the cephalic border of the defect, is designed with the apex of the flap positioned laterally. The inferior border of the flap rests in the alar groove. The superior border extends laterally from the defect to include skin of the nasal sidewall and tapers to meet the inferior border in the alar facial sulcus. The flap is incised to the level of the perichondrium of the lateral crus. The adjacent skin is undermined widely over the nasal tip, dorsum, and sidewall, extending inferiorly beneath the skin of the ala to the level of the caudal border of the defect. Beginning at the cephalic border of the defect, fine scissors are used to undermine beneath the cutaneous island, liberating the distal

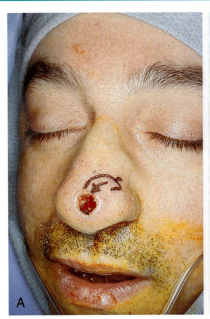
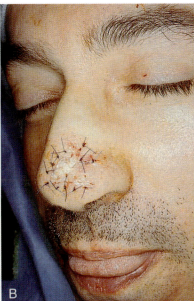
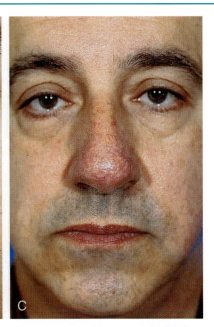

■ **Figure 10–3.** *A,* A rotation flap designed to repair a 1.0-cm superficial skin defect. *B,* The flap is pivoted into place. Z-plasty at the pivotal point eliminated the need to excise Burow's triangle to equalize the length of the wound borders. *C,* A 4-month postoperative view.

third of the island from underlying tissue. Next, the proximal (lateral) third of the flap is dissected in the subcutaneous plane, freeing it from surrounding tissue. The muscle and subcutaneous fat underlying the middle third of the flap are not disturbed and represent the pedicle. It is this zone of tissue attachment, located in the central portion of the alar groove, that provides mobility to the flap so it may be advanced as far forward as the nostril margin. The pedicle is bluntly freed from the upper and lower lateral cartilages sufficiently to permit only the exact degree of flap advancement necessary for wound repair. The vascular supply to the flap is from the alar branch of the angular artery. This branch is readily observed during the dissection; it perforates the deep tissues in the extreme lateral aspect of the alar groove. The vessel is preserved whenever possible to provide the flap with a more axial vascular supply. The flap is secured at the recipient site first, and then the donor site is closed, creating a V-to-Y configuration to the repair. Wound repair is similar to that previously described for nasal cutaneous flaps.

The tissue comprising the flap is immediately adjacent to the defect and provides an excellent color and texture match with no significant thickness discrepancies. If the flap is designed sufficiently wide, there is minimal elevation of the alar margin. Another advantage is the lack of a standing cutaneous deformity and scarring in or parallel to the alar groove.

The V-to-Y island pedicle advancement flap may be used only for small defects confined to the alar groove and lateral nasal tip. The flap cannot extend across the midline or to the supratip region. Some distortion of the nostril margin typically occurs, although the majority of deformation resolves as wound maturation occurs.

Dorsal Nasal Flap

The dorsal nasal flap recruits redundant skin of the glabella and is a pivotal flap that can be used to repair skin defects of the nasal tip, dorsum, and sidewall. Elliott[5] detailed the Banner and bilobe flap for nasal repair, designing them as interpolated flaps that require detachment. Rieger[6] described the basic design of the dorsal nasal flap used currently. The flap utilizes the entire dorsal nasal skin to facilitate repair. Further refinements of the flap were offered by Rigg,[7] who introduced the concept of limiting the area of nasal skin used for construction of the flap. He advocated a backcut of the flap toward the medial canthus. Marchac and Toth[8] designed the flap with an axial vascular pattern by incorporating a constant branch of the angular artery in the pedicle. This enabled a longer descent of the glabellar backcut to the level of the medial canthus. The greater backcut facilitates flap transfer, reducing wound closure tension and distortion of the nostril margin.

The dorsal nasal flap enables the surgeon to repair relatively large lower and midnasal defects measuring 2.5 cm in diameter or less with matching adjacent tis-

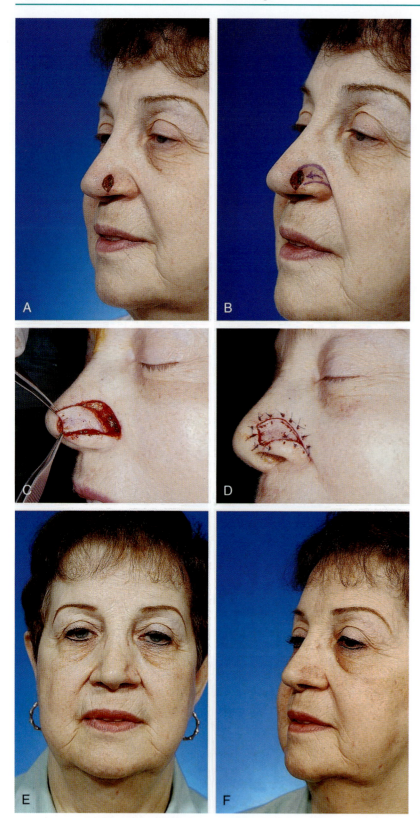

■ **Figure 10–4.** *A,* A 1.5 cm skin defect of the anterior alar groove. *B,* A V-to-Y island advancement flap is designed *C,* The flap is mobilized on the muscle pedicle beneath the center of the flap. The pedicle is freed from the nasal cartilages sufficiently to permit only the exact degree of flap advancement necessary for wound repair. *D,* The flap in position. The donor site is closed in a Y configuration. *E* and *F,* A 2-month postoperative view.

sue. There is insufficient nasal skin to repair larger defects in this manner. The flap is ideally suited for elderly patients for repair of defects located centrally on the tip. By necessity, the flap is large to maximize tissue movement and decrease wound closure tension at the donor site. Distortion of the free margins of the nasal tip and ala is prevented by the compensatory size of the flap, which incorporates the majority of the remaining nasal skin. It is imperative to assess skin laxity and plan for some degree of secondary movement at the free margins of the nasal alae and tip. Skin laxity in the glabella and dorsal nasal regions is best determined by the pinch test, which consists of grasping the skin between the surgeon's thumb and index finger and determining the amount of redundancy.[9] For success, sufficient skin laxity is present when the surgeon can gather 1 to 2 cm of skin on the nasal bridge and glabella. Greater laxity is necessary as the size of the defect increases.

Commonly, the dorsal nasal flap is designed as a laterally based pivotal flap (Fig. 10–5). The pedicle is centered in the region of the medial canthus. A curvilinear line is drawn laterally from the defect to the junction of the cheek and the nose. From this point, the line is directed superiorly, passing 0.5 cm medial to the medial canthus and extending to the superior aspect of the glabella within a glabellar crease. Because the flap is transferred primarily by pivoting, the effective length of the flap diminishes progressively as the flap rotates about its pivotal point (medial canthus). The

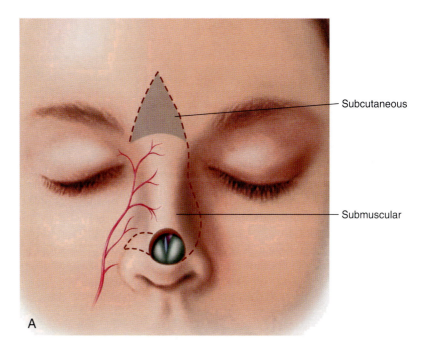

Subcutaneous

Submuscular

A

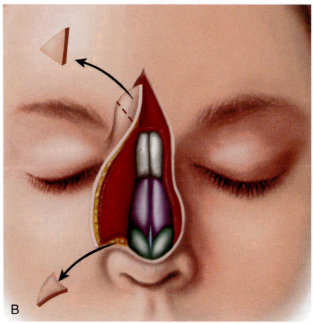

B

■ **Figure 10–5.** *A*, The dorsal nasal flap is a pivotal flap based on the branches of the angular artery. The glabellar portion (shaded) is dissected in the subcutaneous plane. *B*, The nasal portion is dissected beneath the musculature. An SCD is excised in or parallel to the alar groove.

Illustration continued on following page

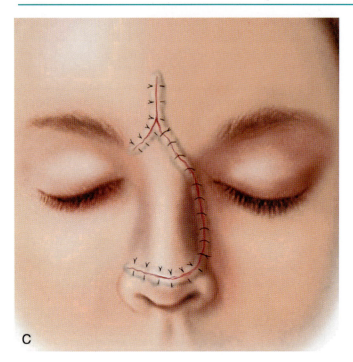

C

■ **Figure 10–5** *Continued. C,* The glabellar donor site wound is closed in a V-to-Y configuration.

height of the flap and thus the arc of pivotal movement must be sufficient to compensate for this shortening. Supplemental flap height is gained from the glabella extension. The higher the extension, the greater the height of the flap, and the easier it will be to close the donor defect. From the nasofrontal angle, the glabellar

extension is approximately 1½ to 2 times the vertical height of the nasal defect. From the superior point of the glabellar extension, a line angles inferiorly toward the contralateral medial canthus, creating a 30- to 45-degree angle backcut. The backcut remains just superior to the level of the medial canthal tendon to protect the axial vessels from the angular artery located inferior to the tendon. Heminasal flaps survive as random flaps, enabling the backcut to extend inferiorly to the medial canthal tendon if necessary. In designing the flap, it is helpful to triangulate the defect by excising the standing cutaneous deformity in such a manner that the excision lies within the alar groove or above and parallel to it. The flap should not extend below the alar groove or obliteration of the concave topography will occur between ala and nasal sidewall.

After injecting the nose with a local anesthesia containing epinephrine, the flap is elevated in a fashion similar to that of other nasal cutaneous flaps. The portion of the flap arising from the glabella is elevated in the subcutaneous plane, and the remaining portion of the flap is dissected beneath the nasal musculature. Nasal skin surrounding the flap is widely undermined, which may include a limited dissection of the medial cheek skin, releasing the fibrous attachment between cheek skin and periosteum along the junction of the cheek with nasal sidewall. Complete mobilization of the pedicle beneath the nasal muscles is necessary for proper tissue movement. The flap is secured with a temporary suture to allow the surgeon to check for discrepancy of skin thickness or distortion of alae or nasal tip. The undersurface of the distal flap may be

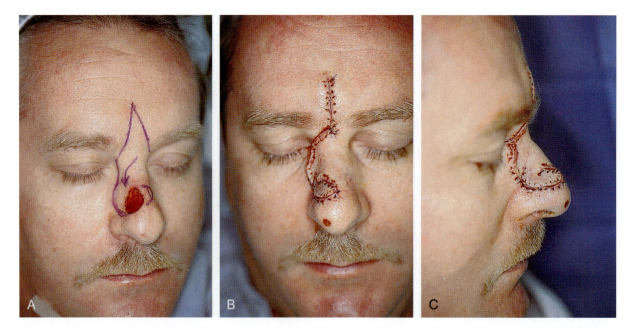

A B C

■ **Figure 10–6.** *A,* A dorsal nasal flap is designed to repair a 2.0 cm skin defect. An SCD is marked on the left side of the defect. *B* and *C,* The flap has been transferred. The distal portion was turned on itself, which reduced the pivot of the flap, eliminating the need to excise the SCD. The flap was thinned to the level of the dermis in the area of the medial canthus.

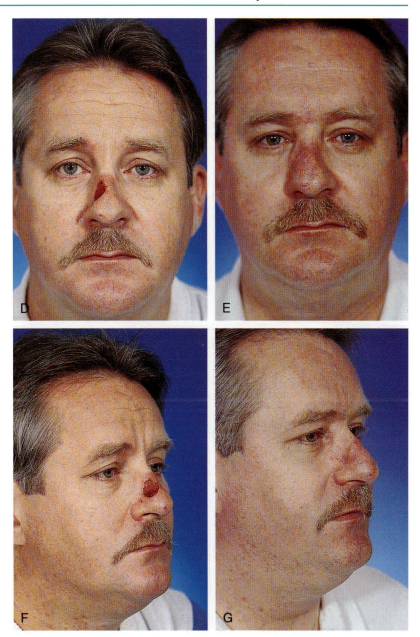

■ **Figure 10–6** *Continued. D–G*, Preoperative view and 6-month postoperative view.

trimmed to maximize thickness match between flap and recipient site. Only three or four deep sutures are necessary to position the flap. Skin incisions are repaired with 5-0 polypropylene vertical mattress cutaneous sutures to evert wound edges.

The donor site in the glabella may be closed by V-to-Y advancement, Z-plasty or, more commonly, primary repair. When primary wound closure is used, the triangular segment of glabella skin that moves with the flap is trimmed for a perfect fit, creating a single glabellar incision line. Thinning of the flap in the area of the medial canthus is critical to improve the mismatch of thickness between the thin skin of the medial canthus and the thicker glabellar skin of the flap (Fig. 10–6).

A common disadvantage of the dorsal nasal flap is cephalic displacement of the nostril margin and nasal tip. In older patients with tip ptosis and a central tip

skin defect, slight elevation of the nasal tip is beneficial. In younger patients, however, elevation of the tip may result in an unacceptable appearance. Repair of lateral nasal defects may result in permanent mild to extreme elevation of the ala in patients with insufficient laxity of the nasal and glabella skin. In spite of aggressive thinning of the flap in the area of the medial canthus, marked discrepancy in thickness between flap and native medial canthal skin is often problematic. This is the greatest disadvantage of using this flap, which precludes its common use by the authors.

We occasionally use a modified design of the dorsal nasal flap for midline skin defects of the upper dorsum (Fig. 10–7). The design is such that the lateral border of the flap remains anterior to the thin skin of the medial canthal region to avoid mismatch in skin thickness. We call this design a dorsal heminasal flap. The

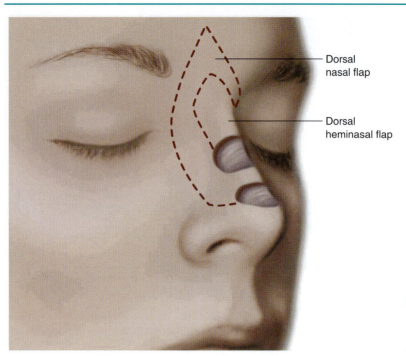

Dorsal
nasal flap

Dorsal
heminasal flap

■ Figure 10–7. Dorsal nasal and heminasal flaps. The heminasal flap is used to repair more cephalad defects. Its borders remain anterior to the thin skin of the medial canthal region.

design limits the arc of tissue movement; the modified flap can be used only for smaller (less than 2 cm) skin defects of the nasal bridge that are 1 cm away from the nostril margin and not below the tip-defining points.[9] The dorsal heminasal flap does not necessarily require a glabellar incision. The lateral incision is along the junction of the nasal sidewall and dorsum and therefore recruits skin only from the nasal bridge.

As discussed earlier in this chapter, reduction rhinoplasty may occasionally facilitate repair of a nasal skin defect by creating a relatively greater amount of skin redundancy. The patient in Figure 10–8 presented with a 3 × 2 cm skin defect of the upper dorsum and a marked convexity and overprojection of the upper and middle nasal vaults.[10] She desired a reduction of the nasal bridge. An aesthetic rhinoplasty was performed concomitant with a modified dorsal nasal flap. Reducing the volume of the bony and cartilaginous skeleton created greater skin redundancy, which enabled partial wound closure by advancing nasal skin medially. This in turn reduced the size requirement of a modified dorsal nasal flap used to repair the remaining portion of the defect. The standing cutaneous deformity resulting from bilateral medial advancement of the nasal sidewall skin was excised in the midline immediately inferior to the caudal border of the transferred flap.

Bilobe Flap

Using modifications of the original design, the bilobe flap is the most useful of the nasal cutaneous flaps. It is

■ Figure 10–8. *A,* A 3.0 × 2.0 cm skin defect of the dorsum. *B,* A reduction of the nasal bridge projection created a relatively greater amount of skin redundancy. The defect is partially closed by medial advancement of the nasal skin. A modified dorsal nasal flap is designed to repair the remaining portion of the defect. *C,* The flap is in position. An SCD resulting from bilateral medial advancement of the nasal sidewall skin was excised in the midline, immediately inferior to the caudal border of the transferred flap. *D–G,* A view before the removal of a skin cancer, which resulted in a dorsal defect; 10-month postoperative view. (Courtesy of Arch Otolaryngol Head Neck Surg 121:634, 1995.)

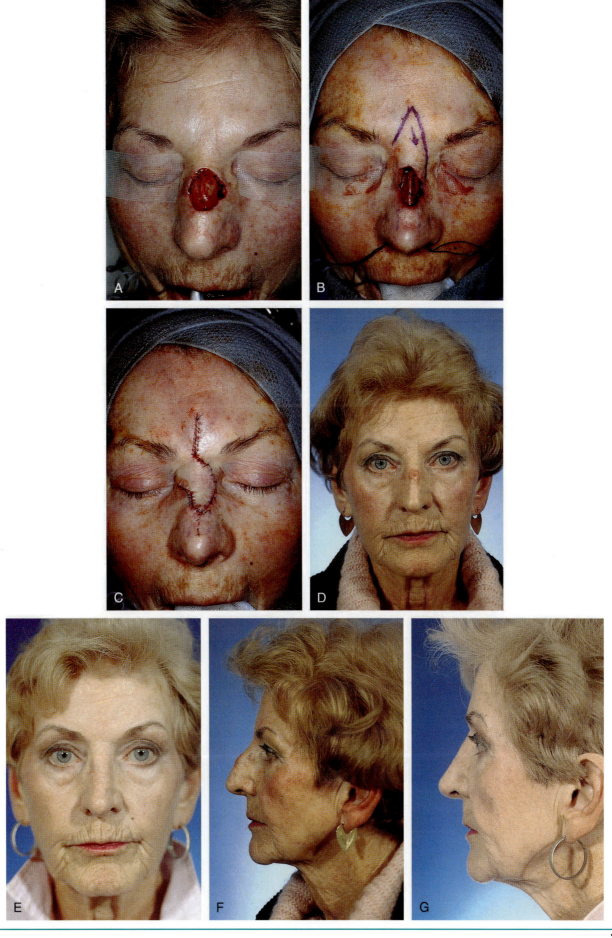

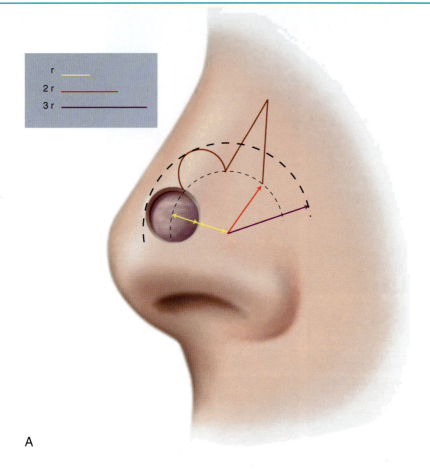

r
2 r
3 r

A

B

45°
45°

Figure 10–9. *A,* A distance equal to the radius of the defect (l × r) is measured from the lateral border of the defect to the pivotal point of the two lobes of the bilobe flap. Two arcs are drawn with their centers at the pivotal point. One arc passes through the center of and the other tangential to the defect. The bases of both lobes arise from the first arc. The height of the first lobe extends to the second arc. The width of the first lobe equals the width of the defect. *B,* The axes of the defect and the two lobes of the flap are approximately 45 degrees apart.

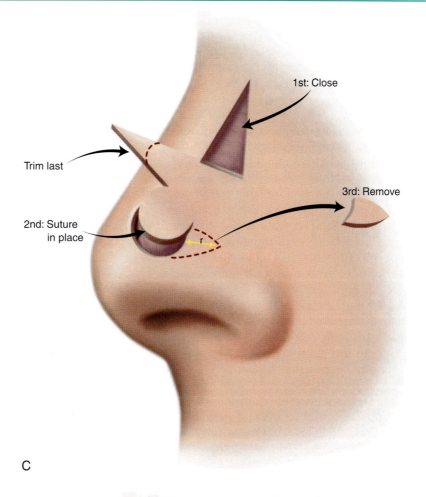

1st: Close

Trim last

3rd: Remove

2nd: Suture
in place

r

C

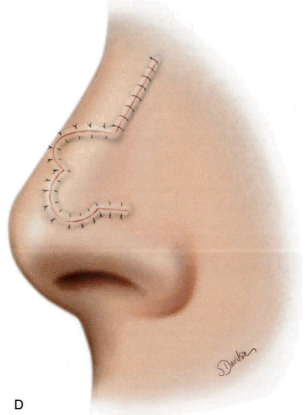

Figure 10–9 *Continued. C,* The donor site of the second lobe is closed first. The first lobe is transposed and the SCD is removed. The second lobe is then transposed and trimmed. *D,* The skin incisions are repaired with vertical mattress sutures.

D

the flap of choice for reconstruction of certain defects of the lower third of the nose. The bilobe flap is a double transposition flap. The primary flap or lobe is used to repair the nasal defect, and a secondary lobe is created to repair the donor site of the primary lobe. The donor site of the secondary lobe is then closed primarily. The original design of the bilobe flap is attributed to Esser,[11] who used it to reconstruct defects of the nasal tip. His design required a 90-degree arc of tissue transfer for each lobe of the flap, resulting in a total transposition of more than 180 degrees. A bilobe flap used to repair a nasal tip defect created the first lobe from skin of the nasal sidewall and the second lobe from the glabella. The wide angles between the axes of each flap created large standing cutaneous deformities and probable trapdoor deformity of both the first and second lobe. These were common sequelae of this flap and an impediment to its use. McGregor and Soutar[12] altered the original design, observing that the arc of tissue transfer could vary greatly from the original 90 degrees between defect and the first lobe of the flap and between the individual lobes. In 1989 Zitelli[13] published his experience using the bilobe flap for nasal reconstruction. He emphasized the use of a limited pivotal arc of 45 degrees between each lobe so that the total pivotal movement occurs over no more than 90 to 110 degrees. This modification greatly limits standing cutaneous deformities and reduces postoperative trapdoor deformities. Burget and Menick[14] confirmed the results using Zitelli's modification. Bilobe flaps expand the use of transposition flaps for repair of the nose. Skin defects that cannot be repaired with a single transposition flap because of wound closure tension may often be repaired with a bilobe flap because wound closure tension is distributed over a greater region.

Whenever possible, the bilobe flap is based laterally. Medial-based flaps are hardy, although the vascular supply is not as abundant as those based laterally. Bilobe flaps are ideally suited for defects less than 1.5 cm in maximum dimension, located on the central or lateral nasal tip without extension to the ala. The defect should be at least 0.5 cm above the margin of the nostril. The flap recruits skin from the mid dorsum and sidewall, where more generous skin laxity allows primary repair of the second lobe donor site. Defects on the upper half of the nose are not suited for reconstruction with a bilobe flap because the flap requires skin from the medial canthus that is thin and immobile. The flap is most useful in patients with thin skin and an amount of laxity along the nasal sidewall. The surgeon may estimate laxity by pinching the lateral nasal skin between the thumb and index finger. Patients with thick sebaceous skin have a higher risk of developing flap necrosis, trapdoor deformity, and depressed scars.

The bilobe flap has a geometrically precise design (Fig. 10–9). The radius of the defect is measured. A point is marked in the alar groove that is one radius from the lateral border of the defect. This point is used for designing both lobes of the flap and also represents the pivotal point for the two lobes. Two arcs are drawn with their centers at the marked point. The first arc passes through the center of the defect, and the other makes a tangent with the most distal border of the defect. Calipers and rulers are not used to draw the arcs because these devices measure straight line distances. In contrast, the topography of the nose is convex in the area of the tip and dorsum; a flexible measuring device is used. A needle with an attached suture is passed full-thickness through the nose at the pivotal point. A knot is tied in the suture inside the nasal vestibule.

The suture is draped from the pivotal point across the defect, and a clamp is applied to the suture at the center of the defect. The clamp with attached suture is then rotated about the pivotal point to indicate the first arc, which is marked with a pen (Fig. 10–10). The clamp is advanced along the suture to the most peripheral point of the defect, and a second arc is drawn tangent to the peripheral border of the defect and parallel to the first arc. The base of the two lobes rests on the first arc. The height of the first or primary lobe extends to the second arc so its height is equal to the distance between the two arcs. The width of the first lobe is equal to the width of the defect. The width of the second lobe is the same or slightly less than that of the first lobe. The height of the second lobe is approximately 1.5 to 2.0 cm greater than the height of the first lobe. The first lobe has the configuration of the defect, and the second lobe is triangular. The axis passing through the center of each lobe is positioned at approximately 45 degrees from each other, with the axis of the first lobe positioned 45 degrees from the central axis of the defect. This orientation of the lobes inevitably positions the axis of the second lobe along the center of the nasal sidewall or at the junction of the sidewall with the dorsum. A Burrow triangle representing the eventual standing cutaneous deformity resulting from the pivot of the first lobe is marked with its apex pointing laterally and one side parallel to or in the alar groove. The base of the triangle is the lateral border of the defect, and the height of the triangle is equal to the radius of the defect.

The flap is elevated using local anesthesia. Like other nasal cutaneous flaps, it is dissected in the plane between the nasal muscles and underlying perichondrium and periosteum. The flap and the remaining skin of the entire nose are completely undermined, sometimes extending the dissection to the cheek a short distance. Wide peripheral undermining of all the nasal skin is essential to reduce wound closure tension, facilitate flap transfer, and minimize trapdoor deformity (Fig. 10–11). The donor site for the second lobe is closed first by primary approximation of the muscle layer. The first lobe is then transposed to the nasal defect and secured

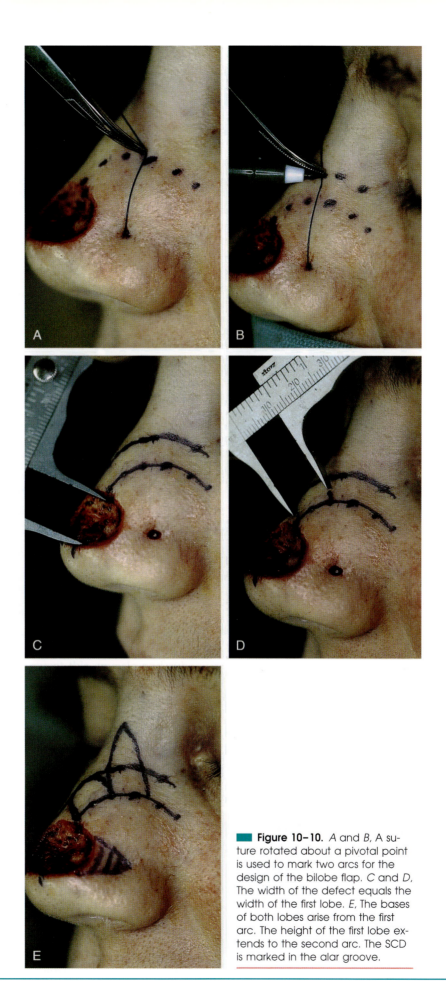

Figure 10-10. *A* and *B*, A suture rotated about a pivotal point is used to mark two arcs for the design of the bilobe flap. *C* and *D*, The width of the defect equals the width of the first lobe. *E*, The bases of both lobes arise from the first arc. The height of the first lobe extends to the second arc. The SCD is marked in the alar groove.

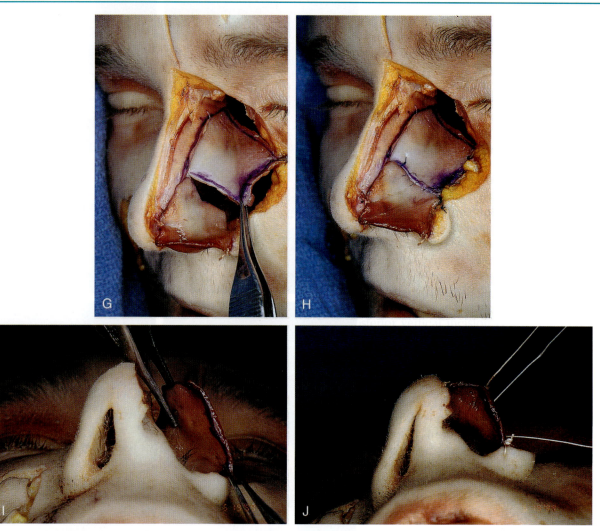

■ **Figure 11–2** *Continued. G,* Flap incised and reflected laterally. *H,* Flaps sutured in position. Caudal edge of contralateral flap is tacked to exposed raw surface of ipsilateral flap to seal off nasal passage from exterior. *I,* Ipsilateral flap is reflected laterally to line lower nasal vault. *J,* Suture suspension of flap to overlying cartilaginous framework (not yet in place) restores arc of nasal vestibule.

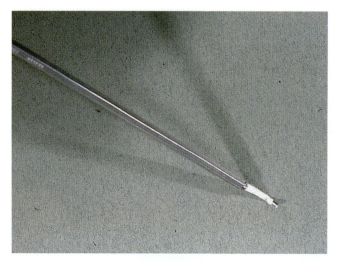

■ **Figure 11–3.** Right-angle scalpel is useful for making posterior vertical mucosal incision.

vertical incision through the caudal septal cartilage, preserving 1.0 to 1.5 cm of cartilage to serve as caudal support to the nose. Contralateral mucoperichondrium and mucoperiosteum are elevated away from the exposed septal cartilage and bone through this incision. The inferior border of the cartilaginous septum is then freed from the nasal crest. An incision is made through the cartilage superiorly, paralleling the dorsal mucosal incision made previously to develop the hinge flap. Of the cartilage, 1.0 to 1.5 cm is left in situ above the incision to maintain a dorsal septal strut providing support to the nasal bridge. Angled turbinectomy scissors are used to make a horizontal cut through the bony septum dorsally. If the bony septum is too thick to be cut, bone-cutting shears or a small rongeur may be used. Inferiorly, portions of the vomer may be included in the specimen by using a 4-mm-wide osteotome to cut

dissec
plane
ing e
dissec
tachm
lage
begin
ues c
encou
of the
The fl
dial a
until
tionec
edge
sional

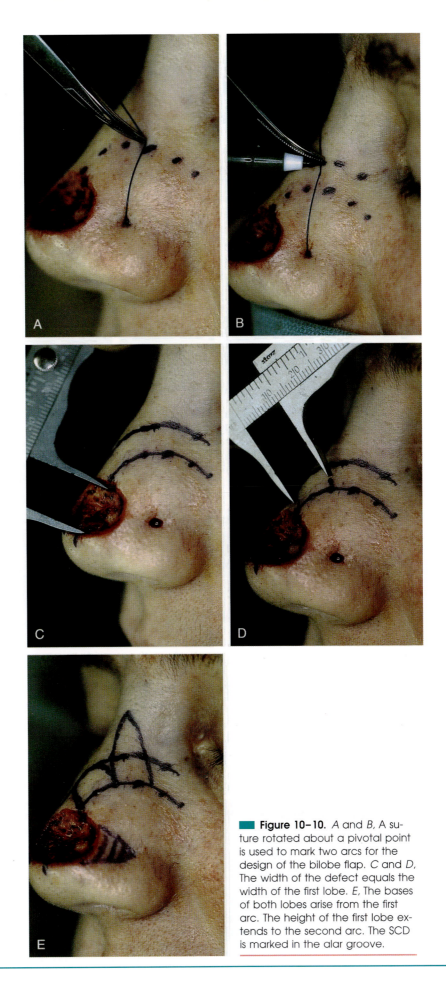

Fig
defec
tween
stage
portec
Acad

Figure 10–10. A and B, A suture rotated about a pivotal point is used to mark two arcs for the design of the bilobe flap. C and D, The width of the defect equals the width of the first lobe. E, The bases of both lobes arise from the first arc. The height of the first lobe extends to the second arc. The SCD is marked in the alar groove.

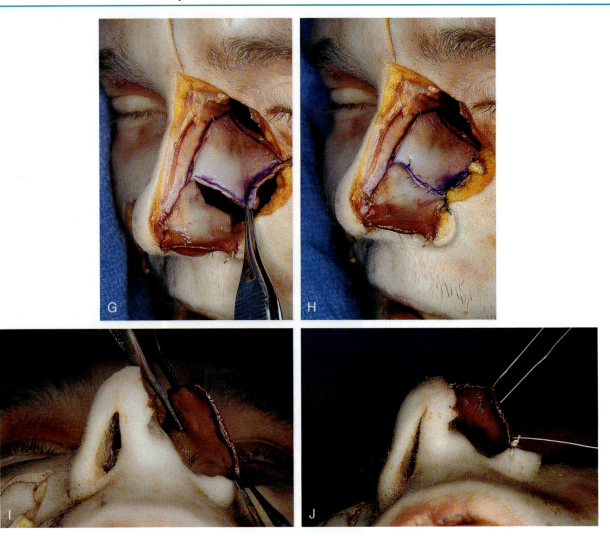

■ **Figure 11–2** *Continued. G,* Flap incised and reflected laterally. *H,* Flaps sutured in position. Caudal edge of contralateral flap is tacked to exposed raw surface of ipsilateral flap to seal off nasal passage from exterior. *I,* Ipsilateral flap is reflected laterally to line lower nasal vault. *J,* Suture suspension of flap to overlying cartilaginous framework (not yet in place) restores arc of nasal vestibule.

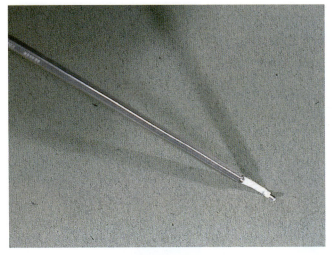

■ **Figure 11–3.** Right-angle scalpel is useful for making posterior vertical mucosal incision.

vertical incision through the caudal septal cartilage, preserving 1.0 to 1.5 cm of cartilage to serve as caudal support to the nose. Contralateral mucoperichondrium and mucoperiosteum are elevated away from the exposed septal cartilage and bone through this incision. The inferior border of the cartilaginous septum is then freed from the nasal crest. An incision is made through the cartilage superiorly, paralleling the dorsal mucosal incision made previously to develop the hinge flap. Of the cartilage, 1.0 to 1.5 cm is left in situ above the incision to maintain a dorsal septal strut providing support to the nasal bridge. Angled turbinectomy scissors are used to make a horizontal cut through the bony septum dorsally. If the bony septum is too thick to be cut, bone-cutting shears or a small rongeur may be used. Inferiorly, portions of the vomer may be included in the specimen by using a 4-mm-wide osteotome to cut

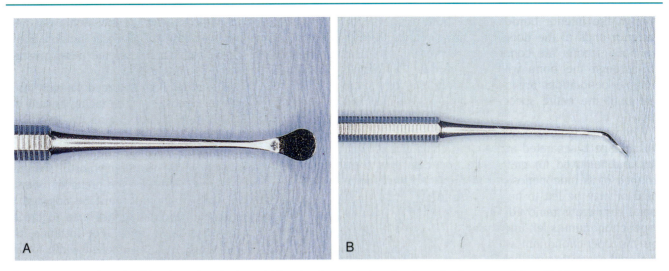

Figure 11–4. *A* and *B*, Woodson elevator is useful in releasing posterior attachments of mucoperichondrial flap.

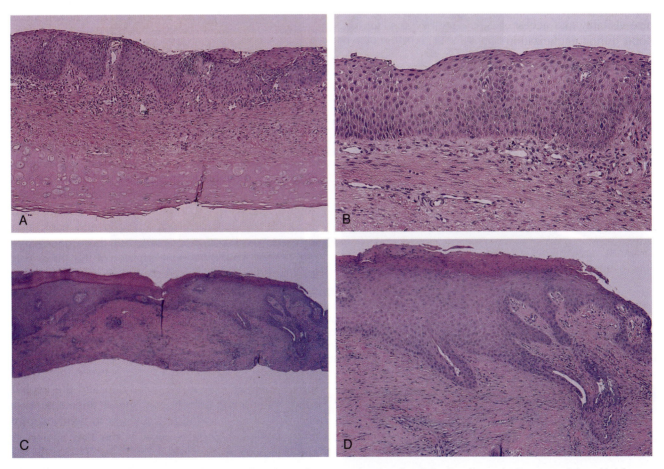

Figure 11–5. *A* and *B*, Biopsy sample of nasal septum after secondary healing following harvest of mucoperichondrial flap where septal cartilage was left in situ. *A*, Note viable chondrocytes in matrix of cartilage. *B*, The septal cartilage is resurfaced with stratified epithelium without glanular elements. *C* and *D*, Septal mucoperichondrial flap 4 months after transfer to lateral ala as lining flap. Biopsy was adjacent to reconstructed nostril margin. The mucosa has undergone squamous metaplasia with hyperkeratosis and parakeratosis. There are remnants of glanular elements.

Contralateral Caudally Based Septal Mucoperichondrial Hinge Flap

There are occasions when the surgeon is confronted with full-thickness loss of the ala or hemitip with extension of the defect into the upper lip and loss of the septal branch of the superior labial artery. The author has been successful in using an ipsilateral septal mucoperichondrial hinge flap for lining the caudal nose in these circumstances in patients who do not use tobacco products. Presumably, sufficient collateral circulation from the contralateral side of the membranous septum is sufficient to support the flap. However, when the ipsilateral septal branch of the labial artery has been ablated, it is probably more prudent to use a contralateral septal mucoperichondrial hinge flap based on the caudal septum (Fig. 11–9). This design precludes the use of a contralateral dorsally based muco-

perichondrial lining flap; such a flap should not be used if that flap will be necessary for reconstructing a more cephalically located area of lining deficit. The flap must be designed sufficiently long to span the distance from the contralateral caudal septum to the most cephalic portion of the lining defect while concommitantly providing an adequate surface area to reline the nasal defect. The flap is dissected in a fashion identical to that for the ipsilateral flap. The exposed septal cartilage may be removed for grafting purposes or left in situ. If left in situ, a strip of cartilage must be removed behind the caudal strut of the septum to allow passage of the flap through the septum to the contralateral side. A vertical incision is made through the septal mucoperichondrium on the side opposite to the flap to accommodate the passage of the flap. The flap is folded on its base and delivered to the defect through the vertical septal fenestra. In contrast to its counterpart, the pedicle must be twisted in order for the raw surface of the mucoperichondrium to face outward. The edges of the flap are sutured to the edges of the lining defect, and

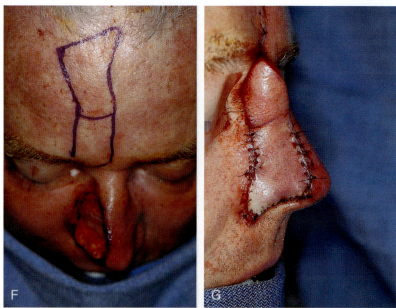

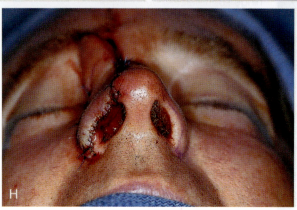

Figure 11–7 *Continued. F* and *G,* Paramedian forehead flap provides covering for reconstructed ala and intermediate zone. *H,* Alar batten graft has restored normal contour to reconstructed nostril.

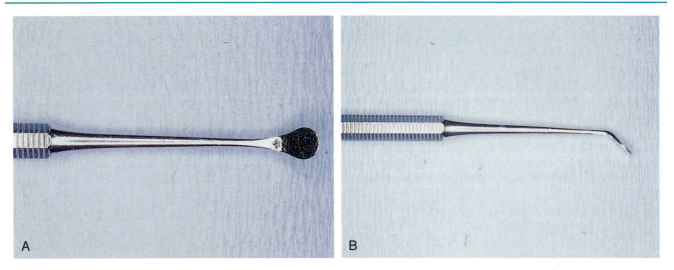

■ **Figure 11–4.** *A* and *B*, Woodson elevator is useful in releasing posterior attachments of mucoperichondrial flap.

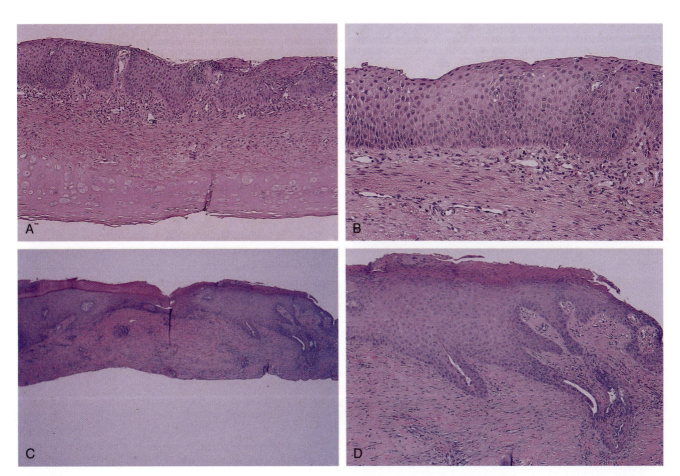

■ **Figure 11–5.** *A* and *B*, Biopsy sample of nasal septum after secondary healing following harvest of mucoperichondrial flap where septal cartilage was left in situ. *A*, Note viable chondrocytes in matrix of cartilage. *B*, The septal cartilage is resurfaced with stratified epithelium without glandular elements. *C* and *D*, Septal mucoperichondrial flap 4 months after transfer to lateral ala as lining flap. Biopsy was adjacent to reconstructed nostril margin. The mucosa has undergone squamous metaplasia with hyperkeratosis and parakeratosis. There are remnants of glandular elements.

through the inferior border of the bony septum. The posterior ends of the dorsal and inferior cuts through the bony septum are connected by making a vertical cut through the bone with a 2-mm-wide osteotome. Multiple perforations are made through the bony septum until the entire specimen can be gently rocked free.

When large grafts are not required, the exposed septal cartilage is separated at the bony-cartilaginous junction and removed for grafts. The bone that has been stripped of its mucoperiosteum may be removed piecemeal or may be left to heal by secondary intention. If septal cartilage is removed, the intact contralateral mucoperichondrium is left undisturbed. The raw surface of the mucoperichondrium will become covered with a thin epithelium through healing by secondary intention (see Fig. 11–5).

The borders of the septal mucoperichondrial incisions are now completely cauterized with an extended insulated electrical cautery. An ideal device for accomplishing this is a Bovie suction device used to perform tonsillectomies (Fig. 11–6). It has a malleable shaft that may be angulated in a desirable configuration to maximize visibility and access. It also enables the suction of blood during cauterization without the need for switching from a suction to cautery device. Achieving near complete hemostasis along the mucosal incision line is imperative because the flap crosses the nasal passage, making nasal packing unfeasible.

The mucoperichondrial flap is turned laterally as a hinge flap, with the mucosal surface facing toward the nasal passage. Most defects requiring an ipsilateral septal mucoperichondrial hinge flap extend through the nostril margin. The distal corners of the rectangular flap are usually sutured to the remaining nostril margins. However, this may not always be the preferred orientation of the flap. Flap positioning must be adjusted to provide the maximum mucosal surface area to the region that requires the most lining. For instance, the distal end of the flap may lack sufficient width to line the entire arc of the nostril margin. The flap is angulated so that a portion of the inferior or superior border of the flap is recruited alongside the distal flap margin to provide the necessary lining along the caudal border of the missing nostril. The flap is secured to the distal peripheral margins of the lining defect, and the more proximal borders are sutured to the edges of the lining defect with interrupted 5-0 or 6-0 polydioxanone sutures. Depending on the shape of the defect, portions of the flap border are occasionally sutured together, creating a cul-de-sac within the reconstructed nasal vestibule (Fig. 11–7).

The septal mucoperichondrial hinge flap is thin and flexible and must be supported by a framework of septal and auricular cartilage grafts carefully crafted to replicate the contour of the missing region of the nose. Similar to the bipedicle vestibular skin advancement flap, the ipsilateral mucoperichondrial hinge flap is suspended to overlying cartilage grafts with 5-0 polydioxanone sutures that pass from the external surface of the grafts through the cartilage and flap and back again. The number of sutures is limited to those necessary to restore the desired internal contour of the lower vault. It is important to protect the cartilage grafts from exposure to the nasal passage by providing complete internal coverage of the grafts. This prevents contamination of the grafts with nasal secretions and provides a source of revascularization of the undersurface of the grafts. Sealing off the grafts from the nasal passage is achieved by placing a few sutures between the exposed submucosal surface of the hinge flap and the cephalic edge of the lining defect. Only two or three sutures are necessary; they are tied in a fashion to lightly approximate the submucosal surface of the flap against the upper margin of the lining defect (Fig. 11–8). Because these sutures are placed across the pedicle of the flap, they have a potential for causing distal necrosis if placed injudiciously. The use of mattress sutures placed perpendicular to the axis of blood flow should be avoided.

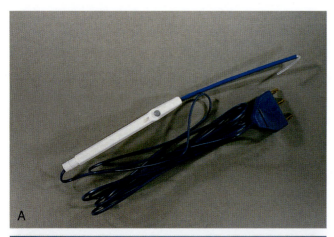

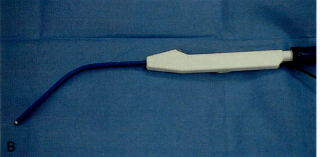

■ **Figure 11–6.** *A* and *B,* Bovie suction is an insulated device useful in cautery of incised borders of nasal septum. Malleable shaft maximizes visibility and access.

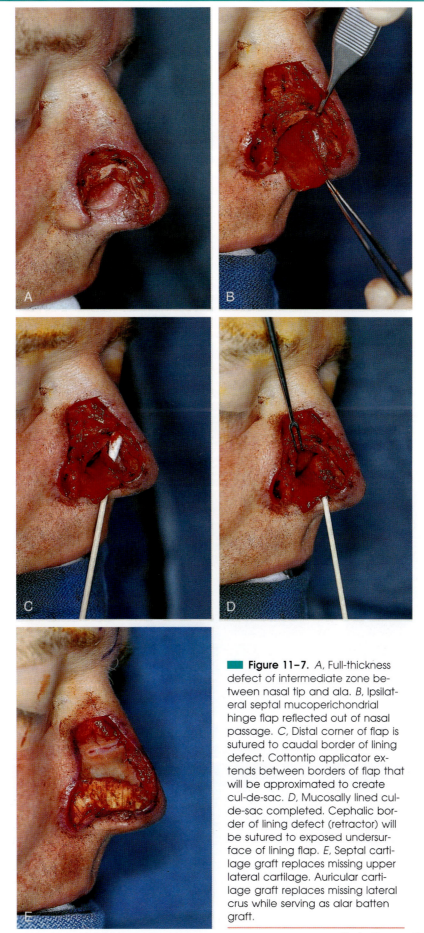

Figure 11–7. *A,* Full-thickness defect of intermediate zone between nasal tip and ala. *B,* Ipsilateral septal mucoperichondrial hinge flap reflected out of nasal passage. *C,* Distal corner of flap is sutured to caudal border of lining defect. Cottontip applicator extends between borders of flap that will be approximated to create cul-de-sac. *D,* Mucosally lined cul-de-sac completed. Cephalic border of lining defect (retractor) will be sutured to exposed undersurface of lining flap. *E,* Septal cartilage graft replaces missing upper lateral cartilage. Auricular cartilage graft replaces missing lateral crus while serving as alar batten graft.

Illustration continued on following page

Contralateral Caudally Based Septal Mucoperichondrial Hinge Flap

There are occasions when the surgeon is confronted with full-thickness loss of the ala or hemitip with extension of the defect into the upper lip and loss of the septal branch of the superior labial artery. The author has been successful in using an ipsilateral septal mucoperichondrial hinge flap for lining the caudal nose in these circumstances in patients who do not use tobacco products. Presumably, sufficient collateral circulation from the contralateral side of the membranous septum is sufficient to support the flap. However, when the ipsilateral septal branch of the labial artery has been ablated, it is probably more prudent to use a contralateral septal mucoperichondrial hinge flap based on the caudal septum (Fig. 11–9). This design precludes the use of a contralateral dorsally based muco-

perichondrial lining flap; such a flap should not be used if that flap will be necessary for reconstructing a more cephalically located area of lining deficit. The flap must be designed sufficiently long to span the distance from the contralateral caudal septum to the most cephalic portion of the lining defect while concommitantly providing an adequate surface area to reline the nasal defect. The flap is dissected in a fashion identical to that for the ipsilateral flap. The exposed septal cartilage may be removed for grafting purposes or left in situ. If left in situ, a strip of cartilage must be removed behind the caudal strut of the septum to allow passage of the flap through the septum to the contralateral side. A vertical incision is made through the septal mucoperichondrium on the side opposite to the flap to accommodate the passage of the flap. The flap is folded on its base and delivered to the defect through the vertical septal fenestra. In contrast to its counterpart, the pedicle must be twisted in order for the raw surface of the mucoperichondrium to face outward. The edges of the flap are sutured to the edges of the lining defect, and

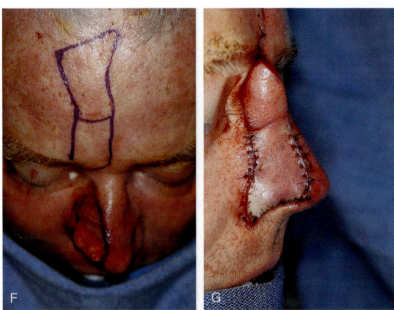

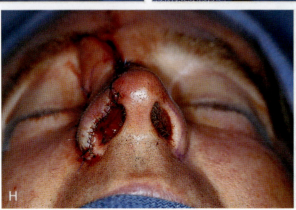

Figure 11–7 *Continued. F* and *G*, Paramedian forehead flap provides covering for reconstructed ala and intermediate zone. *H*, Alar batten graft has restored normal contour to reconstructed nostril.

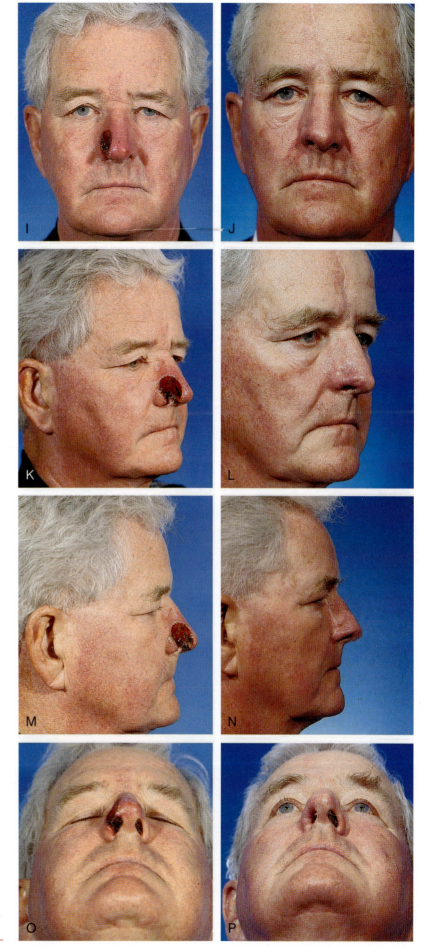

■ **Figure 11-7** *Continued. I–P,* Preoperative and 1 year postoperative. A contouring procedure was performed 3 months following detachment of forehead and lining flaps.

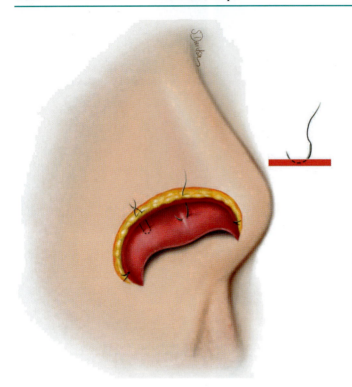

Figure 11–8. Nasal passage is sealed off from exterior by placing sutures from submucosal surface of hinge flap to cephalic edge of lining defect. Sutures pass submucosally to maximize flap vascularity.

the flap is suspended to an overlying framework of cartilage, with mattress sutures placed through the cartilage and flap. The submucosal surface of the flap is tacked to the posterior and cephalic borders of the lining defect in order to completely cover the framework grafts and seal the grafts from the nasal passage. The pedicle of the flap is detached from the septum 3 weeks following transfer.

Bilateral Caudally Based Septal Mucoperichondrial Hinge Flap

A septal mucoperichondrial hinge flap based on the caudal septum may be developed bilaterally (Fig. 11–10). Concurrent bilateral flaps preclude the use of a dorsally based septal mucoperichondrial hinge flap for repair of more cephalically located lining deficits. Bilateral flaps are indicated when a full-thickness defect of the entire nasal tip is present but with an intact columella. In this situation, each flap provides lining for the ipsilateral hemitip and any portions of the adjacent ala that may be absent. The flaps are designed, incised, and dissected in a fashion identical to the methods for a unilateral flap. The exposed septal cartilage is re-

moved as resurfacing of the cartilage by secondary intention healing is unlikely. A 1.5-cm-wide dorsal and caudal strut of septal cartilage is maintained for proper support of the nasal bridge. The borders of the mucosal incisions along the remaining septum at the donor site are carefully cauterized to prevent postoperative bleeding. Each flap is turned laterally and anteriorly in a hinged fashion with the raw surface of the mucoperichondrium turned outward. The flaps are sutured to their respective lining defects and suspended to a framework of cartilage grafts used to restore the structure and topography of the nasal tip and any portions of the ala that may be missing.

Contralateral Dorsal Septal Mucoperichondrial Hinge Flap

A mucoperichondrium hinge flap harvested from the side opposite the nasal defect and based on the nasal dorsum may be turned laterally to resurface the roof and lateral wall of the middle vault of the nose[3] (Fig. 11–11). The flap may be designed to include all of the mucosa covering the cartilaginous septum, except for the mandatory maintenance of the caudal and dorsal strut of the septum. Similar to the mucoperichondrial

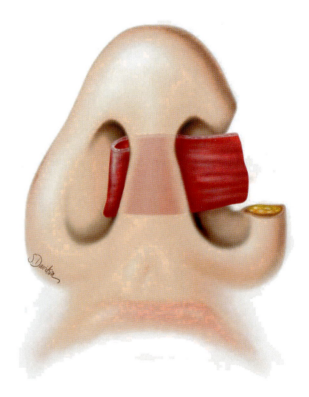

Figure 11–9. Caudally based contralateral septal mucoperichondrial hinge flap is delivered through nasal fenestra to reach lining defect. This flap is used when ipsilateral septal branch of labial artery is absent.

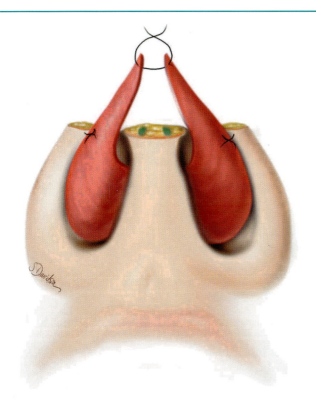

■ **Figure 11–10.** Bilateral caudally based septal mucoperichondrial hinge flaps. These are used to line bilateral full-thickness nasal tip defect with an intact columella.

flap hinged on the caudal septum, the elevation is facilitated by hydrodissection using a solution of local anesthesia injected beneath the perichondrium. Anterior and posterior vertical incisions are made with a right-angled scalpel. Incisions extend from the floor of the nose to within 1 cm of the dorsal septum. The incisions are separated by the distance appropriate for the desired width of the flap. The mucoperichondrium is dissected with a Freer elevator as a bipedicle flap attached to the dorsum above and floor of the nose below. Once the mucoperichondrium has been completely freed from the septal cartilage, it is released from the floor with a scalpel blade attached to an extended handle. The exposed septal cartilage is usually removed for grafting purposes, leaving adequate dorsal support for the nasal bridge. However, the denuded septal cartilage may be left in situ if covered on its other side by mucoperichondrium. If left intact, a linear fenestra extending parallel and below the dorsal strut is created in the septal cartilage and opposing mucoperichondrium to allow passage of the flap. The flap is reflected laterally across the midline toward the side of the lining defect while maintaining its attachment to the contralateral nasal dorsum. This maneuver turns the raw undersurface of the mucoperichondrium outward, away from the nasal passage. The mucosal borders of the donor site are cauterized, and the flap is sutured to the margins of the lining defect. This flap is most commonly combined with an ipsilateral mucoperi-

chondrial flap hinged on the caudal septum. The dorsally based flap passes through the large septal perforation necessitated by the use of the two flaps. The caudal border of the dorsally based flap is sutured to the undersurface of the hinge ipsilateral flap (see Fig. 11–2*H*). This seals off the nasal passage from the exterior portion of the nasal defect, enabling a continuous carpet of mucoperichondrium on which to place an overlying cartilage framework. The flaps are suspended to the framework with mattress sutures so there is intimate contact between the mucoperichondrium and the entire undersurface of the cartilage grafts used for framework.

Usually, the contralateral dorsally based septal mucoperichondrial hinge flap is suspended sufficiently high in the area of the roof of the middle vault that it does not crowd the internal nasal valve. If the lining defect is confined to the lateral wall of the nose and does not extend to the roof of the middle vault, the flap may by necessity span across the internal valve of the nose. In these unusual circumstances, the pedicle of the flap is released from the contralateral dorsal septum 3 weeks subsequent to initial flap transfer. A scalpel on an extended handle is used to release the flap and to excise redundant pedicle mucosa using local infiltrative anesthesia.

Septal Composite Chondromucosal Pivotal Flap for the Tip and Columella

The septal composite chondromucosal pivotal flap is indicated for large full-thickness defects of the central nose, including combined tip and columella defects or the nasal dorsum along with portions of the sidewall. For lower vault defects, the composite flap is only indicated when there is a full-thickness loss of the nasal tip and adjacent columella. In instances of isolated full-thickness tip defects with an intact columella, bilateral septal mucoperichondrial flaps hinged on the caudal septum will suffice for lining the tip and any missing alae. Similarly, large (greater than 75%) isolated full-thickness losses of the columella are best reconstructed with an interpolated cheek or paramedian forehead flap and do not require a lining flap.

When the columella and nasal tip are both missing, the septal composite chondromucosal pivotal flap provides the cartilage necessary for the framework of the columella and the concomitant lining to resurface the area of the membranous septum and nasal domes (Fig. 11–12). The flap is designed with the maximum width possible while still preserving an adequate dorsal septal strut. The flap should extend the entire length of the

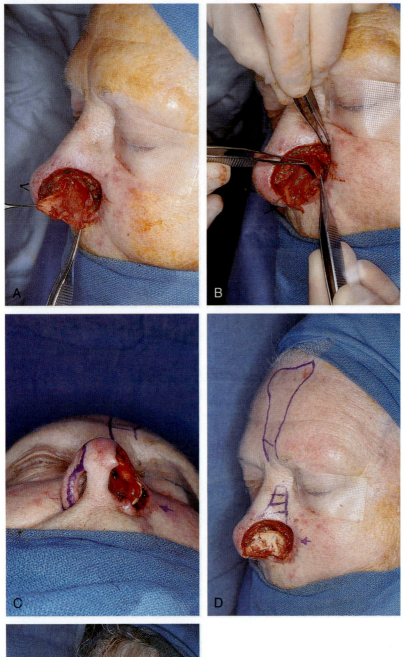

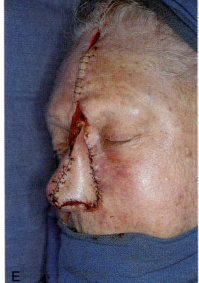

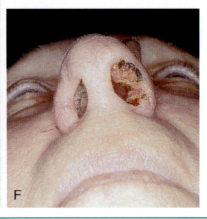

■ **Figure 11–11.** *A,* Ipsilateral septal mucoperichondrial hinge flap held by forceps reflected out of nasal passage to line caudal portion of full-thickness defect of ala and lower portion of nasal sidewall. *B,* Lower forceps are holding contralateral dorsal septal mucoperichondrial hinge flap that will provide lining for the more cephalic portion of defect. *C,* Auricular cartilage graft serves as an alar batten and restores contour to ala. *D,* Paramedian forehead flap designed as covering flap. Cross-hatched area represents remaining skin of sidewall, which was removed. *E,* Forehead flap transposed. *F,* 3 weeks following first stage. Ipsilateral mucosal flap is engorged and crusty. Engorgement regresses and crusting lessens over time as caudal aspect of lining flap undergoes metaplasia (see Fig. 11–5).

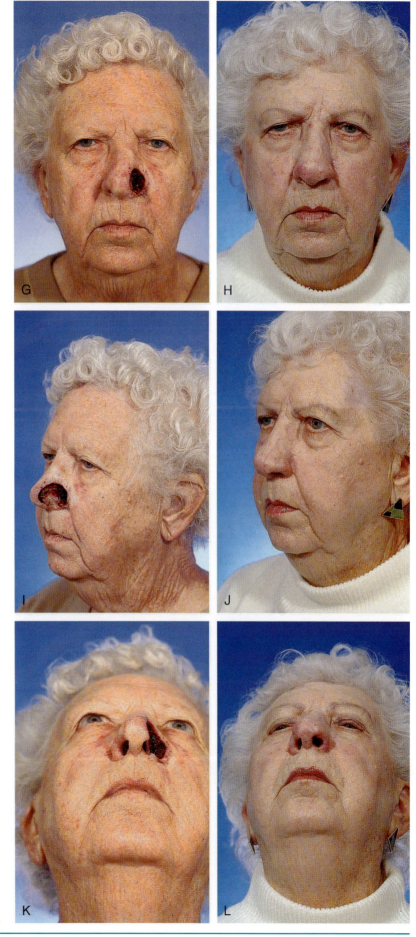

Figure 11–11 *Continued. G–L,* Preoperative and 5 months postoperative. A contouring procedure was performed 2 months following detachment of forehead and ipsilateral lining flap. (Courtesy Facial Plast Surg.[3])

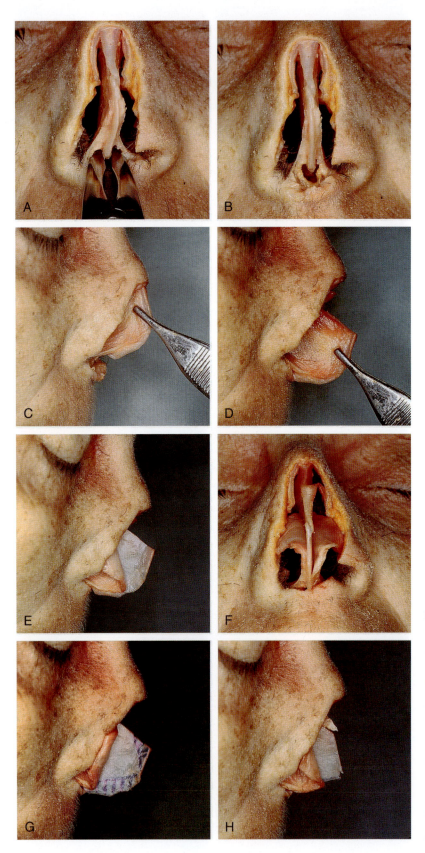

■ **Figure 11–12.** *A* and *B,* Full-thickness columella and nasal tip defect created in dissection specimen. Bilateral septal mucoperichondrial flaps are created adjacent to nasal spine at caudal inferior aspect of defect. Cartilage is removed (with rongeur) from region of posterior and inferior septal angle to facilitate flap transfer. The anterior nasal spine is preserved. *C* and *D,* Composite flap is pivoted anteriorly and caudally and braced against dorsal septum. *E* and *F,* Septal cartilage of pivoted flap provides structural support for construction of columella. Bilateral mucoperichondrial flaps are dissected from distal flap and reflected laterally to line nasal domes. *G* and *H,* Excess cartilage of pivoted flap is trimmed caudally and dorsally to provide desired nasal contour.

cartilaginous septum and usually includes portions of the bony septum. Typically, the flap is 3 cm wide and 5 cm long. Bilateral mucoperichondrial flaps are created with a periosteal elevator along the anterior floor of the nose adjacent to the nasal spine. Access to this dissection is through the anteroinferior margin of the defect near the nasal spine. The dissection is extended superiorly over the lateral aspect of the nasal crest until the septal cartilage is encountered.

A 4-mm-wide osteotome is used to excise a 2-cm-long segment of anterior nasal crest at the pivotal point of the flap while preserving the anterior septal spine. A no. 11 scalpel blade is used to make a full-thickness incision through the cartilaginous septum parallel to and 1.0 cm below the attachments of the upper lateral cartilages to the septum. The incision extends in an anterior direction from the bony perpendicular plate through the exposed margin of the caudal septum. A similar full-thickness incision is made with the same blade along the interface of the cartilaginous septum and the nasal crest, extending anteriorly from the vomer until it is juxtaposed to the previously resected nasal crest. The incision should remain 1.5 cm posterior to the anterior nasal spine to ensure a sufficient vascular pedicle. The pedicle is represented by bilateral mucoperichondrial flaps that are in continuity with the floor of the nose anteriorly and nourished by septal branches of the superior labial arteries.[2] A posterior vertical incision is now made to connect the two previously performed parallel horizontal incisions. If the flap extends only to the bony cartilaginous junction, the incision is made with a right angle scalpel; however, it is usually necessary to include bony septum in the flap to achieve adequate flap length. In these instances, the horizontal incisions are extended posteriorly full-thickness through the bony septum as described for harvesting extended cartilage and bone grafts using heavy-duty angled turbinectomy or bone-cutting scissors. A full-thickness vertical incision is made through the bone connecting the posterior ends of the two horizontal incisions. A curved osteotome is used to gently perforate through bone and mucosa on either side of the septum in multiple sites along the vertical line of the incision. The perforations are connected with a right-angled scalpel or right-angled scissors. It is important to ensure that the superior horizontal incision of the bony septum is completed before making these vertical perforations so that the force of the osteotome is not transmitted to the region of the cribriform plate.

Once the septal incisions are completed, the composite flap is pivoted 90 degrees on its base in an anterocaudal direction until the inferior border of the flap locks in place, bracing it against the remaining dorsal septal strut (Fig. 11–13).[4] It may be necessary to remove a small amount of cartilage in the area of the posterior and inferior septal angles in order for the flap to pivot on the intact anterior mucoperichondrial flaps.

The pivoted flap is secured to the dorsal septal strut using a figure-of-eight permanent 4-0 monofilament suture placed submucosally. After positioning the flap, bilateral septal mucoperichondrial hinge flaps are dissected from the distal portion of the flap's bone and cartilage. The flaps are reflected laterally to provide lining to the nasal domes. Denuded cartilage and bone extending beyond the planned dorsal line is resected and used for framework grafts. The borders of the reflected mucoperichondrial flaps are sutured to the margins of the lining defect. A framework of cartilage grafts is created from septal and auricular cartilage to replace the missing portions of the dome complex and lateral crura. The remaining cartilage of the composite flap serves as the medial crura for the construction and provides support to the columella. It also serves as the foundation of the framework grafts for the nasal domes. These grafts are sutured directly to the cartilage of the composite flap and are then scored and bent in a fashion to restore the contour of the domes. The mucoperichondrial flaps reflected laterally from the composite chondromucosal flap are approximated to the overlying framework grafts with sutures placed through the framework cartilage and underlying flaps. Some of the cartilage of the caudal aspect of the composite flap may require trimming if it causes excessive caudal positioning of the reconstructed columella.

Septal Composite Chondromucosal Pivotal Flap for the Dorsum

There are occasions when a patient presents with an intact nasal tip but has a full-thickness dorsal defect involving loss of cartilaginous dorsum and nasal bones. In these circumstances, the remaining septum may be utilized as a composite chondromucosal pivotal flap to provide a mucosal lining and structural support for the roof of the middle and upper nasal vaults. Usually, the anterior septal angle is missing along with the upper lateral cartilages, and the composite flap is used to resurface the interior of the entire dorsal defect. The flap is harvested in a manner similar to that described for the pivotal flap used to reconstruct full-thickness defects of the tip and columella. The flap pivots only 45 degrees, compared with 90 degrees for repair of the tip and columella, so it is not necessary to remove the anterior nasal crest bone. Working through an endonasal approach as well as through the dorsal defect, a full-thickness horizontal incision is made through the septum along the length of the nasal crest. The anterior extent of this incision remains 1.5 cm posterior to the anterior nasal spine. The length of the incision depends

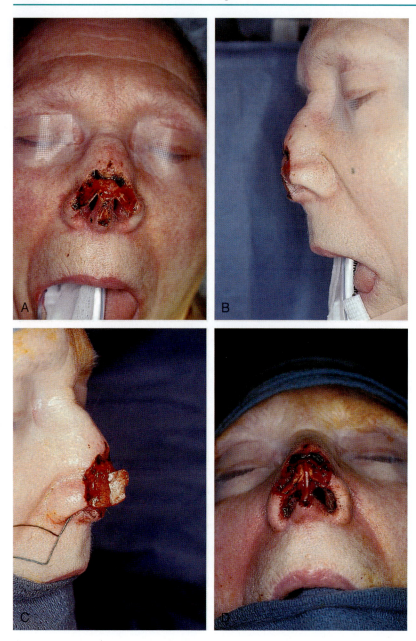

■ **Figure 11–13.** *A* and *B*, Full-thickness defect of nasal tip and columella. Medial and intermediate crura of lower lateral cartilages are absent. *C*, Septal composite chondromucosal pivotal flap turned outward to provide structure and lining. Bilateral septal mucoperiosteal hinge flaps have been reflected from septal bone and sutured to borders of lining defect. *D*, Septal bone has been trimmed from flap. Cartilage of composite flap replaces medial crura, and auricular cartilage grafts replace intermediate and portions of lateral crura. Lining flaps have been sutured to overlying framework. Framework was covered by paramedian forehead flap.

on the defect but usually extends 2 to 3 cm posteriorly through the bony septum. This is usually necessary to ensure sufficient length to enable the flap to engage the frontal bone or remaining nasal bones once it is pivoted in position. A vertical incision is extended from the posterior end of the horizontal septal incision upward to join the most cephalic aspect of the bony or cartilaginous septum exposed by the defect. The flap is delivered from the nasal passage by manually pivoting the flap 45 degrees on its pedicle. It may be necessary to remove cartilage in the area of the posterior septal angle in order to deliver the flap. This should be performed so that the adjacent mucoperichondrium is not damaged; this tissue represents the pedicle for the flap.

The posteroinferior corner of the flap is propped against the persistent nasal dorsum or the frontal bone

if the entire bony dorsum is absent. It is fixed to this stable superior buttress by placing a figure-of-eight permanent suture through holes drilled in the buttress and flap. As the composite flap is pivoted out of the nasal passage, the septal cartilage in the area of the anterior or posterior septal angle may be forced caudally sufficient to distort the infratip lobule or columellar labial junction. If this occurs, a small amount of cartilage is trimmed from the caudal border of the flap in the offending area.

Septal composite chondromucosal flaps used to reconstruct full-thickness tip and columella defects or defects of the nasal dorsum are utilized without delay. Reconstruction of the middle and upper nasal vaults usually requires larger composite flaps than that required for repair of defects of the tip and columella. It

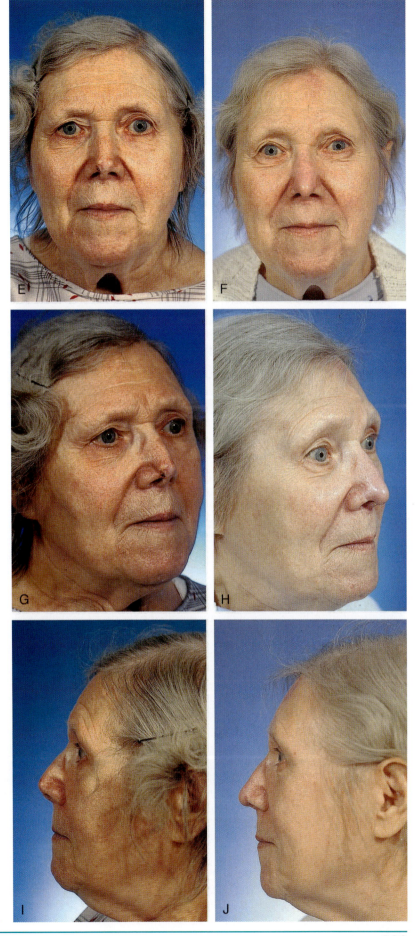

■ **Figure 11–13** *Continued. E–J,* Preoperative
views before Mohs' surgery that resulted in loss
of nasal tip and columella and 1 year postoperative. Reconstructed tip has enhanced projection and contour as compared with preoperative state. (Courtesy Mosby.[4])

may on occasion be prudent to delay the composite pivotal flap when large mucoperichondrial flaps are required to reline the dorsum and sidewalls of the nose. This becomes more important for patients who have received irradiation to the area and patients who use tobacco products. In these circumstances, the pivotal flap is left protruding from the nasal passage for 4 to 6 weeks (first stage). The second stage consists of reflecting bilateral mucoperichondrial and mucoperiosteal flaps away from the cartilage and bone extending beyond the nasal passage. The reflected flaps hinged on the inferior portion of the composite flap are turned laterally and sutured to the margins of the lining defect. The flaps are suspended to a framework of grafts consisting of bone and cartilage with sutures placed through the grafts and underlying flaps.

Septal Composite Chondromucosal Pivotal Flap for the Tip, Columella, and Dorsum

Total and near total nasal reconstruction may utilize the septum for internal lining if sufficient septum remains. This requires incorporating the entire remaining nasal septum in the composite flap. These cases are frequently associated with resection of the caudal cartilaginous septum and loss of the septal branches of the superior labial artery. In these circumstances, the flap is based on the mucoperiostium of the anterior floor of the nose, and delay of the flap is necessary. Three stages are used to line the nose.

Stage one consists of making the previously described inferior horizontal incision along the floor of the nose and vertical incision through the mucosa on either side of the septum but not through the bone and cartilage. Stage two is completed 3 weeks later by making incisions through the cartilage and bone of the septum, following the previous incision lines made in the covering mucosa. The composite flap is delivered from the nasal passage and is pivoted 90 degrees to provide the maximum amount of mucosa for construction of the caudal portion of the nose. If the cephalic portion of the dorsum is missing, there will not be a buttress on which to stabilize the pivoted flap. In this case, nasal packing is used to stabilize the flap. Packing is left in place for 5 days. The flap is left protruding from the nasal passage for 4 to 6 weeks before proceeding with reconstruction of the nasal lining. Stage three consists of creating bilateral mucoperichondrial flaps based on the anteroinferior border of the mobilized composite flap. The flaps are reflected laterally to line the roof and sidewalls of the caudal nose. If the flaps are lacking sufficient tissue to line the cephalic portions of the nasal passage, local turn-in flaps or a paramedian forehead flap is used. The reflected mucoperichondrial flaps are supported by an overlying framework of cartilage and bone that is covered by a paramedian forehead flap.

Turbinate Mucoperiosteal Flap

The middle and inferior turbinates may be used to line limited mucosal defects of the nose. These turbinates are richly supplied by a vascular network arising from a lateral descending branch of the sphenopalatine artery. The main supply to the inferior turbinate from this artery enters 1.0 to 1.5 cm from its posterior border and passes forward, giving off an anastomotic network of vessels. The artery also has anastomotic connections with the anterior blood supply of the turbinate. The anterior blood supply originates from the angular artery and is sufficient to allow the entire turbinate to be pedicled on this source.[5, 6] Murakami et al[7] used the inferior turbinate flap to line full-thickness defects of the ala and nasal tip as well as the middle vault. They also performed cadaver dissections and demonstrated an average flap surface area of 4.97 cm². The average length of the inferior turbinate flap is 2.8 cm, and the average width is 1.7 cm.

Middle and inferior turbinate flaps are harvested by a similar technique (Fig. 11–14). A local anesthetic solution containing a concentration of epinephrine of 1:100,000 is infiltrated along the turbinate, floor of the nose, and middle or inferior meatus, depending on which turbinate is used. The turbinate is medialized with a blunt elevator or the handle of a scalpel to open the meatus below the turbinate. A Cottle elevator or a 2-mm osteotome is placed in the meatus below the turbinate and pushed superiorly to perforate the bony attachment to the lateral nasal wall. Multiple perforations of the bone are made along the length of the turbinate, starting 1 cm posterior to the anterior end of the turbinate. The cutting instrument is maintained in a verticle plane against the lateral nasal wall to maximize the amount of tissue obtained without penetrating the paranasal sinuses. If a dorsal nasal defect allows direct visualization of the turbinate, the structure may more easily be incised from above with an osteotome or angled turbinectomy scissors. Pedicled anteriorly, the posterior aspect of the mobilized turbinate is pivoted toward the nasal defect using Takahaski forceps. The mucoperiosteum is dissected from the underlying concha bone and unfurled. The mucosa along the entire margin of the donor site is meticulously cauterized with

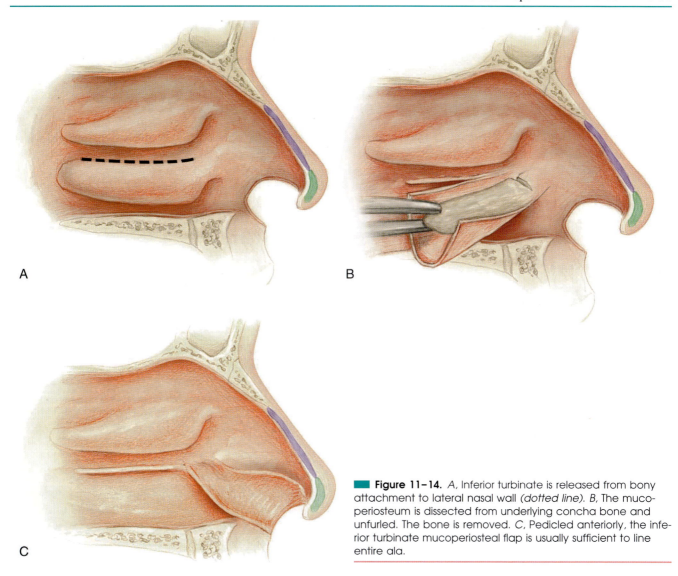

A

B

C

■ **Figure 11–14.** *A*, Inferior turbinate is released from bony attachment to lateral nasal wall *(dotted line)*. *B*, The mucoperiosteum is dissected from underlying concha bone and unfurled. The bone is removed. *C*, Pedicled anteriorly, the inferior turbinate mucoperiosteal flap is usually sufficient to line entire ala.

an extended insulated cautery. A nasal sinus endoscope may be useful for visualization during this step. It may also be prudent to pack the nose lightly for 2 or 3 days. The flap is transferred to the recipient site and sutured in position. If the location of the lining defect is the nasal tip, the pedicle of the flap will by necessity span the nasal passage and partially obstruct the airway. In this case, detachment of the pedicle is accomplished under local anesthesia 3 weeks later.

In cases of total or near total nasal reconstruction, the middle and inferior turbinates may be used in combination with a septal composite chondromucosal pivotal flap to help reline the nose. In these circumstances, bilateral turbinate flaps are delayed at the same time as the pivotal flap. Incisions to release the bony attachment of the turbinates are made, leaving the turbinates in situ, pedicled on their anterior mucosal attachment. The flaps are transferred to the recipient site 4 to 6 weeks later, and the concha bone is re-

moved. Bone is not removed until flap transfer occurs because of contraction of the mucosa, reducing the surface area of the flap. The inferior turbinate flap is usually of sufficient size to line the ala and lateral portions of the nasal dome. The length of the flap often precludes adequate tissue to line more medial aspects of the dome. The middle turbinate can provide sufficient tissue to line the roof of the middle vault or small (2.0 × 1.5 cm) lining defects of the nasal sidewall.

Postoperative Nasal Care

Patients may sniff if they feel the need to clear the nose, but they are instructed not to blow the nose for 1 week after surgery in which intranasal lining flaps have been transferred. Similarly, patients are advised to avoid strenuous activity for 1 week following any surgical procedure including flap detachment and not swim until at least 1 month after all nasal reconstruction is completed.

All of the septal and turbinate mucoperiosteal and mucoperichondrial flaps leave raw internal nasal surfaces. Septal perforations are by necessity the product of all septal composite chondromucosal pivotal flaps and many of the septal mucoperichondrial hinge flaps used to reline the nose. The resulting raw surfaces eventually heal, but crusting is a common sequelae until healing is complete. We have never observed a case of atrophic rhinitis or ozena secondary to the use of any of the intranasal flaps described in this book. Even in patients with perforation of the septum, crusting is not a common long-term complaint. This may be because the perforations created by the various intranasal flaps are very large and, as a consequence, there is less septal surface subjected to drying by nasal airflow. Crusting and discomfort may be minimized by maintaining a simple regimen of nasal hygiene during healing. The surgeon should periodically débride the nose of crust to relieve nasal obstruction during the first few weeks after surgery. In addition, we advise our patients to use saline nasal spray or drops at least once an hour while awake during the first week following detachment of intranasal flaps. Thereafter, saline spray is used five times a day until healing is complete. Saline provides moisture to the nasal cavity, especially during the winter months when the environment is dry. It also assists in flushing the nasal cavity of crust and bacteria, thereby assisting the natural mucociliary mechanism. Saline nasal sprays are available over the counter at most retail drug stores. Some preparations contain a preservative that may cause a slight stinging sensation. Most patients accommodate to this quickly and find that saline helps their nasal symptoms quite significantly. When repair involves unilateral mucoperichondrial flaps only, the corresponding nostril may be plugged with cotton or a dental roll covered by petroleum ointment for 1 week after flap detachment. The plug is changed three times a day, enhancing humidification of the nasal passage and promoting more rapid re-epithelialization of the denuded bone and cartilage.

The rare patient with persistent nasal crusting is advised to spray the nose four times a day with a solution of saline containing glycerin and encouraged to perform a nasal douche of saline once or twice a day. The same therapeutic principles for saline sprays apply to nasal saline irrigations. Irrigations are used when greater volumes of irrigant are required to débride crust and purulence. A bulb syringe, often used to clean the nasal cavities of infants, is used to apply the solution. A dental irrigator may be used in place of the bulb syringe. A volume of 8 to 16 oz of solution may be used in each nasal cavity two or three times a day. Bending over a sink during irrigation of the nose will minimize the amount of solution entering the throat. Only enough pressure is applied to mobilize the crust in the back of the nose so that it may be expelled through the mouth or the nose. Irrigation should not cause significant discomfort. A fresh solution of irrigant is prepared daily and consists of a quarter teaspoon of kosher salt mixed in 8 ounces of warm tapwater. A small amount of sodium bicarbonate (eighth of a teaspoon) may be added to reduce the burning sensation of saline.

Nasal steroid sprays are occasionally administered in the postoperative period to treat the general edema that occurs from nasal reconstruction. Systemic side effects of steroids can be eliminated with topical application of very small amounts of steroid sprays. The only side effects that occasionally occur are nasal dryness, crusting, and epistaxis. These may be prevented by using saline sprays frequently. However, if these problems become persistent, the patient should stop using steroid sprays. Nasal steroid sprays may be used long-term for patients with year-round allergies, polyps, or inflammation of the nasal cavity. If possible, it is advisable to stop steroid sprays for 1 month every 3 to 4 months to allow any dryness or crusting to resolve. This month is best taken during a month of minimal allergy problems. Antihistamines may be helpful during this period. Because steroid nasal sprays do not have an immediate onset of action, dosing should commence approximately 1 to 2 weeks before the patient's allergy season. Regular usage ensures adequate tissue concentration for effectiveness. Some patients are able to wean themselves down to a lower dose than initially prescribed while still maintaining adequate control of symptoms. For nasal steroid sprays, the method of administration is important. Orient the spray away from the nasal septum and toward the nasal sidewall. If the spray is applied primarily to the septum, it may result in dryness and crusting.

Decongestant nasal sprays, such as oxymetazoline and phenylephrine, are occasionally used during the first 3 to 5 days following nasal reconstruction in which intranasal mucosal flaps have been used for lining. These over-the-counter medications have vasoconstrictive properties that may be used to constrict mucous membranes and open the contralateral nasal passage. Postoperative bleeding from raw surfaces of the nasal cavity may also be controlled by topical application of such sprays. It is important to limit the use of spray as rebound hyperemia and dependency may develop rapidly. For the first 3 to 5 days following surgery, the patient is instructed to spray the nose once at bedtime only.

References

1. Fader DF, Baker SR, Johnson TM: The staged cheek-to-nose interpolated flap for reconstruction of the nasal alar rim/lobule. J Am Acad Dermatol 37:614, 1997.

2. Burget GC, Menick FJ: The marriage of beauty and blood supply. Plast Reconstr Surg 84:189, 1989.

3. Baker SR: Nasal lining flaps in contemporary reconstructive rhinoplasty. Facial Plast Surg 14:1, 1998.

4. Baker SR: Reconstruction of facial defects. In Krause CJ (ed): Otolaryngology Head and Neck Surgery, 3rd ed. Philadelphia, Mosby, 1998, p 527.

5. Burnham HH: An anatomical investigation of blood vessels of the lateral nasal wall and their relationship to turbinates and sinuses. Laryngol Otol 50:569, 1935.

6. Padgham N, Vaughan-Jones R: Cadaver studies of the anatomy of arterial supply to the inferior turbinates. Trans Soc Med 84:728, 1991.

7. Murakami CS, Kriet D, Ierokomos AP: Nasal reconstruction using the inferior turbinate mucosal flap. Arch Facial Plastic Surg 1:97, 1999.

12

Subcutaneous Hinge Cheek Flaps

Shan R. Baker

The nasal facial sulcus represents an important anatomic boundary between the aesthetic region of the nasal sidewall and the medial cheek. Inferiorly, the nasal facial sulcus is continuous with the alar facial sulcus, which represents the boundary between the ala, cheek, and upper lip. Skin defects that extend from the ala or sidewall across these boundaries are best resurfaced with separate skin flaps. The cheek and lip are repaired in most cases with cutaneous advancement flaps harvested within their respective aesthetic facial region. The nose is resurfaced with a separate flap or graft so that scars will ultimately be positioned in the nasal facial and/or alar facial sulcus.

Lateral nasal defects involving the ala and sidewall may be reconstructed by a number of surgical approaches. When alar defects extend to the cheek, the cheek component of the defect is commonly repaired with a cheek advancement flap, and the ala is usually repaired with an interpolated cheek flap. The latter flap may be used provided that the vascularity of the superiorly based flap is not compromised by significant loss of soft tissue in the deeper aspect of the medial cheek. Likewise, large lateral defects of the nasal sidewall that extend to the medial cheek are repaired preferably with a cheek advancement flap for the cheek component and a paramedian forehead flap to resurface the nasal sidewall. Lateral nasal defects are not reconstructed with transposition flaps from the cheek because they cause loss of the upper melolabial fold, producing marked asymmetry of the cheeks in the frontal view. In

addition, transposition cheek flaps used to repair the nose pass through the alar facial and/or nasal facial sulcus to reach their destination. This inevitably obliterates the concave topography of these aesthetic junctions between the cheek, lip, and nose. Subsequent revisional contouring procedures are frequently necessary and rarely achieve a completely symmetrical match with the contralateral side.

Although cheek and forehead interpolated flaps are the preferred covering flap for large skin defects of the lateral nose, there are occasions when the patient desires a one-stage, less complex reconstruction, even if the ultimate aesthetic result may be less than that using the preferred surgical approach. In this circumstance, if a cheek component of the defect exists, it is still most simply repaired with a cutaneous advancement flap, but the portion of the defect involving the nose presents more of a challenge. If the nasal defect is superficial, a full-thickness skin graft may be used, understanding that the aesthetic outcome may be compromised. However, full-thickness skin grafts used solely for repair of deep lateral nasal defects result in a noticeable contour deformity. In the case of deep alar defects, skin grafts do not lend any structural support, and their use may lead to collapse of the external nasal valve and compromise of the airway.

Another surgical approach may be appropriate for reconstruction of lateral nasal defects of limited size in patients who want to avoid an interpolated cheek or forehead flap. A hinge flap consisting of subcutaneous tissue and harvested from the cheek may be used to fill the depths of the nasal defect and is covered with a full-thickness skin graft.[1] The flap may also nourish an alar batten graft when required. This approach is useful only for defects of the ala or sidewall that are not full-thickness and that are immediately adjacent to or involve the nasal facial or alar facial sulcus. The technique has the advantage of a one-stage procedure that does not violate the melolabial fold. It avoids the need for an interpolated cheek or forehead flap, and it restores a natural contour to the repair, often achieving comparable aesthetic results. When the nasal defect extends to the cheek, the cheek component is repaired by advancement of cheek skin to the level of the cheek/nose junction. This places scars in the aesthetic junction and restores the sulcus between these structures. Thus, a relatively complex skin defect of the central face that involves two or three facial aesthetic regions may be repaired by dividing the defect into smaller components that are repaired independently in a single-stage procedure.

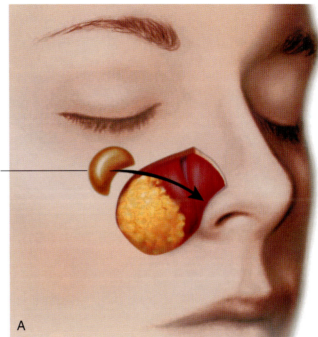

Auricular cartilage alar batten

A

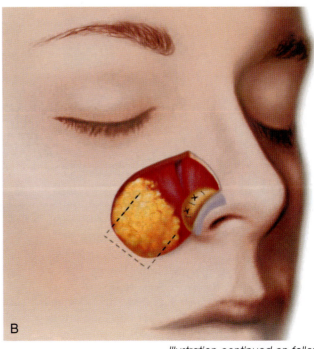

B

■ **Figure 12–1.** *A*, Skin and a soft-tissue defect of the lateral ala and sidewall, with extension to the medial cheek. An alar batten graft is placed along the margin of the nostril. *B*, The *dotted line* represents the incision made for a subcutaneous hinge cheek flap. The pedicle of the flap is based on soft tissue in the depths of the alar-facial and nasal-facial sulci. An auricular cartilage alar batten graft is secured to the vestibular skin with mattress sutures. It supports the nostril margin and prevents cephalic migration.

Illustration continued on following page

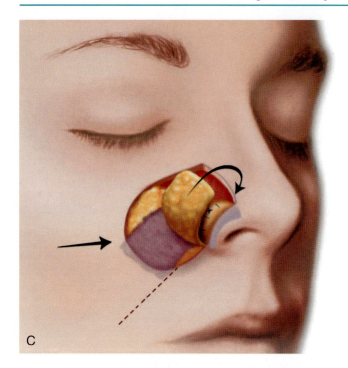

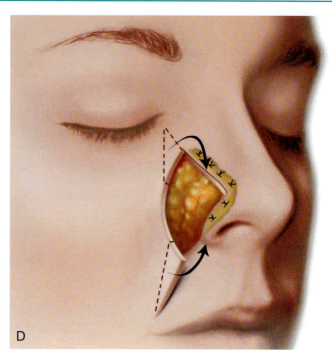

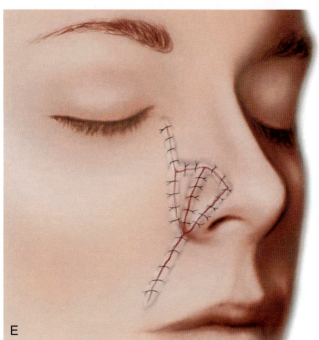

Figure 12–1 *Continued. C*, The hinge flap is turned medially to cover the cartilage graft and fill the soft-tissue void. The *dotted line* in the melolabial sulcus represents the incision necessary to enable medial movement of the cutaneous advancement flap to the level of the nasal-facial sulcus. *D*, The borders of the hinge flap are tucked beneath the nasal skin surrounding the defect. A cutaneous cheek advancement flap repairs the medial cheek defect and is secured into place at the nose-cheek junction. Standing cutaneous deformities are excised at the melolabial sulcus and the nasal-facial sulcus. *E*, Standing cutaneous deformities are used as full-thickness skin grafts to cover the exposed hinge flap.

The subcutaneous hinge cheek flap is based on a pedicle of soft tissue located in the depth of the alar facial and/or nasal facial sulcus. It is always used with a full-thickness skin graft to resurface the nasal defect. It may be used to repair small to medium (1–6/cm) deep lateral nasal defects that involve either or both the ala and nasal sidewall. The technique is best suited for repair of deep soft-tissue defects of the alar base and lower lateral nasal sidewall with extension to the cheek and where internal nasal lining is intact (Fig. 12–1). Skeletal support for the alar base is supplied by an auricular cartilage graft placed beneath the hinge flap (Fig. 12–2).

Although the subcutaneous hinge cheek flap combined with a full-thickness skin graft is useful in repairing skin and soft-tissue defects of the lateral nose, its use is restricted because the results do not consistently provide the best aesthetic outcome. Indications for this method of repair are the following:

1. Deep lateral defects of the ala 1.5 cm or smaller in size with an intact nasal lining.

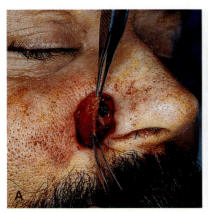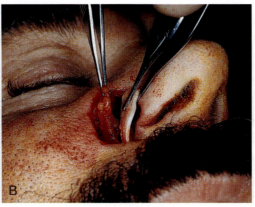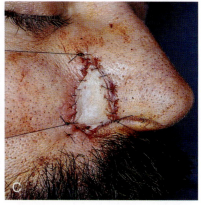

Figure 12–2. *A,* The skin and a soft-tissue defect of the lateral ala, lower sidewall, and medial cheek. A subcutaneous hinge cheek flap has been dissected and is held by forceps. *B,* The auricular cartilage graft is positioned in the alar base and covered by the hinge flap. *C,* The hinge flap is covered by a full-thickness skin graft.

Illustration continued on following page

2. Deep defects of the nasal sidewall with exposure of the nasal skeleton and loss of perichondrium or periosteum.

3. Deep soft-tissue defects of the alar facial or nasal facial sulcus that have limited involvement of ala or nasal sidewall skin. These defects are primarily a tissue volume problem that requires a small area of skin resurfacing but demanding considerable soft-tissue replacement in order to restore proper contour to the area of reconstruction.

4. Patients who are not willing to undergo a multi-staged reconstruction or who will not accept the donor site scar resulting from an interpolated cheek or forehead flap.

Lateral Alar Defect

A template duplicating the configuration of the alar defect is designed with the alar facial sulcus representing the lateral border of the template. If the alar defect is round, it is converted to one with square corners to reduce trapdoor deformity. If the defect involves more than half of the surface area of the ala, the remaining skin of the ala is included in the defect when fashioning the template, and this skin is removed before transferring the flap. The template is placed over the subcutaneous tissues of the medial cheek exposed by the cheek defect. It is oriented so that the portion of the template representing the base of the ala is positioned at the junction of the cheek and nose. The template helps the surgeon estimate the surface area of soft tissue necessary to fill the tissue void and reach the periphery of the nasal defect. The template is oversized in all dimensions by 2 to 3 mm to ensure that the flap is of sufficient size to allow tucking of the edges of the

flap beneath the nasal skin surrounding the defect. It is better to make the flap too large and trim the excess if necessary than to stretch the flap in order for it to reach the distal borders of the defect. When there is an isolated nasal defect that does not extend to the alar facial sulcus, the remaining lateral nasal and adjacent medial cheek skin is elevated in the subcutaneous plane sufficiently to allow placement of the template beneath the skin for designing the hinge flap (Fig. 12–3). In this case, it may be helpful to make a small incision in the nasal alar sulcus to enhance the surgical exposure for developing the hinge flap. The cheek skin is elevated in the superficial subcutaneous plane sufficiently away from the deeper soft tissue to enable the surgeon to incise and dissect the hinge flap in a retrograde direction toward the nose. The pedicle of the hinge flap should extend the full length of the vertical height of the alar defect.

The flap is incised, and a peninsula of soft tissue is elevated from a lateral to a medial direction. The flap consists primarily of fat and occasionally some muscle, depending on the quantity of tissue required to fill the alar soft-tissue deficit. A greater amount of tissue is required if there is loss of soft tissue in the area of the alar facial sulcus. Consideration is given to the thickness of the skin graft and cartilage batten graft that will contribute to the total dimensions of the repair. Generally, a hinge flap used for alar repair is 3 to 4 mm in thickness. The flap is dissected with a scalpel or scissors in such a manner that the base is situated in the alar facial sulcus. Adequate thickness is maintained at the base of the flap to ensure a vascular supply. The thickness of the base typically ranges from 4 to 6 mm, depending on the overall quantity and vascularity of the tissues. It is better to construct the flap too thick and then trim it as necessary than make the flap too thin.

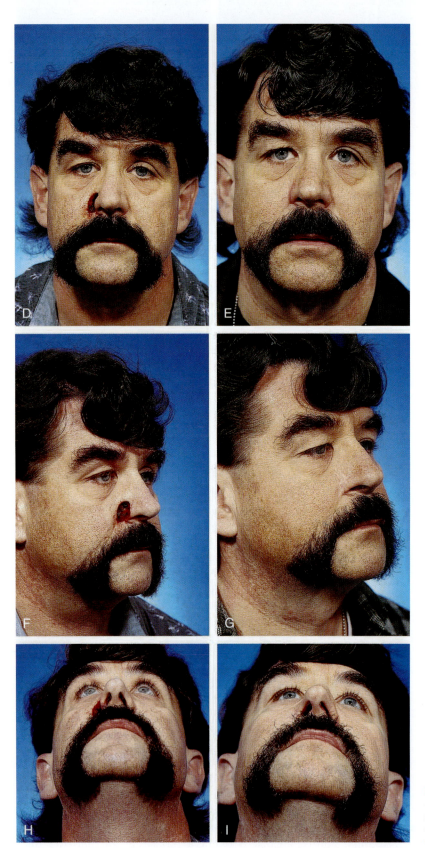

Figure 12–2 *Continued. D–I,* Preoperative and 4-month postoperative views of the reconstruction. The skin graft was dermabraded 6 weeks after reconstruction.

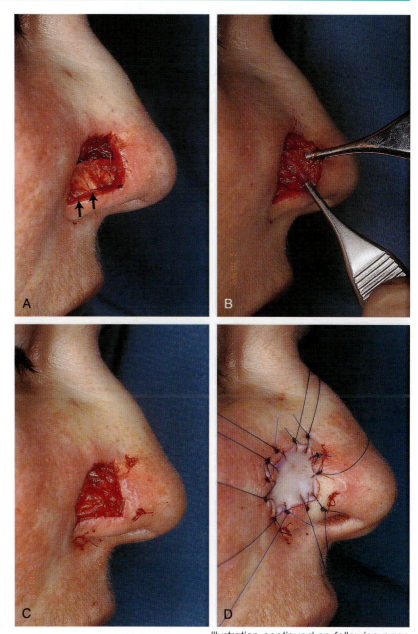

Figure 12–3. *A*, A defect isolated to the ala has been modified to create square corners. An auricular cartilage alar batten graft is in place (*arrows*). *B*, A subcutaneous hinge cheek flap held by forceps is tunneled from beneath the cheek skin to the alar defect. *C*, The hinge flap covers the cartilage graft and is tucked beneath the borders of the skin defect. The flap is secured with two mattress sutures passed through the nasal skin. *D*, The exposed hinge flap is covered with a full-thickness skin graft.

Illustration continued on following page

The margins of the alar defect are freshened, and square corners are created if not present, or the remaining skin of the aesthetic unit is excised if warranted. The nasal skin around the periphery of the defect is widely undermined in the subfascial plane. An auricular cartilage alar batten graft is sculptured and placed along the caudal border of the nostril margin. The cartilage graft should extend from the alar base to a point 0.5 cm anterior to the most anterior border of the skin defect. A few horizontal mattress sutures of 5-0 polydioxanone are used to secure the batten to the underlying vestibular skin.

Following hemostasis, the hinge flap is transferred to the nasal defect by turning it over on itself in a hinge motion, like turning a page in a book. If the defect does not encompass the alar facial sulcus, the flap is tunneled under the cheek skin and delivered to the nasal defect. The flap is layered over the cartilage graft, and the borders of the flap are tucked under the nasal skin around the periphery of the skin defect. The tucked borders are secured in place with horizontal mattress 5-0 polydioxanone sutures that pass from nasal skin through the border of the flap and back again through skin. The knot is tied lightly over the nasal skin adjacent to the defect. This method of securing the flap eliminates the need for quilting sutures between the hinge flap and the deeper tissues of the ala. Such sutures may impair vascularity and the successful revascularization of skin grafts placed on the surface of the flap. It also maintains the free edge of the defect to

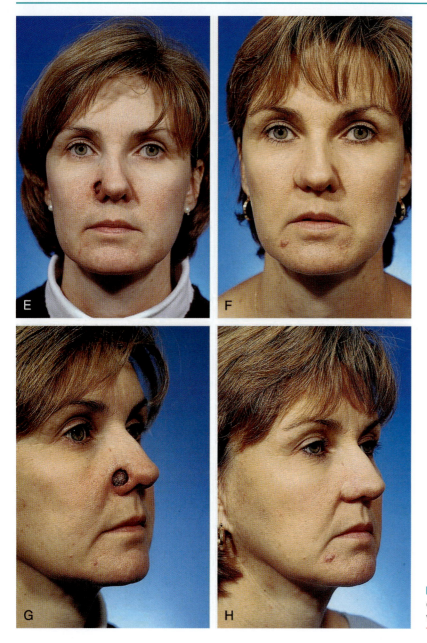

■ **Figure 12–3** *Continued. E–H,* Preoperative and 3-month postoperative views. The skin graft was dermabraded 6 weeks after reconstruction.

which a skin graft is sutured. A full-thickness skin graft is thinned to the level of the dermis and placed over the exposed surface of the flap, covering the defect. The graft is sutured to the nasal skin along the borders of the defect with a continuous 5-0 fast-absorbing plain gut suture. A bolster dressing consisting of 5-0 polypropylene tied-over layered Telfa is used to compress the skin graft lightly against the underlying hinge flap. The dressing is removed in 3 to 5 days.

If the alar defect encompasses the alar facial sulcus, the skin of the adjacent cheek is advanced medially to the level of the sulcus after dissecting and transferring the hinge flap. The advanced cheek skin is secured in place using two or three 4-0 polydioxanone sutures that pass from the leading edge of the advanced skin to the periosteum at the piriform aperture. These sutures must

not pass through the pedicle of the hinge flap. They prevent the cheek skin from migrating laterally during wound healing. Larger medial cheek defects require a cheek advancement flap, which is developed by making an incision along the melolabial sulcus and undermining the entire medial cheek skin for several centimeters. In this case, greater advancement of cheek skin is necessary, and standing cutaneous deformities develop adjacent to the base of the nose and in the superior aspect of the nasal facial sulcus. These are excised in the area of the melolabial sulcus and along the cheek/nose junction (see Fig. 12–1). If sufficiently large, one or both of the standing cutaneous deformities may be used as the source for the full-thickness skin graft used to cover the alar defect. Another preferred source for skin grafts is from the preauricular area. Skin in the preauricular region usually has color and thickness similar to that of the skin of the nasal sidewall, although it matches less well with the alar skin. Skin grafts and the adjacent nasal skin are dermabraded 6 to 8 weeks following reconstruction. This is accomplished in the office and usually aids in blending the color and skin texture of the graft with the nasal skin (Fig. 12–4).

Nasal Sidewall Defect

The subcutaneous hinge cheek flap is used most commonly to repair small but deep lateral skin defects of the ala with or without extension to the alar facial sulcus. The flap may also be used to replace soft-tissue loss in the lower lateral nasal sidewall and in the nasal facial sulcus between the sidewall and the cheek. The technical aspects of developing a hinge flap in this area are similar to those for repair of alar defects. Only minimal subcutaneous fat and muscle naturally occur beneath the skin of the nasal sidewall, so the flap used to fill the soft-tissue void in this area is by necessity thin. There is a greater amount of subcutaneous fat and muscle in the caudal aspect of the nasal sidewall, and deeper nasal defects are observed here. Accordingly, the quantity of tissue included in the flap is adjusted to properly replace the soft-tissue deficit. Lateral defects of the nasal sidewall with loss of perichondrium or periosteum may be resurfaced with a thin subcutaneous

hinge flap from the cheek to cover the exposed cartilage or bone, followed by a full-thickness skin graft.

The most common situation where the subcutaneous hinge cheek flap is used for repair of the nasal sidewall is when the nasal defect extends beyond the nasal facial sulcus to the cheek with loss of some of the abundant subcutaneous soft tissue located immediately lateral to the nose. Fat in the form of a hinge flap is harvested from the exposed soft tissue within the cheek defect, elevating it in such a way that the pedicle of the flap is turned toward and deposited in the depths of the nasal facial sulcus. The flap serves to fill the soft-tissue void at the junction between the cheek and nose while replacing missing subcutaneous tissue of the nasal sidewall. A full-thickness skin graft is used to cover the nasal component of the defect, and a cutaneous cheek advancement flap is used to repair the cheek component of the defect. The cheek advancement flap is designed to convey sufficient subcutaneous tissue to fill the donor site of the hinge flap. This fat is recruited from an area lateral to the cheek defect. Leaving subcutaneous fat attached to the undersurface of the cheek advancement flap may also assist the hinge flap in filling a particularly extensive soft-tissue loss along the nasal facial sulcus. Advancement of the leading edge of the cutaneous cheek flap is limited to the nasal facial sulcus. Several sutures of 4-0 polydioxanone are placed between the deep aspect of the leading edge of the advancement flap and the periosteum along the nasal facial sulcus. This prevents lateral migration of the flap during the healing process. Care is taken to avoid placing these sutures through the hinge flap. The two stand-

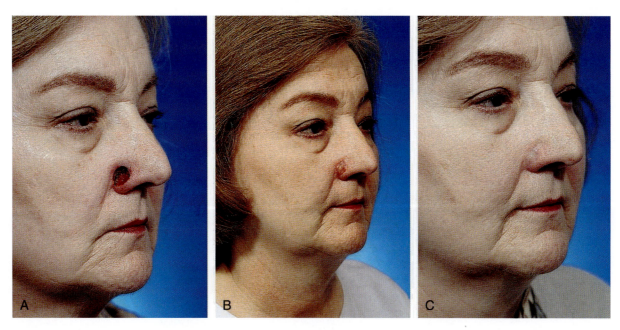

■ **Figure 12–4.** *A,* Skin and a soft-tissue defect of the ala. *B,* View taken 6 weeks after repair with an auricular cartilage alar batten graft, a subcutaneous hinge cheek flap, and a full-thickness skin graft. The skin graft is hyperpigmented. *C,* View taken 8 months after dermabrasion of the skin graft and the adjacent nasal skin. The postinflammatory hyperpigmentation has resolved.

ing cutaneous deformities that result from advancement of the cheek skin are excised, one superiorly along the junction of the lateral nose and cheek and one inferiorly in the alar facial sulcus. The excised skin may be used as full-thickness skin grafts to cover the lateral nasal sidewall defect, provided they are of sufficient size. The cutaneous cheek advancement flap is repaired with a standard two-layer wound closure.

Combined Ala and Sidewall Defect

There are occasions when the surgeon may be confronted with deep lateral nasal defects that involve portions of both the ala and nasal sidewall with or without concomitant extension to the medial cheek (see Fig. 12–1). Lateral nasal defects having a vertical height up to 6 to 7 cm may be repaired by replacing the soft-tissue deficit with a subcutaneous hinge cheek flap and resurfacing the entire nasal area with a full-thickness skin graft. If the nasal defect encroaches on the alar margin (within 5 mm), an alar batten graft is required to support the ala and prevent cephalic migration of the nostril margin during wound healing.

Complications

The subcutaneous hinge flap is not frequently associated with complications. Partial or complete failure of skin graft survival is treated by allowing the wound to heal by secondary intention. Disharmony of skin texture and color match between the graft and the nose may occur. This is particularly true when grafts are obtained from areas other than the medial cheek or when the skin of the nose is thick and unusually sebaceous. Postoperative dermabrasion of the graft and adjacent nasal skin are very effective in reducing this disharmony.

The most common complication with use of this method of nasal repair is mild distortion of the alar facial sulcus. This results from transferring the flap beneath the sulcus. The bulk of the flap's pedicle causes slight fullness in the depths of the sulcus. On occasion, it is necessary to perform a second operation in which subcutaneous tissue is removed from beneath the sulcus. This minor procedure restores the alar facial sulcus to a natural contour.

Reference

1. Johnson TM, Baker SR, Brown MD, et al: Utility of the subcutaneous hinge flap in nasal reconstruction. Dermatol Surg 30:459, 1994.

13

Interpolated Cheek Flaps: Reconstruction of the Alar and Columellar Units

Shan R. Baker

Burget[1] outlined seven principles unique to aesthetic reconstruction of the face. These principles also apply to reconstruction of the nose. Whether repairing a defect of the face or nose, the goal is normal contour. The missing part is restored in its three-dimensional form, replacing each missing layer with like tissue. Templates are used to design grafts and flaps. Scars are camouflaged by placing them along the junction of aesthetic regions or units whenever possible. Entire aesthetic units are resurfaced when practical. In the case of the nose, cartilage grafts are used to create contour, prevent collapse, and resist the forces of wound contraction. Refinement of the repair is accomplished by a contouring procedure consisting of subcutaneous sculpturing. All these reconstructive principles are important, particularly when surgically restoring defects of the ala.

Reconstruction of the Ala

Most nasal cutaneous malignancies occur on the caudal third of the nose. Commonly, following Mohs' surgery, the surgeon is asked to reconstruct the ala. Small skin defects of the tip, dorsum, or sidewall may be left to heal by secondary intention. Although this may at times create an unsightly scar, it rarely results in functional impairment. In contrast, even very small defects (1 cm) of the ala left to heal by secondary intention cause notching of the nostril and may cause partial collapse of the external nasal valve, especially on inspiration. For this reason, essentially all cutaneous defects of the ala require reconstruction.

Cheek (melolabial) flaps are the preferred method of resurfacing most alar defects. Three types of flap design have been used for this purpose. These are transposition, interpolated, and island-pedicled. The transposition flap is popular because of its ease of design and transfer. A transposition flap has a cutaneous pedicle that is developed immediately adjacent to the skin defect. The flap is pivoted toward the defect, and a standing cutaneous deformity develops at the base of the pedicle.

An interpolated flap may have a cutaneous or subcutaneous tissue pedicle. Flaps based on subcutaneous tissue do not develop a standing cutaneous deformity. In contrast to the transposition flap, the base of an interpolated flap is designed at some distance from the defect. The flap is pivoted toward the defect, and the pedicle crosses over or under the intervening skin between pedicle and defect. A second operation is necessary to detach the pedicle and inset the flap. The paramedian forehead flap used for nasal reconstruction is typically designed as an interpolated flap. The pedicle extends from the forehead to the nose, passing over the glabellar skin.

An island cutaneous flap is designed as an island of skin completely isolated on a subcutaneous tissue pedicle. The flap is pivoted toward the defect, and the pedicle remains beneath the cheek skin. In contrast to the interpolated cheek flap, the island flap does not require pedicle detachment. The island flap is the least common form of melolabial flap used for nasal reconstruction.

The melolabial transposition flap has been frequently used for reconstruction of the ala and nasal sidewall. It has the advantage of maintaining a lymphatic drainage route through the pedicle of the flap, which remains in continuity with cheek skin. It also avoids a circumferential scar, which in part accounts for trapdoor deformity. Why not use a transposition instead of an interpolated cutaneous cheek flap for ala repair? Both flaps have the advantage of using skin with color, texture, and sebaceous qualities similar to those of the natural skin of the ala. Both flaps leave an acceptable donor scar in the depth of the melolabial sulcus. The biggest reason for not using a melolabial transposition flap is that it deforms the alar facial sulcus and lateral portion of the alar groove. A portion of the flap by necessity must pass through the superior aspect of the alar facial sulcus, which represents an important topographic junction between the facial aesthetic regions of the nose, cheek, and upper lip. Whenever possible, local flaps should be designed so they do not cross borders that separate aesthetic regions. This is especially true if the border has a concave topography like that of the alar facial sulcus.[2] Too often, this sulcus has been violated by transposition flaps harvested from the cheek to reconstruct lower lateral nasal defects. The flap passes through the sulcus, obliterating the valley between the ala and cheek. When this happens, it is extremely difficult to restore the valley to a completely natural contour. For this reason, an interpolated melolabial flap is recommended for reconstructing the ala. The pedicle of the flap crosses over, not through, the alar facial sulcus. The pedicle may consist of skin and subcutaneous fat or subcutaneous fat only and is detached from the cheek 3 weeks after the initial transfer to the nose. Although 3 weeks is a lengthy period for the patient to endure the deformity caused by the flap, this interval enables the surgeon to thin and sculpture the subcutaneous tissues of the distal flap at the time of flap transfer and the proximal portion of the flap at the time of pedicle detachment and flap inset. On detachment of the flap, the patient is left with a completely natural alar facial sulcus because no incision or dissection has been performed in this region. We recommend the choice of an interpolated design when a pivotal cheek flap is planned for reconstruction of a defect of the ala and the defect does not extend laterally to the alar facial sulcus.[3]

Burget and Menick[4] have shown that an interpolated melolabial flap is ideal for reconstructing the ala. They believe that the skin of the melolabial fold when transferred as a cutaneous flap to resurface the entire ala tends to contract so that the scar pulls the subcutaneous cheek fat into a hemicylindrical shape closely simulating the contour of the natural ala. If used to resurface only a portion of the ala, there is a propensity for the flap to contract into a spherical contour, causing the flap to stand up above the surface of the residual ala, distorting the natural contour. These surgeons have also shown that even when the entire alar aesthetic unit is resurfaced with an interpolated cheek flap, the flap will contract into a spherical rather than a hemicylindrical configuration if a cartilaginous alar batten graft is not used to support the ala. This occurs presumably because of unrestricted wound contraction. Interpolated cheek flaps require detachment of the flap's pedicle from the cheek, which results in a circumferential scar surrounding the entire flap. The circumferential scar, in turn, creates a mild trapdoor deformity as it contracts, but this deformity is limited by the cartilaginous alar batten. Scar contraction is counterbalanced by the support of the alar batten, resulting ultimately in the flap assuming a hemicylindrical configuration as healing progresses.

The nasal alar unit is highly contoured, has a free margin, and functions as the external nasal valve. When reconstructing the ala, consistent results require a cartilage subsurface framework to resist the forces of contraction, provide a stable external valve, and serve as a scaffold for contour. The framework in the form of a cartilage graft must be utilized at the time of the initial reconstructive procedure and requires vascularized tissue superficial and deep to the graft, totally enveloping the cartilage. Adequate function of the nose requires a thin internal layer most appropriately supplied by vascularized mucosa.[5] The external covering flap is provided by an interpolated cheek or forehead flap.

Technique: Interpolated Subcutaneous Pedicled Cheek Flap

Chapters 4 and 11 discuss the methods of providing lining for full-thickness defects of the ala. A brief description is included here to provide a more comprehensive overview of alar reconstruction using a cutaneous cheek flap.

For full-thickness defects limited solely to the ala, a bipedicle vestibular skin advancement flap may be used for lining (Figs. 13–1 and 13–2). This flap is created by making an extended intercartilaginous incision

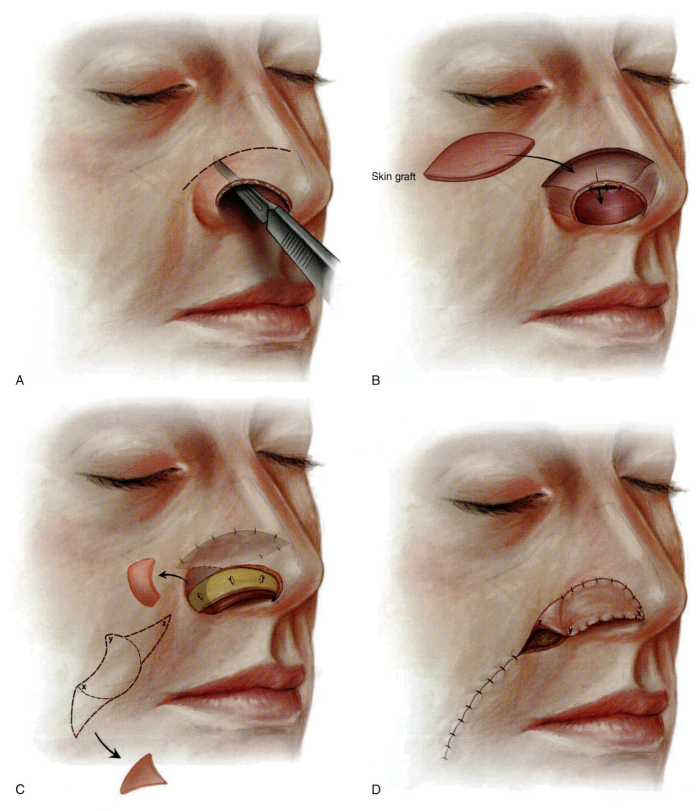

Figure 13-1. *A,* Bipedicle vestibular skin advancement flap may be used to line full-thickness alar or unilateral tip defects that have a vertical dimension of 1 cm or less. An extended intercartilaginous incision between lateral crus and caudal aspect of upper lateral cartilage is made *(dotted line). B,* Remaining vestibular skin is mobilized caudally in the form of a bipedicle advancement flap. Flap donor site is repaired with thin full-thickness skin graft. *C,* Auricular cartilage alar batten graft provides framework for nostril margin. Graft is secured to vestibular skin flap with mattress sutures. Remaining skin of alar base may be discarded. Interpolated cheek flap is designed *(dotted line). D,* Interpolated flap based on subcutaneous tissue pedicle is turned toward midline as covering flap. Note orientation of flap relative to flap design. Cheek donor site is closed primarily following removal of standing cutaneous deformity inferiorly.

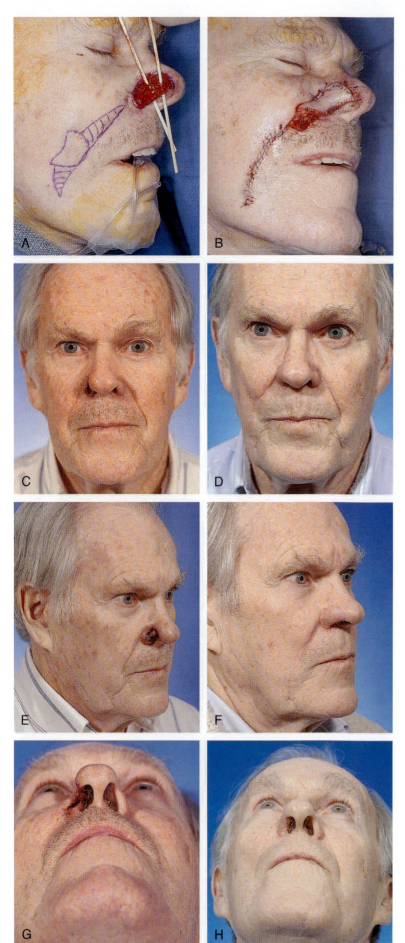

Figure 13–2. *A,* Cottontip applicators are beneath bipedicle vestibular skin advancement flap used to line full-thickness alar defect. Interpolated subcutaneous pedicled cheek flap is designed for external cover. *B,* Cheek flap is used to cover auricular cartilage alar batten graft and resurface skin defect. *C–H,* Preoperative and 3 months following reconstruction.

from the nasal dome to the lateral floor of the vestibule. For a larger flap, the incision is made more cephalad. The skin is then elevated and mobilized inferiorly, suturing the inferior edge of the advancement flap to the caudal border of the covering flap if the defect extends through the alar margin. The superior edge is sutured to soft tissue at the superior aspect of the lining defect. The skin void remaining superior to the bipedicle advancement flap is then repaired with a full-thickness skin graft.[2] This is supplied by excising the standing cutaneous deformity that occurs during primary closure of the interpolated cheek flap donor site. The bipedicle vestibular skin advancement flap yields a limited amount of lining and should not be used for defects larger than the alar unit.

For larger full-thickness defects of the ala, a septal mucoperichondrial hinge flap is used for lining. This flap is based on the septal branch of the superior labial artery, which enters the nose at the level of the nasal spine. If required, most of the mucoperichondrium on one side of the septum may be used for reconstruction. The typical boundaries of the dissection are limited superiorly to 1 cm from the dorsum of the nose, inferiorly to the nasal crest, and as far posteriorly as necessary (usually to the posterior third of the bony septum). The anterior extent of the dissection is 1 cm from the caudal edge of the septum. The flap is created by making the superior and inferior incisions with a sickle-shaped knife or a scalpel on an extended handle and the posterior incision with an angled blade. The flap is then mobilized from anterior to posterior with a Woodson elevator. The flap is reflected laterally toward the defect so the mucoperichondrium faces externally and the mucosa internally. The most distal border of the flap becomes the inferior free margin of the reconstructed ala. Care is taken when harvesting the lining flap. If the distal portion does not survive, the overlying cartilage framework will be exposed, resulting in necrosis and subsequent development of an alar notch. Once the mucoperichondrial flap is elevated, the exposed septal cartilage is removed and used to reconstruct the framework for the ala or missing sidewall. The flap is sutured to the edges of the lining defect; the distal free margin of the lining flap is eventually sutured to the covering flap if the defect extends through the alar margin. When lining is restored to the ala, a cartilage graft is placed over the lining flap to serve as framework for the new ala.

Although septal cartilage may be used as an alar batten, auricular cartilage harvested from the conchal bowl has a configuration that closely resembles the contour of the ala. Cartilage is generally harvested from the contralateral ear through a postauricular incision. Concha cymba and concha cavum are harvested as a single piece, preserving the anterior base of the helix. The incision is closed with 5-0 plain gut using a continuous suture. A bolster consisting of two dental rolls,

one placed postauricular straddling the incision and a second in the corresponding position in the conchal bowl, helps compress the medial and lateral auricular skin in the area of the cartilage void. Three 4-0 polypropylene sutures placed through both medial and lateral auricular skin on either side of the rolls are used to secure them in place. The auricular bolster dressing is tied loosely to minimize donor site pain and accommodate postoperative swelling. The bolster is removed on the first postoperative day. The auricular cutaneous sutures are left to absorb spontaneously.

The cartilage graft is carved to create the appropriate shape, thinned to a thickness of 1.5 mm, scored occasionally to increase its convexity, and sutured in place. The graft typically measures 1.5 cm in width by 3.0 cm in length. The graft is usually of sufficient width to extend 0.5 cm cephalad to the alar groove. This width enables the surgeon to leave a small segment of cartilage above the groove following restoration of the groove at a subsequent contouring procedure. To secure the graft, a small pocket is developed in the soft tissue at the alar base by dissecting medial to the piriform aperture, similar to the placement of an alar batten in aesthetic rhinoplasty. This pocket keeps the cartilage from prolapsing into the airway and prevents lateral migration of the end of the graft. To fix the graft in place, a horizontal mattress 5-0 polydioxanone suture is passed from the nasal vestibule through the lateral end of the cartilage positioned in the tissue pocket. The suture is passed back through the vestibular skin and tied. The cartilage is held in a convex position while it is sutured to the underlying vestibular skin or lining flap. The medial end of the cartilage graft is trimmed to fit snugly in the nasal facet and is sutured to the caudal edge of the lateral crus with 5-0 polydioxanone sutures placed in a figure-of-eight fashion. This prevents the cartilage graft from telescoping over the lateral crus. After the cartilage is secured in place, a skin flap is transposed to cover the cartilage graft and resurface the entire ala.

The porous and sebaceous nature of medial cheek skin closely resembles that of the lower third of the nose, so an interpolated cheek flap is generally the preferred covering flap for alar reconstruction. The flap is based superiorly on the rich vascular supply as described by Herbert[6] in the region of the alar facial sulcus. In this location, perforating branches from the angular artery penetrate the levator labii muscle. Other perforating vessels on both borders of the midportion of the zygomatic major muscle assist in supplying the cheek skin adjacent to the ala. The flap may be designed as a peninsular flap based superiorly on a cutaneous pedicle or as an island based on a subcutaneous tissue pedicle. In most circumstances, we prefer to design the flap as a crescentric-shaped island of skin based on a subcutaneous tissue pedicle. The superior extent of the island remains 5 mm below the alar facial sulcus, preserving this important aesthetic area[2] (see Fig. 13-2).

An exact template of the alar unit is made from the contralateral normal side with a malleable material such as foil or a thin sheet of foam rubber. The template is reversed to design the interpolated cheek flap. When the defect extends beyond the confines of the ala, a template is designed slightly smaller than the defect to accommodate the phenomenon of distraction of the wound margins, which creates an open wound that is larger than the surface area of the skin removed. If excision of additional skin is indicated in order to resurface an adjacent aesthetic unit, the template is fashioned before the remaining skin is removed because of this same phenomenon.

When reconstructing the ala, the entire ala is resurfaced with the cheek flap, except for 1 mm of alar skin just anterior to the alar facial sulcus. This small skin tag preserves the alar facial sulcus and often provides a better scar than when the flap extends to the sulcus. This approach is similar to the method recommended by Sheen and Sheen[7] for performing a type II Weir excision to reduce the size of the nasal base. Maintaining the excision outside of the alar facial sulcus lessens the risk of developing a depressed scar. This approach also avoids the technically challenging requirements of intregrating the flap into the nasal sill at the time of flap inset. When using cheek flaps for repair, we often delay excising the extreme lateral portions of the residual alar skin until the time of pedicle detachment and flap inset. This delay reduces the wound tension on the flap at the time of initial transfer.

The fashioned template is placed on the melolabial fold so that the center of the flap is positioned slightly above the horizontal plane of the lateral oral commissure. The template is positioned over the melolabial fold so that the medial border of the designed flap lies in the melolabial sulcus. This arrangement ensures that the flap is harvested from the cheek, not the lip, and that donor site wound closure will lie within the melolabial sulcus, providing maximum scar camouflage. Patients who do not demonstrate a melolabial sulcus at rest are asked to grimace so that the sulcus may be precisely marked before the patient is sedated or the site is injected. The flap is designed to pivot 90 degrees toward the midline in a clockwise direction when harvested from the left cheek and counterclockwise when harvested from the right cheek. Thus, the template is positioned to design the flap with a specific orientation. As the flap is pivoted and transferred to the recipient site, the in situ medial border of the flap is sutured to the cephalic border of the defect. This in turn causes the in situ inferior border of the flap to join the anterior border of the defect. The lateral border of the in situ flap becomes the inferior border of the reconstructed ala (see Fig. 13-1).

A tracing is made around the template. A triangle of skin is marked superior and inferior to the tracing in order to fashion a crescentric-shaped island of skin. The two triangles extending from the template tracing represent standing cutaneous deformities that will form when the cheek wound is closed. The lower triangle of skin is excised at the time of flap transfer, and the upper triangle is transferred with the skin of the flap and is discarded at the time of pedicle detachment and inset of the flap. The superior triangle of skin is minimized to reduce loss of tissue from the upper melolabial fold where the fold is well developed. Removing skin from the upper portion of the fold may result in considerable asymmetry of the medial cheeks.

The flap is incised, and the distal portion is elevated in the subcutaneous plane. The distal third of the flap is thin, leaving 1 to 2 mm of subcutaneous fat attached to the undersurface. As the dissection proceeds superiorly, the plane extends deeper to facilitate development of the subcutaneous tissue pedicle. The pedicle of fat is freed from the surrounding cheek fat by incising through the borders of the pedicle perpendicular to the surface of the skin (Fig. 13-3). The depth of the incision is carried to the level of the superficial surface of the zygomatic major and levator labii muscles. On reaching the zygomatic major muscle, blunt dissection continues upward on the surface of the muscle, releasing the attachments of the pedicle to deeper structures until the flap can reach the recipient site without undue tension. To aid in reducing tension, it is sometimes helpful to place a 4-0 polypropylene suture between the superior skin edge of the donor incision and the alar base. This has the effect of pulling the pedicle upward toward the ala without the need to place additional traction on the subcutaneous tissue pedicle. The suture is released when the pedicle is divided at the time of flap detachment.

When the alar defect extends to the alar facial sulcus and medial cheek, a cutaneous cheek advancement flap is necessary to repair the cheek component of the defect. The cheek advancement flap is dissected, first exposing the underlying subcutaneous tissues of the cheek. In this circumstance, an island cutaneous flap based on a subcutaneous tissue pedicle is frequently used as covering for the ala. The island flap is dissected, and the pedicle is delivered to the nose beneath the cheek advancement flap. The island flap does not require detachment; however, the pedicle usually causes excessive fullness adjacent to the ala. Thus, a procedure to contour the region is often necessary and is performed 2 to 3 months following flap transfer (Fig. 13-4).

To close the donor wound following transfer of an interpolated cheek flap, the skin adjacent to the incision is undermined peripherally for a distance 2 cm in the superficial subcutaneous plane, and the standing cutaneous deformity that develops inferiorly from the advancement of wound margins is removed. Depending

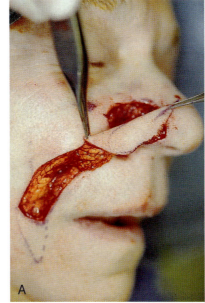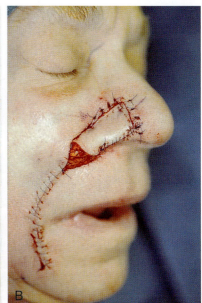

■ **Figure 13-3.** *A,* Subcutaneous tissue pedicle of interpolated flap maintains deep attachment but is freed from adjacent cheek fat. Pedicle is 1.5 to 2.0 cm thick. *B,* Flap is turned toward midline and sutured to recipient site with vertical cutaneous mattress sutures. Subcuticular sutures are not used.

on the shape of the flap, the lateral border of the donor site may be considerably longer than the medial border. If this is the situation, it may be necessary to excise an additional standing cutaneous deformity (Burow's triangle) at right angles to the melolabial closure. This is accomplished at the inferior pole of the wound. The donor wound is repaired with 5-0 subcuticular sutures and a continuous simple 5-0 cutaneous suture. The cheek flap is turned toward the midline and sutured to the nasal skin with 5-0 polypropylene using interrupted vertical cutaneous mattress sutures. A more precise epidermal approximation between the margins of the flap and the adjacent nasal skin is achieved using a continuous 5-0 or 6-0 cutaneous suture. Subcuticular sutures

are not used. The inferior border of the flap is sutured to the vestibular skin or lining flap with a continuous 5-0 suture. If a bipedicle vestibular skin advancement flap has been developed to restore a lining deficit, the standing cutaneous deformity removed from the cheek is defatted to the level of the dermis and used as a full-thickness skin graft to resurface the donor site of the bipedicle flap (see Fig. 13–1). A few interrupted 4-0 chromic sutures are used to secure the graft in place. The graft does not require stenting. A compression dressing is applied to the cheek, positioning it below the pedicle of the flap. This dressing is removed the next day.

Cheek flaps are detached 3 weeks following transfer.

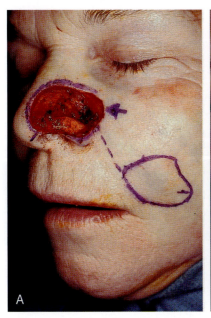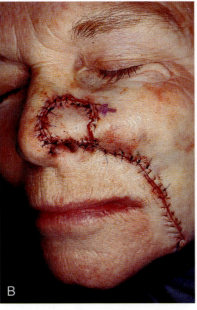

■ **Figure 13-4.** *A,* Skin and soft-tissue defect of ala and nasal sidewall with small extension to cheek. Auricular cartilage alar batten graft is positioned along nostril margin. Subcutaneous pedicled island cheek flap is designed to resurface nasal defect. Diagonal line at corner of flap and defect assist with orientation following release of flap from lower cheek. Cutaneous cheek advancement flap *(dotted line)* is designed for concomitant repair of cheek defect. *B,* Island flap is delivered to nose by transferring its subcutaneous pedicle beneath cheek advancement flap.

Illustration continued on following page

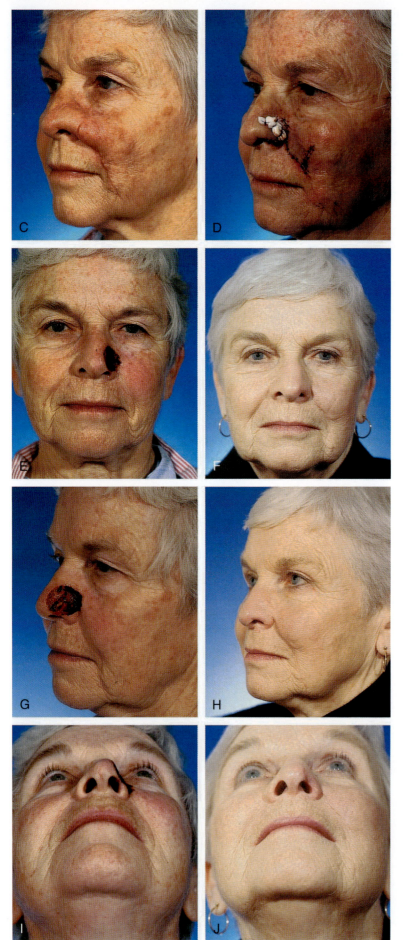

■ **Figure 13–4** *Continued. C,* 1 month following flap transfer. Pedicle of island flap created fullness in area of alar facial sulcus. *D,* Immediately after contouring procedure to restore natural topography to medial cheek and lateral nose. *E–J,* Preoperative and 1 year postoperative. No additional surgical procedures were necessary.

For subcutaneous tissue pedicled flaps, the pedicle is transected at the base, and the cheek skin is undermined for a distance of 2 cm around the periphery of the wound. After freshening the skin margins with a scalpel, the wound is closed by advancing the borders together. As this is accomplished, it is usually necessary to open the superior end of the donor site scar to facilitate excision of redundant subcutaneous tissue and a small standing cutaneous deformity that often forms as the wound margins are approximated (Fig. 13–5). Subcuticular sutures of 5-0 polyglactin followed by a continuous 5-0 polypropylene cutaneous suture complete the repair.

The portion of the flap attached to the nose is released from attachments to the adjacent nasal skin for a distance of 0.5 to 1.0 cm to achieve sufficient freedom to unfurrow the flap. Release enables the surgeon to remove excessive subcutaneous fat not trimmed at the time of flap transfer. The residual skin of the alar unit is excised if present. However, a 1-mm fringe of skin at the junction of the ala and the alar facial sulcus is preserved. The flap is precisely trimmed to fit the skin defect and sutured in place with simple interrupted 5-0 polypropylene cutaneous sutures (see Fig. 13–5). When the alar base is absent, the flap is tailored to replace the missing base and is intregrated with the nasal sill. When the sill requires reconstruction, the flap is trimmed so that it has a tapered end that may serve as the sill. The end is turned medially and sutured to the upper lip.

Subsequent flap contouring and the creation of an alar groove is a necessary third surgical stage in 75% of cases. It is performed 3 months following pedicle detachment (Fig. 13–6). A template of the contralateral normal alar unit is made, reversed, placed over the reconstructed ala, and traced carefully with a marking pen. The superior border of the tracing represents the appropriate location for the alar groove. If the superior border of the flap is no greater than 1 cm superior to the border of the tracing, then the scar marking the juncture of the flap and nasal skin is used as the access incision for contouring the flap. If a larger portion of the sidewall was resurfaced, then a 3-cm incision is made along the superior border of the tracing. The flap is undermined, leaving a few millimeters of subcutaneous fat attached to the dermis. For males, the flap is elevated in a more superficial plane immediately below the dermis in order to expose all of the hair follicles transferred from the cheek. This may require undermining the entire flap caudally to the level of the nostril margin. The exposed follicles are cauterized individually under magnification with a fine-tipped monopolar electrocautery. The power setting of the cautery device is set sufficiently low to prevent damage of the adjacent dermis. To ensure flap survival in patients who use tobacco, it may be prudent to depilate the flap in two stages: the upper part of the flap at the time of flap contouring and restoring of the alar groove and the lower part at a separate time, 2 to 3 months later.

Flap contouring and construction of an alar groove is accomplished by removing scar tissue and the majority of the remaining subcutaneous fat beneath the flap. Excision continues deeply until the cartilage graft used as the alar batten is exposed. A trough of cartilage centered under the planned alar groove is excised from the graft with a scalpel (see Fig. 13–6). The trough typically measures 4 to 5 mm wide and extends along the entire projected length of the groove. Care is taken not to deepen the cartilage trough excessively as this

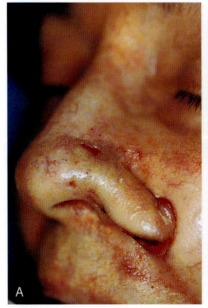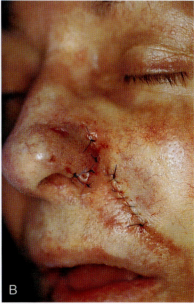

■ **Figure 13–5.** *A,* 3 weeks following transfer of interpolated subcutaneous pedicled cheek flap to ala. *B,* It is usually necessary to open superior end of donor site scar to facilitate excision of redundant subcutaneous tissue and small standing cutaneous deformity that forms as wound margins are approximated.

A

B

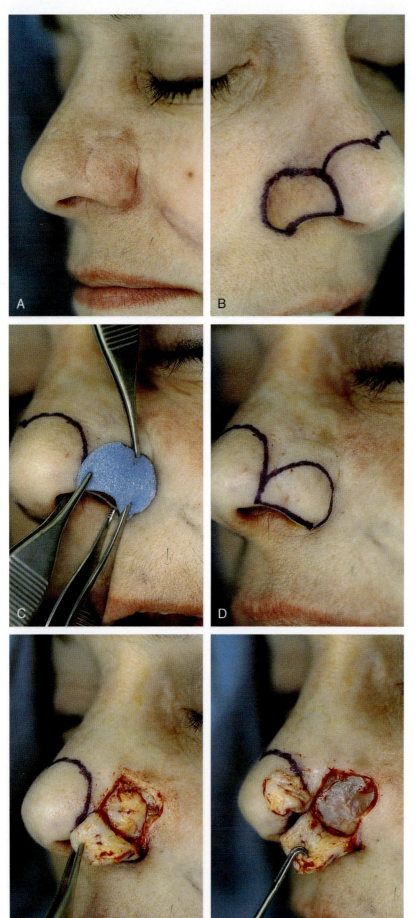

Figure 13–6. *A,* Flap 2 months following transfer to ala to repair full-thickness defect. Septal mucoperichondrial hinge flap was used for lining and septal cartilage for alar batten graft. *B,* Contralateral normal ala is used to design template. *C,* Template is reversed and placed over reconstructed ala. *D,* Using template, alar groove is traced on surface of flap. *E,* Superior border of flap is less than 1 cm from tracing so scar between flap and nasal skin is incised. Flap is dissected in subcuticular plane, leaving fat and scar tissue attached to underlying cartilage graft. *F,* Fat is removed, revealing septal cartilage batten graft.

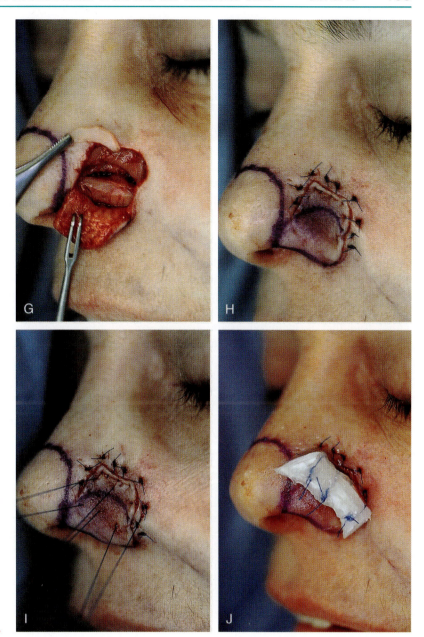

Figure 13-6 *Continued. G*, Alar groove is restored by removing trough of cartilage centered under tracing of groove. Forceps hold crescent of cartilage removed to create trough. As in this case, the alar batten graft is usually made sufficiently wide to allow for cartilage above and below reconstructed groove. *H*, Access incision is repaired with vertical mattress cutaneous sutures. *I*, Interrupted 4-0 sutures are passed full-thickness through nose, straddling reconstructed alar groove. *J*, Bolster is secured with sutures.

may cause a depressed narrow crease to form in place of the shallow valley of the alar groove typically observed in most noses. Some of the cartilage shavings may be replaced if overcorrected. Proper contour is determined by replacing the skin of the flap and compressing it gently. Continued excision of soft tissue and cartilage is performed until the constructed groove has an identical topography to its counterpart. The skin incision is closed with 5-0 polypropylene using interrupted vertical mattress cutaneous sutures. A dental roll is cut longitudinally and used as a bolster. It is secured in place along the length of the constructed groove by passing interrupted 4-0 polypropylene sutures full-thickness through the nose so as to straddle the groove. The sutures are tied lightly over the dental roll. Tight sutures may cause flap necrosis as considerable flap swelling

occurs postoperatively. The roll offers an effective method of obliterating potential dead space, enhancing hemostasis, and maintaining the constructed alar groove. The bolster is removed on the fifth postoperative day along with the cutaneous sutures.

The third stage of contouring the cartilaginous framework and subcutaneous tissues completes the reconstruction of the ala. It has the effect of improving the patency of the reconstructed nasal airway by removing excessive bulk in the area of the internal nasal valve. The width of the alar batten graft typically measures 1.5 cm. This is usually sufficient to ensure the presence of cartilage inferior and superior to the constructed alar groove and helps to stent the internal nasal valve.[8, 9] Prophylactive antibiotics are administered at the first and third stage of alar reconstruction. We have not found it necessary to use antibiotics when detaching the pedicle and inseting the cheek flap.

Technique: Interpolated Cutaneous Pedicled Cheek Flap

This is a peninsular flap with a linear axis based on a cutaneous pedicle that connects the flap to the cheek. This is in contrast to the subcutaneous pedicled (island) flap, which does not have a cutaneous pedicle and is connected to the cheek by subcutaneous tissue. Whether a peninsular or island flap, the pedicle is developed at the superior aspect of the donor site.

In most cases, we prefer to design cheek flaps on a subcutaneous tissue pedicle because this design limits the quantity of skin in the superior aspect of the melolabial fold that is included in the flap or excised to facilitate closure of the donor site. The island design has greater freedom to pivot on its pedicle and may have a better blood supply by incorporating within the pedicle of the flap a greater number of perforating vessels arising from the angular artery. The pedicle of the island flap does not require tailoring and inset following detachment of the flap. The subcutaneous pedicle is simply excised, and the skin edges surrounding the pedicle are freshened and closed primarily. However, harvesting the island flap is technically more difficult than harvesting the peninsular flap because the plane of dissection is considerably deeper, placing the branches of the facial nerve supplying the zygomatic major and minor muscles at greater risk of injury.

The peninsular flap depends on the dermal and subdermal vascular plexes of the cutaneous pedicle to provide vascularity to the distal flap. The cutaneous pedicle must be of sufficient width and depth to ensure this vascularity. When designing a peninsular flap, the orientation of the template remains the same as for designing an island flap. The width of the cutaneous pedicle is approximately the width of the template, although it may be narrower than the template when a wide (more than 2 cm) flap design is required. The peninsular flap is elevated in a subcutaneous plane, maintaining 3 mm of fat on the undersurface of the cutaneous pedicle. This is in contrast to the island design, based on a subcutaneous tissue pedicle that may be as much as 1.5 cm thick. Thus, the plane of dissection for the peninsular flap is considerably more superficial. Like the island flap, the peninsular flap pivots 90 degrees toward the midline and is sutured to the nose in a similar fashion to that described for the island flap. Care is taken not to kink the pedicle on transferring the flap. Like the island flap, the distal half of the flap may be thinned as necessary to replicate the thickness of the recipient site. The proximal portion of the flap bridging

between cheek and nose is not thinned to ensure an ample vascular supply. The cheek wound is closed using a method identical to that for the island flap.

Similar to the island flap, the peninsular flap remains attached to the cheek for 3 weeks to enable the establishment of collateral vascularity. The pedicle is divided at a second stage, and the proximal portion of the pedicle is inset in the cheek by opening the superior portion of the donor site scar for 1 to 2 cm. The wound edges are spread widely, creating a space to accommodate the proximal pedicle. The skin adjacent to the opened wound is undermined for 2 cm. This allows the cheek skin to contract, assisting in enlarging the wound. The pedicle stump is then trimmed to precisely fit the wound and inset in the melolabial fold, creating a V-shaped wound closure (Fig. 13–7). Returning most of the skin of the proximal pedicle to the cheek helps maintain the natural fullness observed in the upper portion of the melolabial fold. Alternatively, the proximal pedicle may be amputated in an eliptical configuration, and the cheek wound is closed primarily. This has the advantage of giving a linear donor site scar positioned in the melolabial sulcus but the disadvantage of restoring less soft tissue and skin to the melolabial fold. The proximal portion of the flap left attached to the nose is thinned and inset with methods similar to those for the island flap. Less aggressive sculpturing of subcutaneous fat is recommended for patients who use tobacco products.

Six weeks following the final contouring procedure, the reconstructed ala and adjacent nasal skin may be dermabraded. This is performed as an office procedure. Two months following flap detachment, the patient is instructed to massage the donor cheek scar and reconstructed nostril several times a day for 6 months. Indurated areas of the donor site are injected with 0.5 to 1.0 mL of a suspension of triamcinolone acetonide in a concentration of 10 mg/mL. This is placed in the deep subcutaneous plane at 6- to 8-week intervals. Two or three injections may be administered.

The greatest advantage of using the melolabial flap for resurfacing the ala in the form of an interpolated rather than a transposition flap is the preservation of the aesthetically important alar facial sulcus. The technique also minimizes flattening of the upper melolabial fold because the majority of skin removed from the cheek is from the middle and lower portions of the fold. Another advantage over the more conventional transposition flap is when necrosis of the distal flap occurs. In this instance, the pedicled flap may be dissected away from the defect, trimmed of devitalized tissue, and reattached to the nose provided there is sufficient tissue to allow for this.

A disadvantage of the interpolated melolabial flap is the necessity for a two- or even three-stage procedure. However, when standard transposition cheek flaps are used to reconstruct the ala, revision surgery is fre-

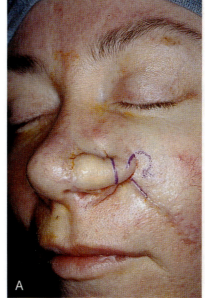 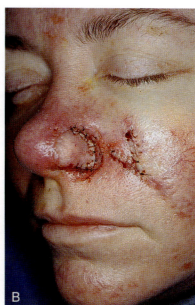

■ **Figure 13–7.** *A,* Interpolated cutaneous pedicled cheek flap used to resurface alar defect. Vertical line indicates location for incision to detach pedicle. *B,* Proximal pedicle is trimmed and inset in upper melolabial fold, creating V-shaped wound closure.

quently necessary to restore the superior portion of the alar facial sulcus and lateral aspect of the alar groove commonly deformed by the flap. This is the case even when the pedicle of the flap is designed well above the sulcus in an attempt not to deform it. A disadvantage of all cheek flaps in males is the transfer of hair-bearing skin to the nose. This is particularly true for the interpolated flap because it is harvested in the hair-bearing lower portion of the melolabial fold. A surgical procedure is nearly always required in males to remove the hair follicles; it is performed concomitant with restoration of the alar groove.

Cheek Versus Forehead Flap

In analyzing an alar defect, the surgeon is often faced with the decision whether to select the forehead or cheek as the donor site for the external flap. This decision is influenced by a number of factors. One factor is the laxity of skin in the medial cheek and the size of the melolabial fold. To the trained eye, the use of a cheek flap invariably results in some asymmetry of the melolabial fold. This asymmetry is typically represented by a flattening of the inferior aspect of the fold. The asymmetry may be corrected by excision of skin and fat from the contralateral fold; however, most patients do not notice or are not bothered by the asymmetry. A relative indication for the use of a paramedian forehead flap is the young patient with little cheek laxity and no melolabial sulcus. In this patient, cheek donor site scars

may remain conspicuous even a year after surgery. In contrast, properly closed forehead donor sites rarely result in an unsightly scar, even when complete primary closure is not possible. Forehead scars have the added advantage of being able to be camouflaged with certain hairstyles. In males, the cheek flap transfers hair-bearing skin to the nose and necessitates a surgical stage to depilate the flap. This factor may make the forehead the preferred donor site if the patient has dense facial hair. The most important factor influencing the selection of the covering flap is the size of the defect. In most instances, defects limited to the ala are reconstructed with interpolated cheek flaps. This is because cheek skin provides a better textural match with adjacent nasal skin, compared with forehead skin (Figs. 13–8 and 13–9). Defects that extend beyond the ala to the nasal sidewall more than 1 cm are best resurfaced with a paramedian forehead flap. Likewise, when alar defects encompass significant portions of the hemitip, the forehead is selected as the donor site for the covering flap.

The selection of a donor site for the covering flap is also influenced by the social and economic situation of the patient. An interpolated cheek flap is usually used for patients who express a strong desire to continue to work at their employment between the first and second stage of reconstruction. Paramedian forehead flaps often preclude the ability of the patient to work during the 3-week interval between transfer and pedicle detachment. Flaps from the forehead make it difficult to wear eye and safety glasses properly, and covering the flap with a bandage obstructs the vision. In contrast, an interpolated cheek flap may easily be covered with a

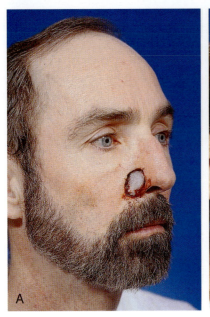
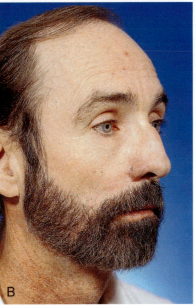

■ **Figure 13–8.** *A* and *B*, Preoperative and 1 year postoperative following alar repair with interpolated cheek flap.

bandage, keeping it from the sight of persons working with the patient. The cheek flap does not impair the use of eyeglasses.

Another social issue to consider is the patient's use of tobacco. In patients who smoke cigarettes, cheek flaps are more likely to manifest necrosis of the distal portion as compared with paramedian forehead flaps. This is because cheek flaps have a more random vascularity compared with the well-developed axial vascular pattern of the paramedian forehead flap. We are inclined to select the forehead as the preferred donor site for reconstruction of the ala in persons who smoke one or more packs of cigarettes daily.

Complications

All surgery is subject to complications. The most frequent complication encountered in reconstruction of the ala is partial necrosis of lining flaps (15%) in patients with full-thickness defects.[10] Smokers are at a greater risk for this. When a septal mucoperichondrial hinge flap has been used for lining, and necrosis of a portion of the flap occurs, trimming the necrotic tissue and advancing the hinge flap to cover the wound are usually not successful. Management consists of delaying

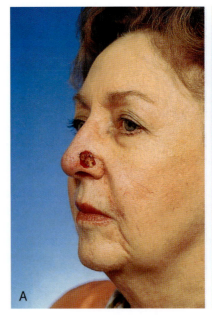
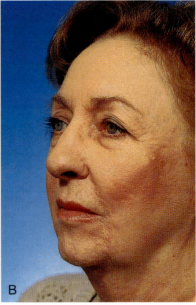

■ **Figure 13–9.** *A* and *B*, Preoperative and 6 months postoperative following alar repair with interpolated cheek flap.

detachment of the flap from the septum and allowing the necrotic tissue to separate spontaneously from viable tissue as the wound heals by secondary intention. Wound care consists of daily cleaning and the application of an ointment containing a topical antibiotic. An oral antibiotic is also administered. Once complete healing has occurred, the lining flap is detached from the septum. Fortunately, partial necrosis of the lining flap is usually limited to a small area along the alar margin. In this instance, postponement of detachment of the pedicle of the covering flap is not necessary.

When necrosis of a lining flap occurs, it results in exposure of the overlying cartilage graft that serves as the framework for the reconstructed ala. Small areas of necrosis will heal by secondary intention without impairing the survival of the graft. However, larger areas of necrosis (greater than 1 cm^2) ultimately result in loss of a portion of the exposed cartilage. Subsequent notching of the nostril margin is inevitable. Correction of the notch is not performed until all healing is complete. A small notch may be repaired with a Z-plasty. More commonly, it is necessary to place a cartilage graft along the nostril margin to bridge the notched area. This may be performed concomitant with construction of an alar groove during the third-stage contouring procedure. The trough of cartilage removed to create the alar groove is placed along the alar margin in the area of the notch and secured to the surviving cartilage framework with sutures.

The second most common complication encountered in reconstruction of the ala using cheek flaps is partial necrosis of the distal portion of the covering flap (8%).[10] Typically, only the distal border of the flap is lost. In all cases in which necrosis has occurred, we have been successful in remedying the problem by detaching the flap from the recipient site, trimming the necrotic skin and reattaching it. The subcutaneous pedicle is gently mobilized sufficiently to enable the flap to cover the entire alar defect. The procedure is accomplished as soon as the area of necrosis is delineated (2 to 3 weeks following transfer). Detachment of the flap's pedicle is delayed for 3 weeks following reattachment of the flap. The ability to adequately manage this complication prevents these setbacks from becoming poor results.

Reconstruction of the Columella

The columella is the most difficult aesthetic unit of the nose to reconstruct. This is partly due to the distant location of this structure from the cheek and forehead and partly due to the nature of the columella. The columella is the most delicate external structure of the nose and is characterized by fragile medial crural cartilages covered with extremely thin skin lacking subcuta-

neous fat. Replication of similar skin and topography is impossible. The goal of reconstruction is to provide cartilaginous support to the nasal tip covered by skin that does not cause excessive bulk and distortion. Because of the difficulty in duplicating the delicate nature of the columella, many elaborate operative techniques requiring multiple stages have been suggested. Various composite grafts from the ear and lip have been described, but these have been of most value in repairing partial losses of the columella. Composite grafts are unreliable and often contract, with loss of tip support. Surgeons have used mucosal flaps from the inner aspect of the upper lip combined with skin grafts, but scar contraction causes loss of vertical height. Intranasal vestibular skin flaps based on the floor of the nasal vestibule have been used for columellar reconstruction; this technique provides only limited tissue and requires the presence of the membranous septum.[11]

Puterman et al[12] used a unilateral septal mucoperichondrial flap for resurfacing the columella. This approach places mucosa, rather than skin, on the exterior of the nose and is not advised. Composite flaps consisting of skin, cartilage, and mucosa have been transferred to the columella from the transition region between the ala and nasal sidewall.[13] The flap is based on the vestibular skin of the nasal dome and is transferred to the region of the columella in a one-stage procedure. Although the approach simultaneously restores skin and cartilage to the columella, it inevitably results in alar retraction and may constrict the internal nasal valve. Bilateral medially based nasal skin flaps developed along the nostril margins have been transferred to the columella.[14] This may be combined with a cartilage graft for structural support, but it is only useful for limited defects of the columella and when the nostril margins are sufficiently thick to provide a donor site for the flaps.

Interpolated melolabial flaps have been used for repair of the columella by passing the pedicle of the flap through an opening created between the ala and nasal sidewall.[15] This route serves as a shortcut between the cheek and columella, but requires repair of the nasal fistula following pedicle detachment. Bilateral inferiorly based subcutaneous tissue pedicled interpolated flaps tunneled under the skin of the upper lip may be used to reconstruct defects limited to the columella.[16] The flaps are based on the angular artery, a branch of the anterior facial artery. By necessity, the pedicles must be of sufficient size to ensure flap vascularity. This in turn creates a distortion of contour of the upper lip and base of nose. Likewise, superiorly based interpolated subcutaneous tissue pedicle flaps delivered to the nose beneath lip skin have been successful in reconstruction of the columella.[17] Like its inferiorly based counterpart, the pedicles cause permanent distortion of the upper lip unless a secondary lip contouring procedure is performed.

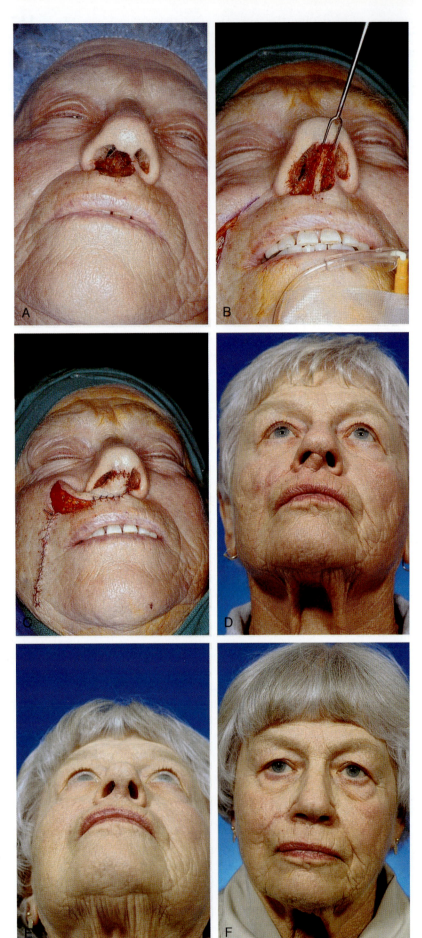

Figure 13–10. *A,* Loss of columella and portion of upper lip filtrum. *B,* Septal cartilage graft is anchored to caudal septum. Graft replaces medial crura and provides support to nasal tip. *C,* Interpolated subcutaneous pedicle cheek flap serves as covering flap. *D,* Appearance following second stage (pedicle detachment). Flap is excessively large and bulky. *E* and *F,* Appearance 5 months after third-stage contouring procedure.

Technique: Interpolated Subcutaneous Pedicled Cheek Flap

The length required of a flap to span the distance from the cheek to the nasal tip often proves excessive for the vascularity of cheek flaps. Distal flap necrosis is not uncommon in such circumstances. Thus, when defects of the nasal columella include portions of the tip, repair is best accomplished with a paramedian forehead flap. However, an interpolated cheek flap based on a cutaneous or subcutaneous tissue pedicle transferred over intervening tissue is our preferred method of repairing isolated columellar defects and those with limited extension toward the infratip lobule. A three-stage procedure is recommended (Fig. 13–10). The first stage consists of replacing any missing medial crura with cartilage grafts harvested from the nasal septum or auricle. Cartilage grafts usually take the form of single or dual pieces of cartilage that serve to replace any portion of one or both medial crura and are of sufficient length to span the distance from the nasal spine to the intermediate or lateral crura, depending on the cartilage deficit. The graft is covered by a unilateral interpolated cheek flap transferred over the upper lip. The technical aspects of dissecting and transferring the flap are identical to those for repair of the ala. The flap is sufficiently large to cover the cartilage graft and replace all missing skin of the columella. Depending on the amount of the columellar soft-tissue loss, the flap is designed large enough to easily wrap around the cartilage graft and reach the membranous septum. When the membranous septum is absent, a wider flap is created so it may be folded on itself and sutured to either side of the caudal septum, completely encasing the restored cartilage framework. The narrow bridge of skin connecting the nasal tip to the upper lip and representing the cutaneous portion of the columella is not initially replaced with a like-sized cheek flap, because such a narrow flap is unlikely to survive. In contrast to flaps used to cover other aesthetic units of the nose, cheek flaps used to repair the columella are oversized in order to ensure adequate vascularity of the skin of the flap. This transfers excessive tissue to the nasal base, which requires another surgical stage to tailor the flap.

Like those used for repair of the ala, interpolated cheek flaps are detached 3 weeks following initial transfer to the columella. When the columellar defect extends to the upper lip, the flap is inset by developing a turndown skin flap hinged on the upper lip at the lip/columellar junction. The hinge flap is sutured to the inferior border of the cheek flap at the recipient site. The turndown flap helps integrate the transition between reconstructed columella and lip and provides an enhanced surface area for contact with the flap. When a limited central portion of the upper lip is missing in conjunction with an absent columella, more of the cheek flap may be left at the recipient site to assist in repair of the filtrum. However, defects of the upper lip that extend beyond the upper half of the filtrum are repaired independently and before the columella is reconstructed. Reconstructing the upper lip provides a stable foundation for subsequent construction of the columella.

When using an interpolated cheek flap for reconstruction of the columella, a third surgical stage is performed 2 months following pedicle detachment and flap inset. This stage requires removal of all subcutaneous fat from beneath the skin of the flap. If hair-bearing skin has been transferred with the flap, the hair follicles are destroyed at this stage. Sufficient skin is removed from the flap to reduce bulk and restore appropriate size and contour to the constructed columella. Excision and contouring are usually accomplished by removing a vertically oriented ellipse of skin from the center of the flap.

References

1. Burget GC: Aesthetic restoration of the nose. Clin Plast Surg 12:463, 1985.

2. Baker SR, Johnson TM, Nelson BR: The importance of maintaining the alar-facial sulcus in nasal reconstruction. Arch Otolaryngol Head Neck Surg 121:617, 1995.

3. Fader DJ, Baker SR, Johnson TM: The staged cheek-to-nose interpolated flap for reconstruction of the nasal alar rim/lobule. J Am Acad Dermatol 37:614, 1997.

4. Burget GC, Menick FJ: The superiorly based nasolabial flap: Technical details. In Burget GC, Menick FJ (eds): Aesthetic Reconstruction of the Nose. St. Louis, Mosby–Year Book, 1994, p 93.

5. Burget GC, Menick FJ: Nasal support and lining: The marriage of beauty and blood supply. Plast Reconstr Surg 84:189, 1989.

6. Herbert DC: A subcutaneous pedicled cheek flap for reconstruction of alar defects. Br J Plast Surg 31:79, 1978.

7. Sheen JH, Sheen A: Aesthetic Rhinoplasty, 2nd ed. St. Louis, CV Mosby, 1987, p 255.

8. Robinson JK, Burget GC: Nasal valve malfunction resulting from resection of a cancer. Arch Otolaryngol Head Neck Surg 116:1419, 1990.

9. Constantian MB: The incompetent external nasal valve: Pathophysiology and treatment in primary and secondary rhinoplasty. Plast Reconstr Surg 93:919, 1994.

10. Driscoll BP, Baker SR: Reconstruction of nasal alar defects. Arch Facial Plast Surg 3:91, 2001.

11. Vecchione TR: Columella reconstruction using internal nasal vestibular flaps. Br J Plast Surg 33:399, 1980.

12. Puterman M, Pitzhaza N, Leiberman A: Reconstruction of columella and upper lip by septal flap. Laryngoscope 95:1272, 1985.

13. Bianchi A, Galli S, Ferroni M: Personal technique for columella reconstruction. Laryngoscope 94:1613, 1984.

14. Saad MN, Barron JN: Reconstruction of the columella with alar margin flaps. Br J Plast Surg 33:427, 1980.

15. Georgiade NG, Mladick RA, Thorne FL: The nasolabial tunnel flap. Plast Reconstr Surg 43:463, 1969.

16. Kaplan I: Reconstruction of the columella. Br J Plast Surg 25:37, 1972.

17. Yanai A, Nagata S, Tanaka H: Reconstruction of the columella with bilateral nasolabial flaps. Plast Reconstr Surg 77:129, 1986.

14

Interpolated Paramedian Forehead Flaps

Shan R. Baker

Median forehead flaps were first described in an Indian medical treatise, the *Sushruta Samita*, approximately in 700 BC.[1-3] The operation was performed by members of a caste of potters known as the Koomas. The need for this operation arose from the common Indian practice of amputating the tip of the nose as punishment for a variety of crimes, ranging from robbery to adultery.[4, 5] The first reported use of the median forehead flap outside of India was by Antonio Branca of Italy. Based on an Arabic translation of the *Sushruta Samita*, Branca performed a nasal reconstruction using the mid–forehead flap in the 15th century.[6, 7] In the 16th and early 17th centuries, little advancement was made in the use of the median forehead flap because plastic and reconstructive surgery fell into disrepute.[4, 5, 7] The flap had a revival in 1794, when J.C. Carpue read an editorial in the *Gentlemen's Gazette of London* describing the flap's use for nasal reconstruction.[8-10] Initially, Carpue practiced the median forehead flap operation on cadavers. Twenty years passed before he performed the operation on two patients; he reported his successful results in a monograph entitled "An Account of Two Successful Operations for Restoring a Lost Nose From the Integuments of the Forehead." His article was widely circulated throughout Europe and served to popularize the operation.[6, 9] In the 1830s, Ernst Blausius, Chief of Ophthalmologic Surgery of Berlin; Johann Friedrich Dieffenbach, Chief of Surgery at Munich Hospital; and Natale Petrali of Milan simultaneously reported on uses and variations of the median forehead flap for reconstruction of the

face and nose. Based on their influence as respected surgeons at large European teaching hospitals, the use and popularity of the forehead flap grew.[6] In the late 1830s, use of the median forehead flap for nasal and facial reconstruction crossed the Atlantic when J.M. Warren performed the operation in the United States.[4, 11]

By the early 1900s, the forehead flap was used to reconstruct losses of the nose secondary to battle, scrofula, syphilis, and cancer. Many American surgeons, such as Pancoast, Mutter, Buck, Davis, and Fomon, wrote about the use of the forehead flap in nasal reconstruction. Little modification of flap design, use, harvest, or donor site closure occurred until articles authored by Kazanjian appeared in the plastic surgery literature of the 1930s. This pioneer plastic surgeon was the first to determine that the primary blood supply of the flap was from the supratrochlear and supraorbital arteries. Kazanjian described a forehead flap designed precisely in the midline, allowing primary closure of the donor site. This technical modification minimized the forehead donor scar, which up to that point represented the major morbidity risk of the operation. Prior to Kazanjian's modification, the donor site had either been skin-grafted or left open to heal secondarily by granulation and wound contraction. This practice commonly left the patient more scarred and disfigured than before the reconstructive surgery.[12]

Kazanjian carried incisions from the hairline to a point immediately above the level of the nasofrontal angle. By his time, surgeons had recognized that the use of unlined forehead flaps to repair full-thickness

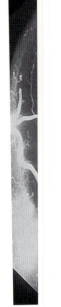

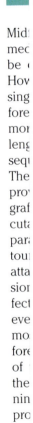

nasa
flap
of th
strict
on t
surge
desig
tiona
inter
izont
flap
he c
tion
supra
tion
verse
pedic
the s
to in
tiona
Unfo
of th
the f
flap
cause
sis of

In
medi
latera
The
bital
scrib
const
outco

Lal
foreh
supra
proxi
ately
This
from
lengt
Milla
foreh
that
glabe
desig
narro
ment
effec

In
tendi
below
often
ing s
tip. T
chlea

F
jectic
supro
Note
Kevir

Midl
mec
be
How
sing
fore
mor
leng
sequ
The
pro
graf
cuta
para
tou
atta
sion
fect
eve
mo
fore
of
the
nin
pro

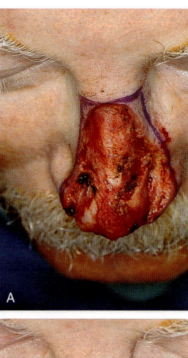

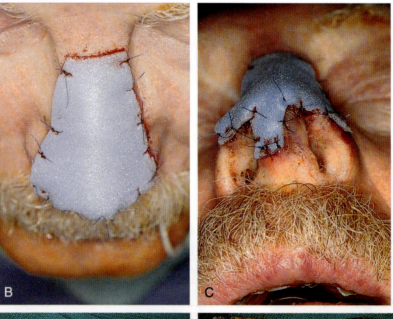

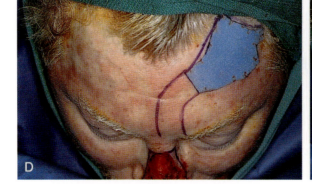

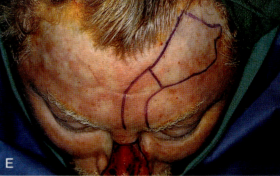

■ **Figure 14–7.** *A*, Final defect to be resurfaced is marked on nasal skin, outlining additional removal of remaining cutaneous portions of aesthetic unit. *B* and *C*, Thin foam rubber is used to fashion template that is carefully shaped to conform to defect. Caudal septum is markedly deviated to patient's left, distorting the view. *D* and *E*, Template is used to design oblique paramedian forehead flap in patient with low anterior hairline.

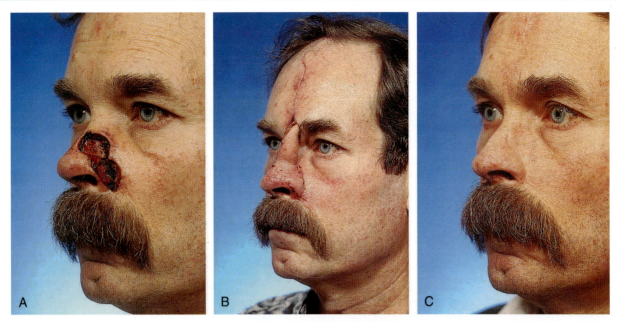

■ **Figure 14–3.** *A,* Skin defect of ala and lower sidewall. *B,* 1 week following transfer of paramedian forehead flap, which was thinned to level of subdermal fat. Thinness of flap allows it to reflect contour of underlying alar batten graft used for alar support. *C,* 9 months postoperative. Patient required contouring procedure as a third stage.

vision of the pedicle and inset of the flap, another procedure is performed to eliminate the hair. The portion of the flap bearing hair is elevated in the subdermal plane where the follicles of scalp hair are located. Exposed follicles are removed or cauterized with a fine-needle tip cautery, using magnification to assist in visualization (Fig. 14–4). Sometimes a third depilation may be required. Even with this persistent approach, a few hair follicles may survive and are treated individually with electrolysis. The hair bulb that is responsible for hair regeneration is located in the subcutaneous fat just beneath the dermis. In some instances, there may be remnants of the bulb left in the dermis after removal of the follicle during surgical depilation. These remnants

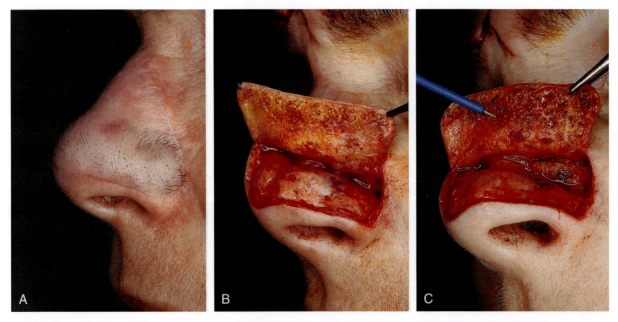

■ **Figure 14–4.** *A,* Paramedian forehead flap used to reconstruct ala and tip defect. Distal flap is covered with hair transferred from scalp. *B,* Flap is elevated in subdermal plane. Note underlying auricular cartilage graft serving as alar batten and exposed hair follicles on undersurface of flap. *C,* Exposed follicles are individually cauterized under magnification.

may have sufficient germinating potential to cause breakthrough hair growth in spite of aggressive removal of exposed hair follicles.

The fine vellus hair that is prominent in some patients just in front of the forehead hairline is even more difficult to eliminate from a forehead flap because the hair follicles are not visible by the human eye and are located in the dermis rather than in the subdermal plane. This hair may be treated by electrolysis with limited success. The best treatment is to have the patient periodically use a depilatory cream for removal. Laser hair removal may be used in place of electrolysis for scalp hair, but it is not effective for vellus hair.

To avoid multiple procedures directed at depilation, whenever possible design paramedian forehead flaps not to include scalp hair. Avoiding scalp hair may be possible by extending the incision for the pedicle through the brow to the level of the bony orbital rim. The pedicle is skeletonized on the soft tissue surrounding the supratrochlear artery as it exits the orbit. This requires complete sectioning of the corrugator supercilii to achieve free tissue movement. If this step is unlikely to lend sufficient length to the flap, another helpful approach is to obliquely angle the flap from the midline laterally toward the temporal recession just beneath the hairline[27, 28] (Fig. 14–5). This modification in design of the paramedian forehead flap is only possible for smaller flaps measuring less than 3 cm in maximum width. For flaps 3 cm or greater, removal of skin from the lateral portion of the forehead may occasionally cause more apparent scars than centrally located donor sites. It may also cause excessive upward displacement

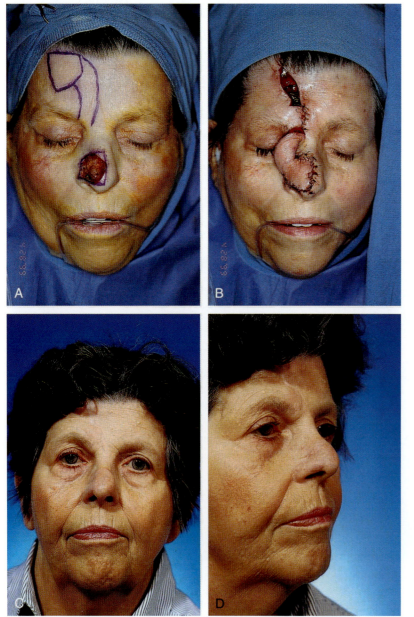

■ Figure 14–5. *A,* Heminasal skin defect in patient with extremely low anterior hairline. Forehead flap is angled obliquely to avoid transferring hair with flap. *B,* Flap transferred. Donor site partially closed. *C* and *D,* 1.5 years following reconstruction. Patient had contouring procedure 2 months following flap detachment.

of the central portion of the eyebrow on the donor side. Thus, flaps wider than 3 cm are usually extended to the hair-bearing scalp rather than designed in an oblique fashion when the length of the flap calls for such extensions. When using the oblique forehead design, the distal portion of the flap does not have the advantage of an axial vascular pattern. However, we have been successful in transferring forehead skin based on a supratrochlear artery but positioned several centimeters lateral to the axis of the artery. This success is related to the rich vascular anastomotic network in forehead skin.

Historically, the paramedian forehead flap has been used for reconstruction of larger defects of the nose. It is the preferred method for covering nasal defects too large to repair with full-thickness skin grafts, nasal cutaneous flaps, composite auricular grafts, or interpolated melolabial flaps.[4, 5, 12] In general, nasal defects larger than 2 cm in width in the horizontal plane are best repaired with a paramedian forehead flap.[12] Additionally, nasal defects with exposed bone and cartilage deficient of periosteum or perichondrium, and in instances where the central face has been irradiated, are best repaired using this flap.[5, 12]

Reconstruction of a nasal defect with a paramedian forehead flap requires planning and preparation. Preoperative assessment includes measurement of the defect and consideration of the required length and width of the flap. Attention is given to the height of the hairline and amount of forehead skin laxity. Patients are counseled concerning their appearance during the staged reconstruction. They are shown photographs of patients who have had similar surgery after the first stage and following flap detachment. Wound care of the pedicle, donor site, and recipient areas and information regarding realistic expectations and goals of the reconstructive procedure are discussed.

Surgical Technique

The paramedian forehead flap is usually harvested using a combination of a short-acting local anesthetic (lidocaine 1% with epinephrine 1:100,000 concentration) and a long-acting local anesthetic (bupivacaine 0.25%) with intravenous sedation. Thirty minutes before skin incision, a prophylactic antistaphyloccal antibiotic of the surgeon's choice is administered intravenously if cartilage or bone graft is required. The patient is placed supine on the operating room table in 20 to 30 degrees of a reverse Trendelenburg position. This position decreases venous pooling, causing less intraoperative blood loss during flap harvest and transfer. The eyes are protected by covering them securely with moist eyepads. The full face and scalp, from midvertex to

submentum, are prepared using a sterilization solution of the surgeon's choice. A sterile head drape is placed, and full-body draping is completed in the usual sterile fashion.

The flap may be designed with the assistance of a Doppler probe to localize the supratrochlear artery, but we have not found this to be necessary. The base of the pedicle is centered over the supratrochlear artery on the same side as the majority of the defect. The vertical axis of the supratrochlear artery is 2 cm lateral to the midline, which corresponds to the medial border of the eyebrow. Therefore, the base of the flap is centered over the medial border of the brow. The base width is 1.5 cm wide and is not flared as this restricts the pivotal movement of the flap.

The cutaneous defect is outlined by squaring off the corners of the defect with a skin marker. Giving the flap angular rather than curvilinear borders reduces the propensity for developing trapdoor deformity. If the defect occupies more than 50% of the surface area of a given aesthetic unit, the remaining border of the unit is marked for removal. An exception to this is the dorsum, where the thin skin of the rhinion is never removed unless required for tumor ablation. The intrinsic thickness of the forehead skin is greater than that of the skin covering the rhinion in most patients. Even with removal of all the subcutaneous tissue from the flap, the thickness of the flap will not match the delicate nature of the in situ skin and muscle of the rhinion. In this region, contour outweighs the advantage of placing the borders of the flap along the junction of aesthetic units. It is wiser to leave this skin intact and resurface only the lower dorsum than resurface the entire dorsal nasal aesthetic unit.

Similar to the rhinion, the skin of the nasal facets is delicate and thin. It is supported only by fibroconnective tissue. Forehead skin cannot replicate the delicate nostril margin in this area of the nose. Nasal tip defects requiring a forehead flap as a cover should be enlarged only to a line along the upper border of the facet. This line corresponds to the caudal border of the intermediate crura of the lower lateral cartilages.

A three-dimensional template exactly duplicating the surface area and contour of the region to be resurfaced is fashioned from foil or a thin sheet of foam rubber. We prefer foam rubber because it has the flexible qualities of skin and easily conforms to the convex and concave contours of the nasal framework (Figs. 14–6 to 14–8). The final defect to be resurfaced is marked on the nasal skin, outlining additional skin removal to square off the corners or remove remaining cutaneous portions of the aesthetic unit. The template is designed before the defect is enlarged because, once the additional skin is removed, the wound will spread and the defect will appear larger than it is. For this reason, if the nasal defect involves an aesthetic unit that has an intact counterpart, the intact unit is used to design the

Text continued on page 184

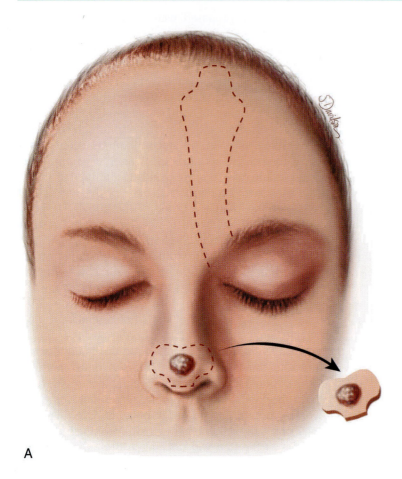

A

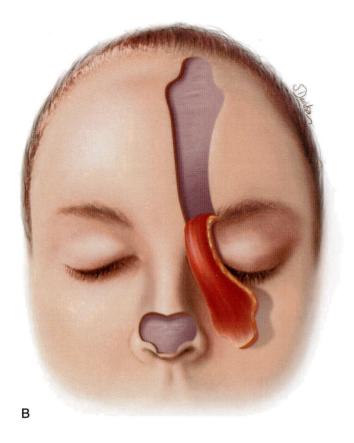

B

■ **Figure 14–6.** *A,* Base of paramedian forehead flap is 1.5 cm wide centered over medial end of brow. Axis of pedicle is vertical and 2 cm from midline. *B,* Flap is elevated from underlying periosteum.

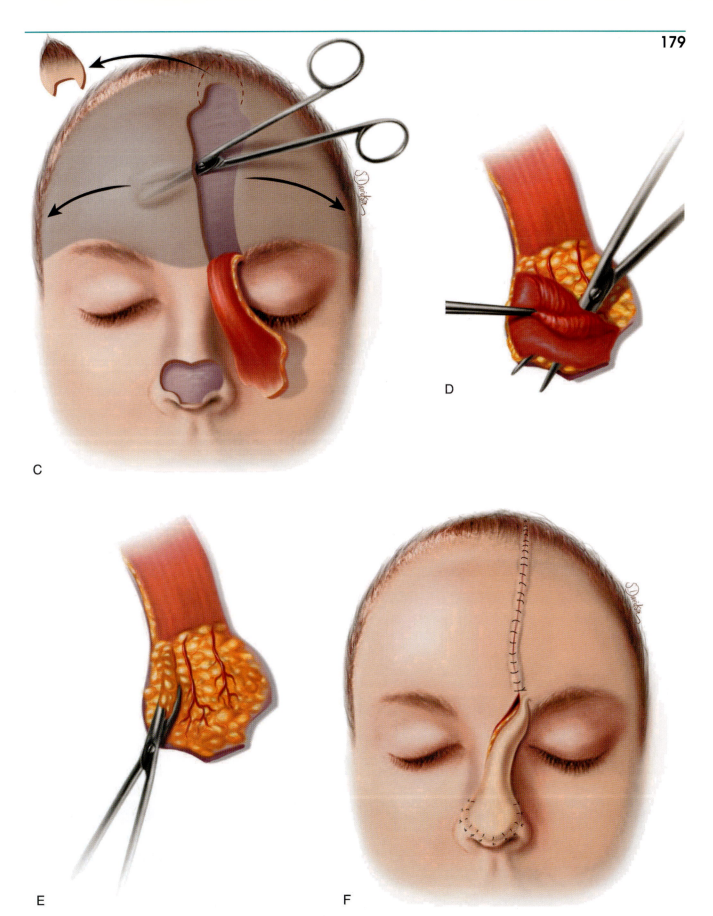

C

D

E

F

■ **Figure 14–6** *Continued. C,* Donor site closure is achieved by undermining in subfascial plane from one temporalis muscle to the other. Standing cutaneous deformity of scalp from advancement of forehead skin is removed vertically. *D,* Galea and frontalis muscles are completely removed from distal flap. *E,* Majority of subcutaneous fat is removed from distal flap. *F,* Flap is sutured at recipient site with vertical mattress cutaneous sutures. Subcuticular sutures are not used. Forehead donor site is closed in two layers: interrupted suture approximation of muscle and galea and continuous cutaneous suture.

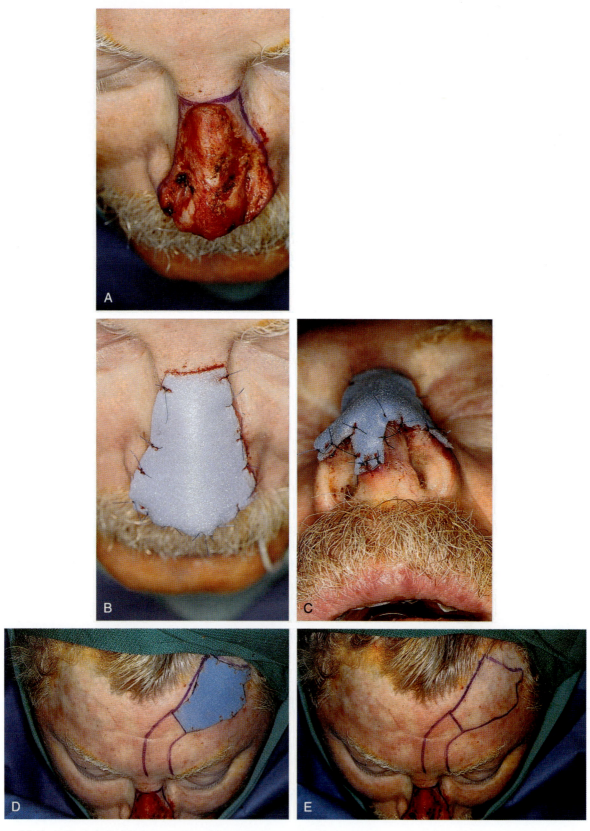

■ **Figure 14–7.** *A,* Final defect to be resurfaced is marked on nasal skin, outlining additional removal of remaining cutaneous portions of aesthetic unit. *B* and *C,* Thin foam rubber is used to fashion template that is carefully shaped to conform to defect. Caudal septum is markedly deviated to patient's left, distorting the view. *D* and *E,* Template is used to design oblique paramedian forehead flap in patient with low anterior hairline.

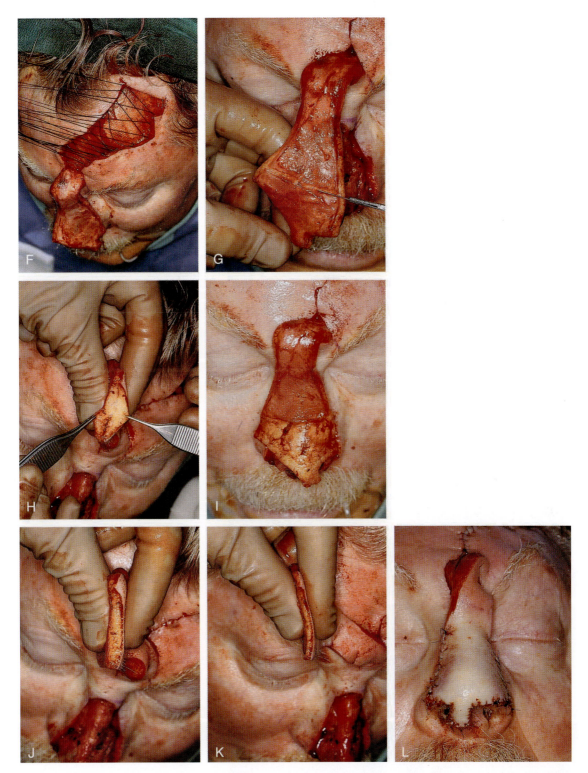

■ **Figure 14-7** *Continued. F,* Flap is elevated superficial to frontal bone periosteum. Sutures to approximate muscle and galea of donor site are left untied until all sutures are placed. Skin approximation is with continuous cutaneous suture. *G,* Flap is thinned by making incision through galea and muscle and completely removing them from distal flap. *H,* Subcutaneous fat of distal flap is split, leaving thin layer beneath dermis. *I,* Thinning of flap completed. Distal vasculature is seen immediately beneath dermis. *J* and *K,* Cross-section of distal flap before and following removal of subcutaneous fat. *L,* Donor site partially closed. Flap in place.

Illustration continued on following page

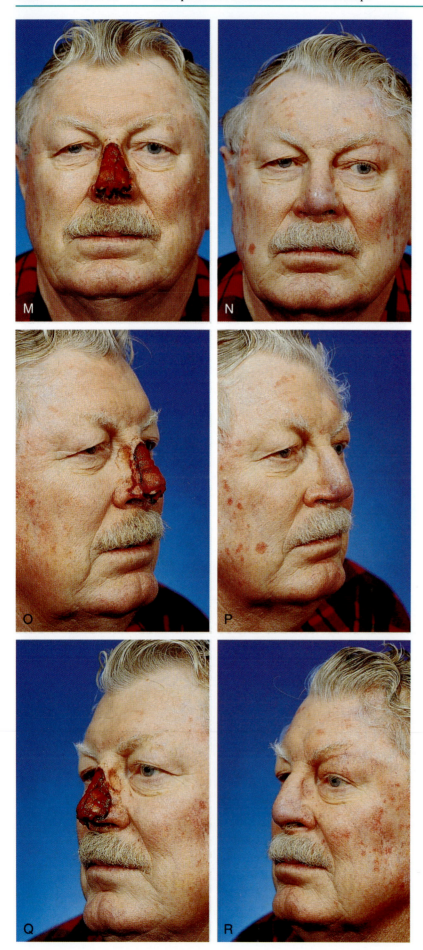

Figure 14–7 *Continued. M–T,* Preoperative and 6 months postoperative of same patient in *A–L.*

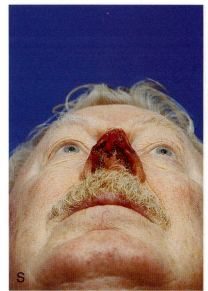
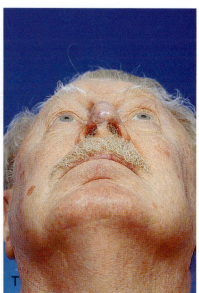

■ **Figure 14–7** *Continued.*

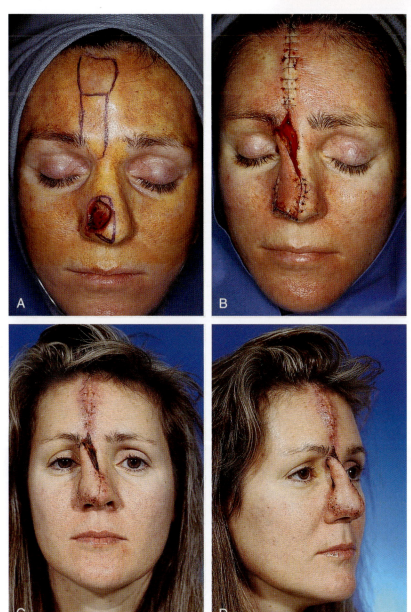

■ **Figure 14–8.** *A,* Skin defect of nasal dome. Defect is enlarged to encompass hemitip. Paramedian forehead flap designed for resurfacing half of aesthetic tip unit. *B,* Flap transferred to nose. Donor site closed primarily. *C* and *D,* 1 week following flap transfer.

Illustration continued on following page

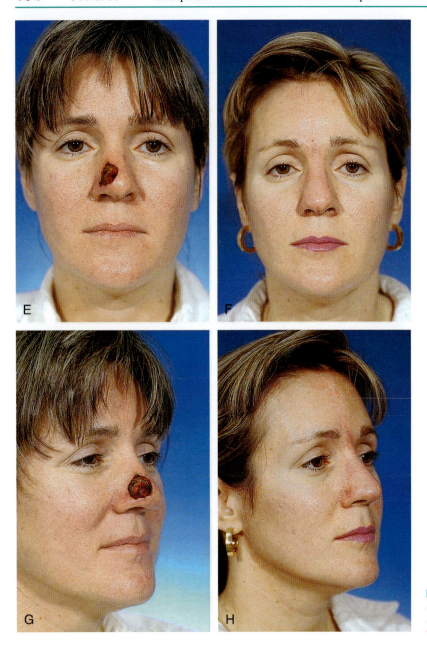

template because it will give a more accurate measurement of surface area. The template is then reversed to design the flap. When the defect involves an aesthetic unit that is unpaired, the template is designed as an ideal size for the specific patient. When dealing with large surface defects, it is helpful to suture the rubber foam template to the margins of the anticipated defect to fashion the template more precisely. Cartilage grafts are required to replace missing framework, and the template is designed after the grafts are in place. Templates should not be oversized, but tailored exactly.

The template is used to create the flap design on the forehead skin (see Fig. 14–7). The center of the template is positioned approximately 2 cm lateral to the midline. At a minimum, the upper border of the template is positioned at the frontal hairline unless the patient has a receding hairline or frontal balding. The length of the flap is measured by a length of suture extending from the distal end of the positioned template to the level of the medial eyebrow. Holding it at the brow, the suture is rotated 180 degrees toward the midline in the coronal plane to the most distal recipient site on the nose. If the suture does not reach this point, the template must be repositioned higher on the forehead, or the pedicle base must be lowered by extending it below the level of the eyebrow. By using this method of determining flap length, a decision can be made concerning the necessity of placing a portion of the template over hair-bearing scalp. The flap is then precisely outlined on the forehead with a skin marker, following the exact shape of the template.

One percent lidocaine with 1:100,000 concentration

of epinephrine is injected circumferentially and deeply about the surgical defect. The entire forehead from the level of the lateral canthus to its counterpart is injected with 15 mL of similar anesthetic solution. The skin along the entire length of the supraorbital rim is infiltrated to the level of the periosteum. Particular attention is given to a broad band of skin vertically along the axes of the supratrochlear and supraorbital nerves. The anesthetic is injected into the subcutaneous plane because this is the location of the nerves and vessels supplying the forehead. The base of the flap and skin over the root of the nose is also injected. Intravenous Anzemet is administered to control postoperative nausea, a common result of the procedure. The margins of the nasal defect are made perpendicular with a scalpel. If indicated, the remaining skin of the aesthetic unit is removed to the level of the perichondrium or periosteum. Until the pedicle of the flap is detached and the flap is inset, it is not necessary to excise the skin of the more extreme cephalic portion of the dorsum and sidewall aesthetic units when defects involve these units. The skin bordering the nasal defect is undermined below the muscular layer for 1 to 2 cm. Undermining of adjacent nasal skin helps prevent trapdoor deformity.

To avoid oversizing the flap, incisions are made inside the lines of the marked pattern. The flap is incised through the skin, subcutaneous tissue, muscle, and fascia. The flap is elevated from superior to inferior in the subfascial plane, just superficial to the periosteum of the frontal bone. Rapid dissection may be performed in this plane until the corrugator supercilii muscle is encountered, at which point the muscle is dissected away from the underlying periosteum bluntly with scissors or a periosteal elevator. If it is necessary to extend incisions for the pedicle below eyebrow level, that is accomplished with a scalpel through skin only. Blunt dissection by spreading tissue with a hemostat is then done to mobilize the pedicle away from the medial bony orbit. The supratrochlear artery can sometimes be identified visually in the area on the deep surface of the frontalis muscle just as it exits over or through the corrugator supercilii muscle and before passing deep to the orbicularis oculi muscle to enter the orbit. Adequate flap mobilization usually requires complete sectioning of the corrugator muscle to achieve sufficient flap length. Blunt and sharp dissections are used to continue flap elevation downward onto the root of the nose or until sufficient pedicle length and flap mobility have been attained to allow tension-free wound closure. Hemostasis along the border of the flap is achieved with an electrocautery applied judiciously.

The forehead flap is covered with a damp sponge and reflected downward to allow repair of the donor site. Donor site closure is accomplished by extensive undermining of the forehead skin in the subfascial plane from the anterior border of one temporalis muscle to the other (see Fig. 14–6). A few parallel vertical galeotomies 2 to 3 cm apart may be made to facilitate primary repair of the upper portion of the donor site. These should be made just through the galea to the level of the muscle and well removed from the vertical corridor of the supraorbital and supratrochlear nerves. The deep branch of the supraorbital nerve can readily be seen through the galea as it travels upward just medial to the temporal line, and it should be protected when performing galeotomies.

Horizontal incisions along the hairline to facilitate closure of the donor site are not performed. This would increase anesthesia of the anterior scalp by cutting through the distal branches of the supraorbital nerves and create an additional visible scar on the forehead. As the wound edges are advanced, a standing cutaneous deformity of scalp tissue occurs at the apex of the closure. This is excised completely by extending an incision sufficiently superior in the scalp to enable excision of the tissue cone (see Fig. 14–6).

The muscle and galea of the forehead are approximated as a single layer with 2-0 polyglactin suture. These are left untied until all have been placed (see Fig. 14–7). The skin incision is repaired with a simple running suture of 5-0 polypropylene. No drain is employed. Primary approximation of the lower forehead wound is rarely a problem because the pedicle width is less than 2 cm wide. However, more superior portions of the donor site may not close completely. Any remaining open wound is filled with an antibacterial ointment. The patient is instructed to keep the wound moist with petroleum ointment until healing is complete. Healing by secondary intention takes 4 to 6 weeks.

The forehead donor site wound is repaired before the flap is sutured in place. The thickness of the flap is tailored by thinning the distal portion. This usually requires removal of the muscle and most of the subcutaneous fat in order to match the thickness of the nasal skin (see Fig. 14–7). When necessary, all but the fat immediately attached to the dermis may be removed. If the vertical height of the nasal defect is less than 2 cm, the portion of the flap covering the entire defect may be thinned at the time of initial transfer. For larger defects, the proximal flap covering the more cephalic portion of the defect is left with all of its muscle and subcutaneous fat intact and is thinned at the time of pedicle division. If necessary, the muscle and galea can be removed from the entire length of the flap beginning 1 cm above the point at which the supratrochlear artery pierces the frontalis muscle. Any hair follicles transferred with the flap should be individually cauterized with a fine-pointed electric cautery or removed manually. The distal flap, appropriately thinned, will be sufficiently supple and thin to conform to the nasal framework and manifest its contour.

The practice of removing the frontalis muscle and the majority of subcutaneous fat from a paramedian forehead flap used to cover the nose begs the question of why the frontalis muscle is transferred with the flap. Including the muscle in the flap inferiorly near the eyebrow protects the supratrochlear artery as it ascends from the eyebrow between the muscle and skin. The superior aspect of a paramedian forehead flap can be dissected in the deep subcutaneous plane, leaving the frontalis muscle in place. However, elevation in the subcutaneous plane causes more bleeding than when elevating beneath the muscle and places the axial blood supply to the distal flap at some risk for injury. Unfortunately, leaving the frontalis muscle in situ when transferring a paramedian forehead flap to the nose does not preserve the supratrochlear nerve, which must be sacrificed when dividing the pedicle of the flap. Removing the muscle beneath the flap does not impair the motor function of the more lateral aspect of the forehead. Removal of the muscle facilitates subgaleal dissection of the remaining forehead skin during closure of the donor wound. Because most donor wounds of paramedian forehead flaps are closed primarily, any muscle preserved in the depths of the donor wound would require excision to prevent bunching and redundancy of the muscle during advancement of the remaining forehead skin. For all of these reasons, the frontalis muscle is included in the flap during dissection.

After thinning, the flap is pivoted in an arc toward the midline and reflected downward toward the nasal defect. The distal flap is sutured in position with interrupted 5-0 polypropylene vertical mattress cutaneous sutures. Deep dermal or subcuticular sutures are not used. Following placement of vertical mattress sutures, a single running 5-0 polypropylene suture on a fine-tipped needle is used to precisely approximate the epi-

dermis by placing the suture in the superficial plane of the skin. It is not possible to approximate the extreme cephalic border of the nasal defect to the flap until pedicle detachment.

Upon completion of flap transfer, the entire forehead is infiltrated with a solution of 0.25% Marcaine (bupivacaine) injected in the subcutaneous plane, with particular attention given to the vertical corridors of the supraorbital and remaining supratrochlear nerves. This helps control postoperative pain and nausea for up to 8 hours. The raw borders of the proximal portion of the flap are cauterized along their entire length to control postoperative bleeding, a common occurrence during the first 12 hours after surgery. Patients may be discharged home the day of surgery or admitted for overnight observation and wound care. Most patients are admitted for an overnight stay because postoperative nausea and vomiting are common. This is the result of donor site repair, which causes headache for 24 to 36 hours and reflex nausea. These are not unlike the symptoms in patients undergoing forehead lifting. Postoperative pain during the first 24 hours can be debilitating and not always controlled by oral analgesics. Prescriptions on discharge usually include an antistaphylococcal oral antibiotic (in case of cartilage or bone graft), a mild pain reliever (acetaminophen with codeine), antiemetic (Promethazine or trimethobenzamide), suppositories, and a topical antibacterial ointment (bacitracin).

Postoperative wound care consists of cleansing the suture lines with hydrogen peroxide and application of the antibacterial ointment twice daily for 3 days, after which the ointment is changed to petroleum ointment. The patient is allowed to shampoo and shower on the first postoperative day. Following the shower, ointment

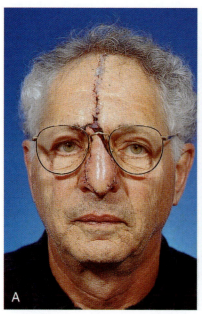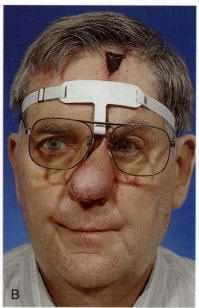

■ **Figure 14-9.** *A,* Patients are allowed to wear eyeglasses during interval between flap transfer and pedicle detachment. *B,* An appliance worn around the head may be used to support eyeglasses when forehead flap prevents proper positioning.

is reapplied to the suture line and exposed raw edges of the proximal flap. On the sixth to seventh postoperative day, sutures are removed. The wound is carefully checked for flap viability and signs of infection. If all appears well and healing is occurring as expected, the patient is scheduled for pedicle detachment approximately 3 weeks following the date of initial flap transfer. Although the pedicle can be safely divided 2 weeks postoperatively, the shorter interval may limit the ability to thin the proximal flap remaining at the recipient site. Patients are allowed to wear their eyeglasses if necessary (Fig. 14–9); however, proper positioning may be problematic. Eyeglasses may require temporary readjustment by an optometrist. Devices are also available for suspending eyeglasses from the forehead, circumventing the need to rest them on the nose (see Fig. 14–9).

Pedicle separation is accomplished under local anesthesia. One percent lidocaine containing epinephrine is injected into the base of the pedicle and circumferentially around the recipient site followed by the usual sterile preparation and draping. The pedicle is separated with a scalpel at the superior margin of the defect or higher if additional nasal skin is to be removed from the superior aspect of the aesthetic unit (Figs. 14–10 and 14–11). An incision is made in the cephalic portion of the old scar between the flap and adjacent nasal skin. The extent of this incision should be such that it releases the cephalic quarter of the flap from the nose. This is necessary to provide sufficient exposure for thinning and proper trimming and inset of the flap. The skin margins surrounding the skin defect created by the flap release are undermined 1 cm. Thinning is performed of any portion of the flap left attached to the recipient site that was not adequately thinned at the initial transfer. In the case of reconstructing skin-only nasal defects that involve the rhinion, it may be necessary to remove all subcutaneous fat in order to more accurately replicate the naturally thin skin of the rhinion. It is often necessary to remove early scar tissue under the flap to facilitate proper tailoring. Deep-layer closure is unnecessary because there is no wound closure tension. The flap is inset using interrupted vertical mattress and simple 5-0 polypropylene cutaneous sutures. An overnight compression dressing is applied.

The base of the pedicle is returned to its donor site in such a fashion to restore the normal intereyebrow distance. Just as with the inset of the flap at the recipient site, it is often necessary to remove early scar deposition in the donor area to enable the pedicle to lie flat between the eyebrows. The medial aspect of both eyebrows is undermined for several centimeters to release all contractions (see Fig. 14–11). This maneuver enables the surgeon to position the medial aspect of the eyebrows in proper relationship to each other and to the supraorbital bony rims. Typically, the medial aspect of

the eyebrow on the donor side is displaced inferiorly as a result of secondary movement from flap transfer. The brow must be mobilized sufficiently to correct malposition. This is accomplished by converting the proximal pedicle into a small triangular flap incorporating in its base the medial aspect of the eyebrow on the donor side. To accommodate for scar contraction and inferior migration of the eyebrow during healing, the flap is mobilized upward until the medial eyebrow is positioned 2 mm above the level of the opposite eyebrow. Excess pedicle tissue above the portion of the triangular flap necessary for securing the medial eyebrow in proper position is resected and discarded. Tissue should not be returned to the forehead above the level of this point. To facilitate superior advancement of the triangular flap, it is sometimes necessary to excise a small crescent or triangular segment of skin just lateral to the base of the triangle along the superior medial border of the eyebrow on the donor side (see Fig. 14–10). This maneuver removes the standing cutaneous deformity that forms from advancement. This in essence serves as a direct browlift limited to the portion of the eyebrow immediately lateral to the triangular flap. The muscle on the deep aspect of the triangular flap is preserved to prevent a depressed postoperative contour. It is often helpful to create a tongue of muscle and subcutaneous tissue extending 0.5 cm beyond the apex of the triangular flap. This tissue is tunneled under the most inferior portion of the forehead scar where it meets the apex of the triangle. The tissue tongue prevents contour depression at this point. The deep layers of the wound are closed with 4-0 absorbable sutures, and the skin is closed with 5-0 or 6-0 polypropylene sutures placed in vertical mattress fashion.

Postoperative care following pedicle detachment consists of local wound cleansing with a hydrogen peroxide solution and application of an antibacterial ointment twice daily for 3 days, followed by petroleum ointment for another 3 days. Sutures are removed in 5 to 7 days. Full physical activities may be resumed 1 week after surgery. The patient is advised to avoid sunlight exposure to the forehead and face region for 3 months to prevent postinflammatory hyperpigmentation of the scars. Patients are instructed that extremes of heat or cold may cause temporary color changes in the flap skin at the recipient site for several months. Revision surgery such as thinning of the flap is delayed 3 to 4 months to allow complete wound healing, wound contracture, and the beginning of scar maturation. Revision surgery is occasionally necessary to create or refine an alar groove or to remove persistent hair follicles transferred from the scalp. These revisions are accomplished using local anesthesia. We have not found it necessary or advantageous to perform an intermediate stage consisting of more proximal thinning of the flap before pedicle division. Although an intermediate stage may be advisable for a patient addicted to tobacco, in

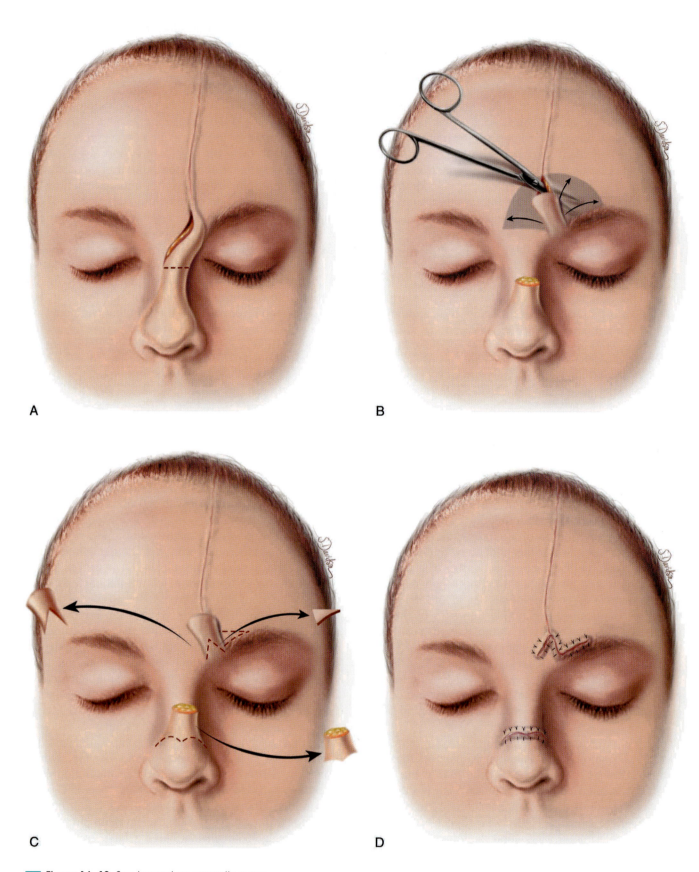

A

B

C

D

Figure 14–10 *See legend on opposite page*

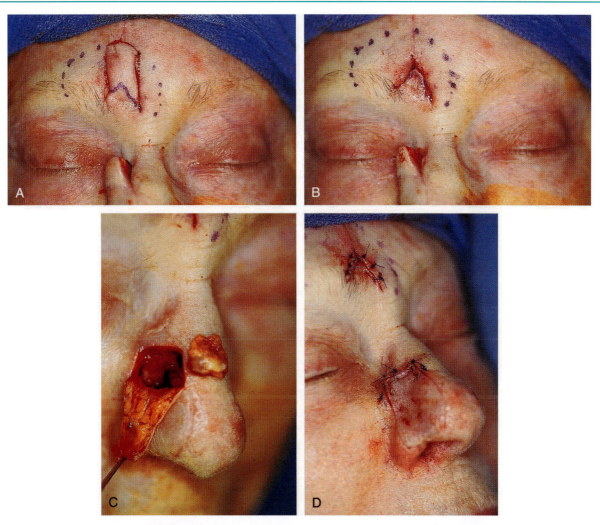

Figure 14–11. *A,* Dotted line indicates area of undermining prior to final trimming of proximal pedicle. Triangular flap is marked on detached pedicle. *B,* Pedicle is converted to triangular flap, with base centered over medial end of brow. Flap is advanced superiorly to position brow at same level as its counterpart. *C,* Cephalic fourth of distal flap is released from nose. Flap is trimmed of excess skin before undermining adjacent nasal skin. Early scar deposition and any excess subcutaneous fat not removed at time of flap transfer are trimmed. Trimmed subcutaneous tissue has been placed on nasal dorsum. *D,* Inset is accomplished using vertical mattress cutaneous sutures. No subcuticular sutures are used.

most patients it is not necessary and does not enhance the final aesthetic appearance of the reconstruction. Depending on the circumstance, the majority of the distal portion of a paramedian forehead flap may be thinned to the subdermis at the time of flap transfer and the remainder at the time of pedicle division. Leav-ing the pedicle attached and performing a debulking procedure as an intermediate stage subjects the patient to another 2 to 3 weeks of enduring the deformity resulting from the flap crossing from the eyebrow to the nose. This delays the patient from returning to work and resuming social activities.

Figure 14–10. *A,* Flap pedicle is separated 3 weeks following flap transfer. *B,* Lower donor site wound is opened and area between eyebrows is widely undermined to release wound contracture. *C,* Proximal pedicle is converted to small triangle flap that is advanced superiorly to restore original position of brow. To accomplish this, it is sometimes necessary to excise a Burow triangle immediately above medial brow. Flap is inset in nose by trimming redundant tissue. *D,* Wound repair is accomplished with vertical cutaneous sutures. A few subcuticular sutures are used in forehead wound repair.

Special Case

■ The Paramedian Forehead Flap as a Lining Flap

Forehead skin is rarely required for lining full-thickness nasal defects. Septal mucoperichondrium and turbinate mucosa are preferred for this purpose and are generally in adequate supply. However, in total or near-total nasal defects that include the nasal septum, the surgeon must look to other sources of lining. A microsurgical flap of skin or temporoparietal fascia is one source of major internal lining. Another alternative is the simultaneous use of two paramedian forehead flaps. One flap provides internal lining, and the other provides external cover (Fig. 14–12). Bone from the calvarium and cartilage grafts from rib or auricle are placed between the two flaps to provide a supporting framework. A template is fashioned that will provide ample skin to line the reconstructed nose, including the dorsum, sidewalls, tip, and alae. Unlike the forehead flap used for covering the exterior of the nose, the lining flap is incised and hinged downward without pivoting the base of the flap. This enables the raw undersurface of the flap to face outward. The pedicle is usually tunneled under the glabellar skin and delivered to the

nasal defect in such a fashion that it will not prevent the plating of bone grafts to the nasal process of the frontal bone. When the nasal bones are intact, the flap is presented to the nasal defect from a lateral approach, which necessitates a temporary nasal fistula. The sidewall dehiscence allowing the admittance of the lining flap is closed in layers when the pedicle of the flap is detached. The entire lining flap, except for the base of the pedicle, is thinned to the level of the subcutaneous plane.

An incision is made at the mucocutaneous junction around the perimeter of the nasal defect. Adjacent skin is reflected sufficiently to expose the bone of the frontal processes of the maxillae. This provides access for attaching bone grafts for skeletal support of the upper vault. The mucosa along the perimeter is reflected sufficiently to provide a flap of tissue. The mucosal margins are approximated to the margins of the forehead lining flap with 3-0 running polyglactin suture. Bone grafts are shaped and contoured to provide a framework for the dorsum and sidewalls. A dorsal bone graft is plated to the frontal bone at the level of the planned nasal frontal junction. This creates strong stable skeletal support for the upper and middle nasal vaults. Additional cranial bone is fashioned into two rectangular grafts. The length of the grafts is sufficient to extend from the maxilla to the level of the lower nasal vault. The grafts

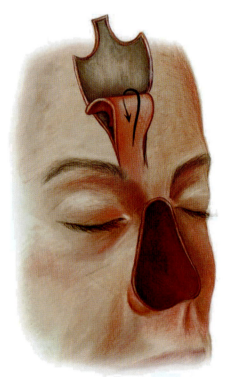
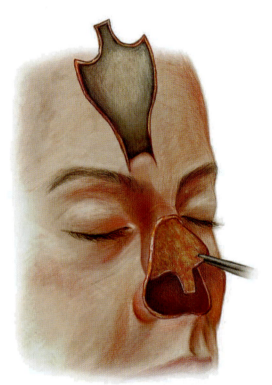

■ **Figure 14–12.** In cases of total or near total loss of nose where nasal septum is absent, a paramedian forehead flap may be used to provide internal nasal lining.

are plated to the dorsal bone graft and to the adjacent maxillae and serve as the framework for the nasal sidewalls. Several holes are drilled through the bone grafts, and horizontal mattress polyglactin sutures are placed through the holes and the lining flap to approximate the exposed raw surface of the flap against the undersurface of the bone grafts. Cartilage grafts are then used to create the framework for the lower nasal vault. The grafts can be stabilized to the caudal end of the bony sidewall grafts with sutures passed through holes drilled in the bone. Once the framework for the lower vault has been constructed, mattress sutures are used to approximate the forehead lining flap against the undersurface of the cartilages. It is important that the lining flap completely cover the undersurface of the bone and cartilage grafts so they are not exposed to the nasal passage.

When the framework has been constructed and secured to the maxillae, a template is fashioned to design a covering flap using a second paramedian forehead flap based on the contralateral supratrochlear artery. The second flap is pivoted toward the midline, and the distal two-thirds of the flap is thinned and used to cover all of the framework. The caudal border of this flap is sutured to the caudal border of the lining flap, completely enveloping the cartilage grafts used for the lower vault framework. The lateral borders of the covering flap are sutured to the surrounding skin edges of the nasal defect. A few bolster sutures passing through both the covering and lining flap may be used to coapt the undersurfaces of the two flaps together and reduce dead space. The forehead donor site is large and can only partially be closed. The remaining forehead wound is allowed to heal by secondary intention.

When dual paramedian forehead flaps are used to provide lining and cover, pedicle detachment is delayed for 2 months as both flaps depend on vascularization across a circumferential scar at the perimeter of the reconstructed nose. The pedicle of the lining flap is detached first, and the nasal fistula is closed. It is important to remove all of the skin of the portion of the pedicle that is beneath the covering flap and not exposed to the reconstructed nasal passage in order to prevent development of skin line cysts and subsequent infection and drainage. The covering flap is detached 2 months following detachment of the lining flap.

Forehead Expansion

Tissue expansion of the forehead in anticipation of using a paramedian forehead flap is not recommended because of the additional morbidity risk of the expansion process. In addition, forehead donor wounds that cannot be closed primarily heal by secondary intention and result in an acceptable appearing scar. However, tissue expansion may have a role in patients who require dual paramedian forehead flaps, which will require removal of the majority of the central forehead skin.[29] The patient must be informed that expansion of the forehead will be an additional surgical procedure and will cause an increasingly noticeable deformity of the forehead for several weeks before nasal reconstruction can be initiated.

Tissue expanders are Silastic balloons with self-sealing valves or reservoirs that are inserted beneath the skin. They are available in many different sizes and shapes such as round, rectangular, and elliptical and in volumes ranging from a few cubic centimeters to several thousand cubic centimeters. Tissue expanders are implanted by performing a ring block using 1% lidocaine and epinephrine (1:100,000 concentration). An access incision for placement of the expander is oriented vertically 3 cm behind the hairline in the paramedian position. The length of the incision should be limited to approximately half the length of the width of the expander. A recipient pocket is created by blunt dissection between the periosteum and the deep fascia of the frontalis muscle. The pocket should be large and extend inferiorly to the level of the supraorbital bony rims. An endoscope may be inserted through a separate scalp incision to assist in visualizing the dissection. The pocket is irrigated with a solution containing an antibiotic. A 250-mL rectangular tissue expander is folded on itself and inserted into the pocket through the access incision. The expander is unfolded within the pocket and manipulated until the base lies flat against the frontal bone without kinking. The injection port is tunneled posteriorly beneath the parietal scalp. Anchoring sutures to prevent migration of the expander are not necessary. The expander is partially expanded (approximately 25 mL for a 250-mL expander) with saline before wound closure to concomitantly obliterate dead space and assist with hemostasis. The incision is closed in layers with permanent sutures to approximate both the galea and the skin.

Inflation begins 2 weeks after implantation of the expander. After preparing the injection site with an alcohol swab, saline is infused by percutaneous puncture of the injection port with a 23-gauge scalp needle attached to a 50-mL syringe. The volume of injection depends on the tensile strength and tension of the skin overlying the expander and the amount of patient discomfort. If not precluded by the patient's discomfort, the forehead should be expanded until slight blanching is observed in the skin overlying the expander. Saline should then be withdrawn until the blanching disappears. However, tightness or pain is usually the limiting factor. Usually 25 to 30 mL of saline can be injected into a 250-mL volume expander on a weekly interval. The discomfort from inflation resolves within 24 to 48 hours, and the patient remains comfortable until the next inflation. Inflation is conducted once a week as more frequent expansion is associated with a greater risk of expander extrusion.

The volume of injected saline is recorded with each inflation. If weekly visits to the office for inflation are not possible, the patient or a family member may be taught the inflation technique. In-home expansion is facilitated by a written list of instructions. A small amount of methylene blue dye may initially be injected into the expander. Before inflation, the person doing the inflation may aspirate a small quantity of saline through the injection port. Proper placement of the needle has been achieved if blue solution is returned.

As expansion proceeds, the dermis becomes thinner, and a capsule forms around the expander. This often results in a reversible blue or red hue of the expanded skin. Dilated subcutaneous veins are frequently observed. The presence of the veins is not an indication of cyanosis or infection. Expansion continues until the circumference of the dome of the expanded skin measures two or three times the width of the proposed defect. For nasal reconstruction, 6 to 8 weeks of expansion are required to achieve this goal.

The second surgical stage requires removal of the expander and proceeding with reconstruction. The expander is deflated and removed through one of the incisions used to create the two paramedian forehead flaps. The capsule surrounding the expander provides an excellent blood supply to the flaps and is not disturbed unless thinning of the flap is necessary to achieve optimal results. A suction drain tube is employed at the donor site that can usually be closed primarily. Wound closure and postoperative care are similar to those used for standard flap surgery. It is important that the expanded forehead skin be supported by a rigid nasal framework to prevent flap contraction and loss of contour. The flaps should not be oversized but designed to reflect accurately the exact surface area required of the lining and cover for the missing nose.

Complications

Complications arising from the use of the paramedian forehead flap are rare as this is the "golden" flap of nasal reconstruction. The superficial axial blood supply of the flap provides ample nourishment, making distal flap necrosis unlikely. The superb vascularity of the flap also markedly reduces the risk of wound infection. However, this vascularity accounts for the most common complication observed with the paramedian fore-

head flap: the development of small hematomas under the distal flap. These develop at the time of initial flap transfer. The rich vascularity of the flap creates a tendency for the undersurface of the portion of the flap thinned of its muscle and subcutaneous fat at the time of transfer to bleed postoperatively. The potential dead space between the flap and the underlying nasal framework will accommodate small hematomas; there are no adhesions or sutures that adhere the covering flap to the framework. To reduce hematomas from developing, careful hemostasis is achieved over the entire raw undersurface of the thin portion of the flap. This portion requires special attention because it may ooze blood continually for a few hours after surgery. Compression dressings secured with a few bolster sutures passing full-thickness through the nose to the nasal passage and back again may be placed judiciously if bleeding is profuse. Bolster dressings, however, are not used routinely because they risk impairing the circulation to the distal flap.

Hematomas that do develop beneath the distal portion of the flap frequently cause a greater amount of swelling than expected and give the appearance of early trapdoor deformity. Usually, hematomas are not discovered until the pedicle of the flap is detached and the flap is inset. The exposed hematoma is managed by evacuating the accumulated blood and sharply scraping and débriding the fibrinous tissue deposited over the nasal framework.

Advantages

The advantages of the excellent blood supply of the paramedian forehead flap far exceed the problems of an occasional postoperative hematoma beneath the flap. One hundred forty-seven patients undergoing forehead flap repair of nasal defects following Mohs' surgery were reviewed from the University of Michigan Mohs database from 1993 to 1999.[30] Secondary procedures following pedicle detachment were performed in 79 patients (54%), with 1 procedure in 56, 2 procedures in 22, and 3 procedures in 1. These procedures consisted of contouring the flap in 68 patients, dermabrasion in 40, Z-plasty scar revision in 11, additional cartilage grafting in 2, and suspension suture for opening the nasal valve in 1. High aesthetic and functional goals were achieved in all patients (Figs. 14–13 and 14–14). No tumor recurrence or significant episodes of local bleeding or infection occurred. Perhaps the most significant finding of this study was that not a single case of significant flap necrosis occurred. Two (1%) patients did develop superficial partial-thickness necrosis. One case was related to a combination of a lengthy flap that was markedly thinned for the purpose of destroying hair follicles in an extended portion of the flap used to cover the columella. The other case occurred in an oblique forehead flap that was harvested 3 to 4 cm lateral to the axis of the supratrochlear artery. Epidermolysis and superficial necrosis occurred in the center of the distal flap. Fortunately, the area healed without impairing the appearance of the reconstructed nose.

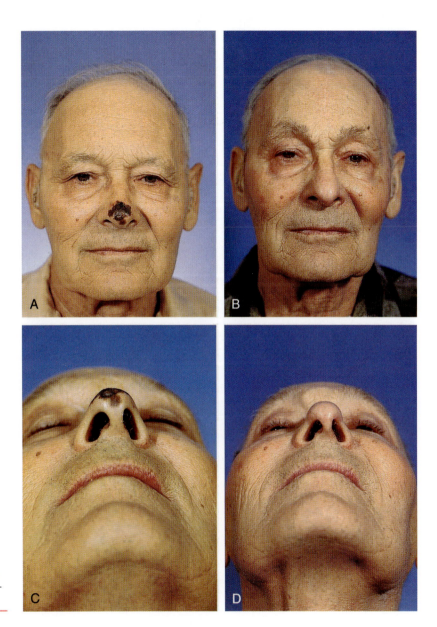

■ **Figure 14–13.** *A–D,* Preoperative and 2 years following excision of lentigo maligna and repair with forehead flap. No contouring procedure was necessary.

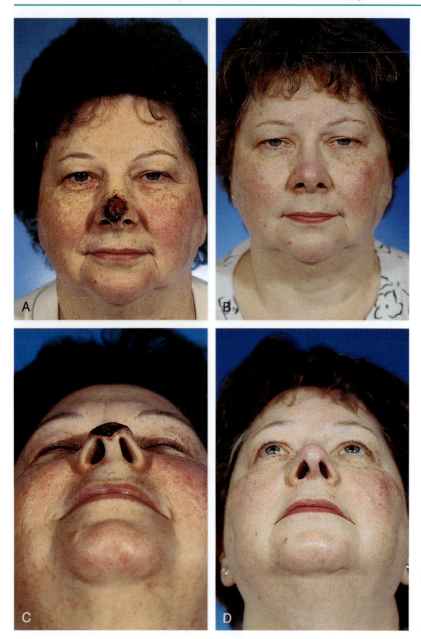

Figure 14–14. *A–D*, Preoperative view of skin defect and 7 months following repair with forehead flap. No contouring procedure was necessary.

References

1. Burget GC, Menick FJ: Nasal support and lining: the marriage of beauty and blood supply. Plast Reconstr Surg 84:189, 1989.

2. Conley JJ, Price JC: Midline vertical forehead flap. Otolaryngol Head Neck Surg 89:38, 1981.

3. Jackson IT: Local flaps in head and neck reconstruction. St. Louis, Mosby, 1985.

4. Converse JM: Reconstructive Plastic Surgery. Philadelphia, WB Saunders, 1964, p 797.

5. Converse JM: Reconstructive Plastic Surgery, 2nd ed. Philadelphia, WB Saunders, 1977, p 694.

6. Mazzola RF, Marcus S: History of total nasal reconstruction with particular emphasis on the folded forehead flap technique. Plast Reconstr Surg 72:408, 1983.

7. Menick FJ: Aesthetic refinements in use of the forehead flap for nasal reconstruction: The paramedian forehead flap. Clin Plast Surg 17:607, 1990.

8. Baker SR: Regional flaps in facial reconstruction. Otolaryngol Clin North Am 23:925, 1990.

9. McDowell F, Valone JA, Bronn JB: Bibliography and historical note on plastic surgery of the nose. Plast Reconstr Surg 10:149, 1952.

10. Shumrick KA, Smith TL: The anatomic basis for the design of forehead flaps in nasal reconstruction. Arch Otolaryngol Head Neck Surg 118:373, 1992.

11. Millard DR: Total reconstructive rhinoplasty and a missing link. Plast Reconstr Surg 37:167, 1966.

12. Kazanjian VH: The repair of nasal defects with the median forehead flap: Primary closure of the forehead wound. Surg Gynecol Obstet 83:37, 1946.

13. Gillies HD: Plastic Surgery of the Face. London, Frowde, Hodder, Stoughton, 1920, p 270.

14. Converse JM: Reconstructive Plastic Surgery, 2nd ed. Philadelphia, WB Saunders, 1977, p 1209.

15. Millard DR: Hemi-rhinoplasty. Plast Reconstr Surg 40:440, 1967.

16. Labat M: De la Rhinoplastic, Art de Restaurer ou de Refaire Completement la Nez [Dissertation]. Paris, Thesis, 1834.

17. Burget GC, Menick FJ: The subunit principle in nasal reconstruction. Plast Reconstr Surg 76:239, 1985.

18. Burget GC: Aesthetic reconstruction of the nose. Clin Plast Surg 12:463, 1985.

19. Burget GC, Menick FJ: Nasal reconstruction: Seeking a fourth dimension. Plast Reconstr Surg 78:145, 1986.

20. Mangold V, Lierse W, Pfeifer G: The arteries of the forehead as the basis of nasal reconstruction with forehead flaps. Acta Anat (Basel) 107:18, 1980.

21. McCarthy JG, Lorenc ZP, Cuting L, et al: The median forehead flap revisited: The blood supply. Plast Reconstr Surg 76:866, 1985.

22. McCarthy JG: Acquired Deformities of the Nose in Plastic Surgery, 3rd ed. Philadelphia, WB Saunders, 1990, p 1925.

23. Burget GC: Current Therapy in Plastic and Reconstructive Surgery. New York, BC Decker, pp 400–412, 1989.

24. Barton FE: Aesthetic aspects of nasal reconstruction. Clin Plast Surg 15:155, 1988.

25. Hart NB, Goldin JM: The importance of symmetry in forehead flap rhinoplasty. Br J Plast Surg 37:477, 1984.

26. Converse JM, Wood-Smith D: Experiences with the forehead island flap with a subcutaneous pedicle. Plast Reconstr Surg 31:521, 1963.

27. Baker SR: Oblique forehead flap for total reconstruction of the nasal tip and columella. Arch Otolaryngol Head Neck Surg 111:425, 1985.

28. Baker SR, Alford EL: Mid-forehead flap. Op Tech Otolaryngol Head Neck Surg 4:24, 1993.

29. Baker SR, Swanson NA: Tissue expansion of the head and neck: Indications, techniques and complications. Arch Otolaryngol Head Neck Surg 116:1147, 1990.

30. Boyd CM, Baker SR, Fader DJ, et al: The forehead flap for nasal reconstruction. Am J Derm 136:1365, 2000.

15

Refinement Techniques

Sam Naficy

Nasal reconstruction begins with transfer of tissue of volume and surface area similar to those of the missing tissues. Depending on the nature of the defect and the type of flap used, some amount of sculpting of the subcutaneous tissues of the covering flap is usually necessary. With increasing experience and skill of the surgeon, a greater level of refinement may be achieved in the initial stages of reconstruction. However, for complex nasal repairs, it is often necessary to perform additional staged procedures aimed at improving the final aesthetic outcome.

Contouring of Flaps

There are three stages at which thinning and contouring of covering flaps may be performed. Sculpting of the restored nasal framework and overlying flaps and grafts begins at the time of initial repair. Depending on the type used, the flap may be thinned of accompanying muscle and fat when initially dissected (forehead flap) without compromising survival. This initial contouring will at times be sufficient and eliminate the need for additional procedures. However, there are limits to the extent of thinning and debulking that may be performed at the initial stage. Excessive contouring may compromise the vascularity of the flap, leading to necrosis. This is especially true for smokers or individuals who have peripheral vascular disease, as in cases of diabetes or following irradiation. When an interpolated flap is used as a covering flap, the distal portion is contoured at the initial transfer. Three weeks later,

when the pedicle is detached from the donor site, the more proximal portion of the flap is sculpted so that flap thickness matches the adjacent nasal skin. The 3-week interval between flap transfer and pedicle division and flap inset enables the surgeon to safely thin the proximal portion of the flap. By this time the distal portion of the flap has developed adequate collateral circulation to support the proximal portion. Interpolated paramedian forehead and cheek flaps are thinned in this staged manner. When necessary, a third contouring of the flap is performed. This is delayed for 2 or 3 months following pedicle detachment. By then, the flap has acquired an adequate blood supply from its periphery and underlying soft tissues and is capable of withstanding more aggressive removal of subcutaneous fat.

Contouring procedures are performed under local anesthesia with or without intravenous sedation. An intravenous dose of an antistaphylococcal antibiotic is given preoperatively if bone or cartilage grafting was performed at the initial reconstructive procedure. The incision and area of planned contouring are infiltrated with lidocaine 1% with 1:100,000 concentration of epinephrine. Excessive infiltration of local anesthetic is avoided as it may distend tissues, making contour analysis difficult. The face is prepared with Betadine and draped appropriately.

Interpolated Paramedian Forehead Flaps

Interpolated paramedian forehead flaps used to repair skin-only defects of the nasal tip and dorsum may be thinned to the fat immediately beneath the dermis at the time of flap transfer (see Chapter 14). For individuals who do not use tobacco products, it is safe to initially thin the distal 2 to 3 cm of the flap to this level. If the flap is more than 3 cm in vertical height, it is prudent to maintain the galea and frontalis muscle in the more proximal portion of the flap and delay the thinning of this area until the time of pedicle division. The flap is thinned at initial transfer by placing it, skin side down, on a moistened 4 × 4 sponge. A no. 15 scalpel blade is used to make an incision parallel to the skin surface along the distal borders of the flap in the superficial subcutaneous plane. This incision controls the amount of subcutaneous tissue maintained under the dermis so that the overall thickness of the flap will match the thickness of the recipient site. The galea, frontalis muscle, and deep subcutaneous fat are removed from the central portion of the distal flap. Varying amounts of subcutaneous fat are left attached to the undersurface of the flap laterally to match the thicker skin of the nasal alae. Generally, bolsters or compression dressings are not used at the time of initial flap transfer and distal thinning as this may compromise the vascularity of the flap.

When the flap is used to cover the tip and is sutured to the thin skin of the facet or columella, all subcutaneous fat is removed from the caudal border of the flap. This provides a better match in thickness between flap and nasal skin. It is sometimes even necessary to remove some of the deeper dermis along the caudal border with a beveled excision. This maneuver facilitates an improved skin-thickness match with the extremely thin skin of the infratip and facets. Thinning and beveling of the dermis may be accomplished with the convex side of curved iris or tenotomy scissors.

When dividing the pedicle and insetting the flap, incisions are made through the scar between the proximal flap and the nasal skin to release the cephalic fourth of the flap from the nose. This provides the necessary exposure for contouring the proximal portion of the flap not thinned at the time of initial transfer. This portion of the flap is elevated and sharply thinned to the appropriate level. In the case of repairing skin-only nasal defects that involve the rhinion, it may be necessary to remove all subcutaneous fat in order to more accurately replicate the naturally thin skin of the rhinion. The nasal skin surrounding the area where the flap was released from the nose is undermined 1 cm. It is often necessary to remove early scar tissue under the flap to facilitate proper tailoring. Deep-layer closure is unnecessary, because the flap is trimmed so there is no wound closure tension. The flap is inset with interrupted vertical mattress or simple 5-0 polypropylene cutaneous sutures. A light compression dressing is applied overnight.

Interpolated Cheek Flaps

The blood supply and perfusion pressure of cheek flaps are not as robust as those of the paramedian forehead flap. More prudence is exercised in thinning of this flap at the time of initial transfer. Cheek flaps are most commonly used for repair of defects of the ala and, as a general rule, require a flap with thicker skin and more subcutaneous tissue than skin flaps used to repair other areas of the nose. Thinning of the entire flap to the plane of the superficial subcutaneous fat may not be necessary. However, some thinning of the flap is always necessary. When initially transferred to the nose, the distal one-third to one-half of an interpolated cheek flap may be safely thinned to the appropriate subcutaneous plane required to match the depth of the defect.

Interpolated cheek flaps are detached from the cheek and inset 3 weeks following transfer (see Chapter 13). The portion of the flap attached to the nose is released from the adjacent nasal skin for a distance of 0.5 to 1 cm to achieve sufficient freedom to unfurrow the more proximal portion of the flap. The distal half to third of the flap, which was thinned at the time of initial transfer, is not dissected in order to maintain the distal blood supply. The proximal flap is elevated in a subcutaneous plane, and excessive subcutaneous fat is trimmed with a no. 15 scalpel blade. In males, hair-bearing flaps are dissected in a more superficial plane so as to expose hair follicles that are destroyed with pinpoint electrocautery using magnification (Fig. 15–1).

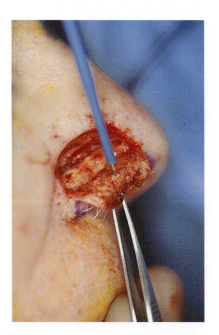

■ **Figure 15–1.** Hair follicles are exposed in subdermal fat and destroyed with pinpoint electrocautery.

Nasal Cutaneous Flaps

Pivotal flaps are based on the skin and soft tissue adjacent to the defect. The bilobe flap is the most common pivotal flap used for nasal reconstruction (see Chapter 10). At the time of transfer, the flap may be safely thinned to the ideal thickness. When the skin adjacent to the defect is quite thin, the first lobe of the flap is thinned of its underlying muscle and fascia to avoid a disparity in thickness.

Secondary Contouring

Three months following pedicle division and inset of an interpolated covering flap, consideration needs to be

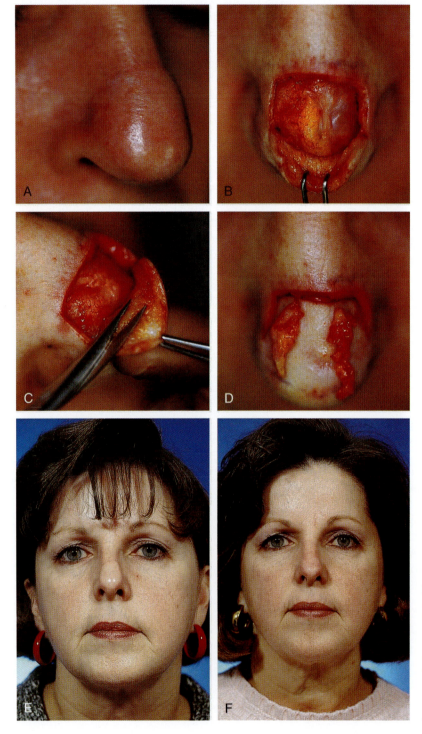

■ **Figure 15–2.** Contouring of paramedian forehead flap used to resurface nasal tip. *A,* Note fullness of flap prior to contouring. *B,* Flap elevated in superficial subcutaneous plane. Fat attached to underlying nasal cartilages will be removed. *C,* Additional subdermal fat is removed from flap with iris scissors. *D,* Fat removed on completion of contouring. *E* and *F,* Before and 3 months following contouring of paramedian forehead flap used to resurface nasal tip.

given to contouring the flap. This procedure is performed if the covering flap appears thickened and does not accurately reflect the topography of the underlying nasal framework. In these circumstances the flap is elevated in the superficial subcutaneous plane to expose deeper scar and subcutaneous fat. The underside of the flap is thinned of fat using fine scissors, and the deeper scar and subcutaneous fat are completely removed to expose the nasal framework (Fig. 15–2).

A contouring procedure to create an alar groove is a necessary third surgical stage in 75% of cases of alar reconstruction. This is performed 3 months following detachment of the pedicle of the interpolated cheek or forehead flap used for resurfacing the ala. The procedure is necessary whenever the defect extends cephalic to the alar groove. A template of the contralateral normal alar unit is made, reversed, placed over the reconstructed ala, and carefully traced with a marking pen (Fig. 15–3). The superior border of the tracing represents the appropriate location for the alar groove. If the superior border of the flap is no greater than 1 cm superior to the border of the tracing, then the scar marking the juncture of the flap and nasal skin is used as the access incision for contouring the flap. If a larger portion of the sidewall was resurfaced, a 3-cm incision is made in the flap, along the superior border of the tracing. The flap is undermined, leaving a few millimeters of subcutaneous fat attached to the dermis. In males, the flap is elevated in a more superficial plane immediately below the dermis in order to expose the hair follicles transferred from the cheek. This may require undermining the entire flap caudally to the level of the nostril margin. The exposed follicles are individually cauterized under loupe magnification with a fine-tipped monopolar electrocautery. The power setting of the cautery device is set sufficiently low to prevent damage to the adjacent dermis. To ensure flap survival in patients who use tobacco products, it may be prudent to depilate the flap in two stages: (1) the upper portion of the flap at the time of flap contouring and restoration of the alar groove and (2) the lower portion 2 to 3 months later.

Flap contouring and constructing an alar groove is accomplished by removing scar tissue and the majority of the remaining subcutaneous fat beneath the flap. Excision continues deeply until the cartilage graft used as the alar batten is exposed. A trough of cartilage centered under the planned alar groove is excised from the graft with a scalpel. The trough typically measures 4 to 5 mm wide and extends along the entire projected length of the groove. Care is taken not to deepen the cartilage trough excessively, as this may cause a depressed narrow crease to form in place of the shallow valley of the alar groove typically observed in most noses. Some of the cartilage shavings may be replaced if overcorrected. Proper contour is determined by replacing the skin of the flap and compressing it gently.

Continued excision of soft tissue and cartilage is performed until the constructed groove has a topography identical to its counterpart. The skin incision is repaired with 5-0 polypropylene interrupted cutaneous sutures. A dental roll is cut longitudinally and used as a bolster. It is secured in place along the length of the constructed groove by passing interrupted 4-0 polypropylene sutures full-thickness through the nose in such a manner to straddle the groove (see Fig. 15–3). The sutures are tied lightly over the dental roll. Tight sutures may cause flap necrosis as considerable flap swelling occurs postoperatively. The roll offers an effective method of obliterating potential dead space, enhancing hemostasis, and maintaining the constructed alar groove. The bolster is removed on the fifth postoperative day along with the cutaneous sutures.

Excessive thickness of the nostril margin may result from reconstruction of full-thickness defects involving the alar margin, causing noticeable differences in thickness of the two alae. This is particularly problematic in patients with delicate nostrils. Thinning of the alar margin from the superior approach is not always expedient and may warrant a direct approach along the margin of the reconstructed ala. In these cases, the ala is thinned by excision of underlying soft tissue through an incision at the free margin of the thickened ala. Excision of a narrow ellipse of flap skin may be necessary at the alar margin to achieve sufficient narrowing. Skin excision may also be necessary on rare occasions to elevate the alar margin when it is positioned more caudally than desirable. The site of the excision or incision is repaired in one layer with 6-0 nylon or polypropylene suture. The dead space between the lining and external skin of the ala is eliminated by placement of an intranasal pack consisting of a single dental roll positioned inside the nasal vestibule with a light external compression dressing. The dressing is removed the first postoperative day.

Alar Base Reduction

Discrepancy in nostril size may result after reconstruction of full-thickness defects of the ala. This asymmetry is usually due to the reconstructed side being smaller that its counterpart. In most instances, as long as the native nostril is not excessively narrow, it may be reduced in size by a unilateral full-thickness alar base reduction (Fig. 15–4). Approximately 1 mm of ala is maintained medial to the alar-facial sulcus. The triangular area to be removed is marked with a surgical marker and excised with a no. 11 scalpel blade. A single deep 5-0 polydioxanone suture is used to approximate the wound. The nasal base is checked for symmetry, and the repair is completed with multiple 5-0

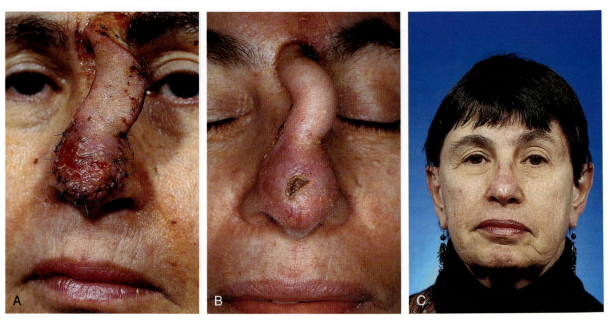

Figure 16–2. *A,* Epidermolysis of paramedian forehead flap. *B,* Detachment delayed until flap was healed. Partial-thickness necrosis of central flap is present. *C,* 6 months following pedicle detachment. Revision surgery was not required.

over concave areas of the nasal sidewall and alar groove. When necrosis of lining flaps occurs, the involved area is débrided, and exposed cartilage and bone are covered with petroleum-based topical antibiotic ointment. This facilitates granulation tissue formation. The patient is also treated with oral antibiotics. This complication is of minimum consequence when the involved area is small and removed from the nostril margin. However, it may result in notching and deformity if it occurs near the alar margin.

Necrosis of a large portion of a cutaneous flap is very rare and is more likely to occur in heavy smokers. It may also be caused by obstruction of vascular inflow or outflow secondary to a twisted or excessively narrow pedicle. This complication requires a salvage operation to prevent loss of the underlying grafts or contracture of the underlying lining tissue. The necrotic flap is excised, the edges of the defect are freshened, and a second cutaneous flap is designed to provide cover. When 1 cm^2 or greater exposure of a cartilage graft occurs, the graft will absorb or die unless another covering flap is used in a timely fashion. The cartilage graft will remain viable as long as the underside of the graft is nourished by vascularized lining tissue. Prior to covering the cartilage graft with a second flap, a thin layer of cartilage may be shaved from the exposed surface of the graft. The salvage flap should be designed with a wider pedicle than usual, and initial thinning should be minimized. In patients who use tobacco products, it may be prudent, when possible, to delay the covering flap for 10 days before flap transfer.

Skin Graft Necrosis

Skin or composite grafts undergoing partial necrosis are best kept dry and allowed to form an eschar of the necrotic segment. The eschar remains as a biological dressing. As the surrounding and underlying tissues heal around the eschar, the edges of the eschar will separate from the wound and may be trimmed. The entire eschar is removed when epithelialization is complete beneath it.

Complete full-thickness loss of skin grafts may be due to heavy tobacco use, infection, an excessively thick graft, or an inadequate bolster dressing. The necrotic graft is allowed to form an eschar, and the wound bed heals by secondary intention, sometimes with satisfactory results. Dermabrasion usually improves the appearance of the scar (Fig. 16–4).

Alar Retraction

Alar retraction or notching is the most common complication of reconstructing full-thickness alar defects. It is usually due to necrosis of the lining or covering flap. This exposes the alar batten graft, which subsequently absorbs, resulting in retraction or notching of the nostril (Fig. 16–5). Minor notching of the nostril is corrected

given to contouring the flap. This procedure is performed if the covering flap appears thickened and does not accurately reflect the topography of the underlying nasal framework. In these circumstances the flap is elevated in the superficial subcutaneous plane to expose deeper scar and subcutaneous fat. The underside of the flap is thinned of fat using fine scissors, and the deeper scar and subcutaneous fat are completely removed to expose the nasal framework (Fig. 15–2).

A contouring procedure to create an alar groove is a necessary third surgical stage in 75% of cases of alar reconstruction. This is performed 3 months following detachment of the pedicle of the interpolated cheek or forehead flap used for resurfacing the ala. The procedure is necessary whenever the defect extends cephalic to the alar groove. A template of the contralateral normal alar unit is made, reversed, placed over the reconstructed ala, and carefully traced with a marking pen (Fig. 15–3). The superior border of the tracing represents the appropriate location for the alar groove. If the superior border of the flap is no greater than 1 cm superior to the border of the tracing, then the scar marking the juncture of the flap and nasal skin is used as the access incision for contouring the flap. If a larger portion of the sidewall was resurfaced, a 3-cm incision is made in the flap, along the superior border of the tracing. The flap is undermined, leaving a few millimeters of subcutaneous fat attached to the dermis. In males, the flap is elevated in a more superficial plane immediately below the dermis in order to expose the hair follicles transferred from the cheek. This may require undermining the entire flap caudally to the level of the nostril margin. The exposed follicles are individually cauterized under loupe magnification with a fine-tipped monopolar electrocautery. The power setting of the cautery device is set sufficiently low to prevent damage to the adjacent dermis. To ensure flap survival in patients who use tobacco products, it may be prudent to depilate the flap in two stages: (1) the upper portion of the flap at the time of flap contouring and restoration of the alar groove and (2) the lower portion 2 to 3 months later.

Flap contouring and constructing an alar groove is accomplished by removing scar tissue and the majority of the remaining subcutaneous fat beneath the flap. Excision continues deeply until the cartilage graft used as the alar batten is exposed. A trough of cartilage centered under the planned alar groove is excised from the graft with a scalpel. The trough typically measures 4 to 5 mm wide and extends along the entire projected length of the groove. Care is taken not to deepen the cartilage trough excessively, as this may cause a depressed narrow crease to form in place of the shallow valley of the alar groove typically observed in most noses. Some of the cartilage shavings may be replaced if overcorrected. Proper contour is determined by replacing the skin of the flap and compressing it gently.

Continued excision of soft tissue and cartilage is performed until the constructed groove has a topography identical to its counterpart. The skin incision is repaired with 5-0 polypropylene interrupted cutaneous sutures. A dental roll is cut longitudinally and used as a bolster. It is secured in place along the length of the constructed groove by passing interrupted 4-0 polypropylene sutures full-thickness through the nose in such a manner to straddle the groove (see Fig. 15–3). The sutures are tied lightly over the dental roll. Tight sutures may cause flap necrosis as considerable flap swelling occurs postoperatively. The roll offers an effective method of obliterating potential dead space, enhancing hemostasis, and maintaining the constructed alar groove. The bolster is removed on the fifth postoperative day along with the cutaneous sutures.

Excessive thickness of the nostril margin may result from reconstruction of full-thickness defects involving the alar margin, causing noticeable differences in thickness of the two alae. This is particularly problematic in patients with delicate nostrils. Thinning of the alar margin from the superior approach is not always expedient and may warrant a direct approach along the margin of the reconstructed ala. In these cases, the ala is thinned by excision of underlying soft tissue through an incision at the free margin of the thickened ala. Excision of a narrow ellipse of flap skin may be necessary at the alar margin to achieve sufficient narrowing. Skin excision may also be necessary on rare occasions to elevate the alar margin when it is positioned more caudally than desirable. The site of the excision or incision is repaired in one layer with 6-0 nylon or polypropylene suture. The dead space between the lining and external skin of the ala is eliminated by placement of an intranasal pack consisting of a single dental roll positioned inside the nasal vestibule with a light external compression dressing. The dressing is removed the first postoperative day.

Alar Base Reduction

Discrepancy in nostril size may result after reconstruction of full-thickness defects of the ala. This asymmetry is usually due to the reconstructed side being smaller that its counterpart. In most instances, as long as the native nostril is not excessively narrow, it may be reduced in size by a unilateral full-thickness alar base reduction (Fig. 15–4). Approximately 1 mm of ala is maintained medial to the alar-facial sulcus. The triangular area to be removed is marked with a surgical marker and excised with a no. 11 scalpel blade. A single deep 5-0 polydioxanone suture is used to approximate the wound. The nasal base is checked for symmetry, and the repair is completed with multiple 5-0

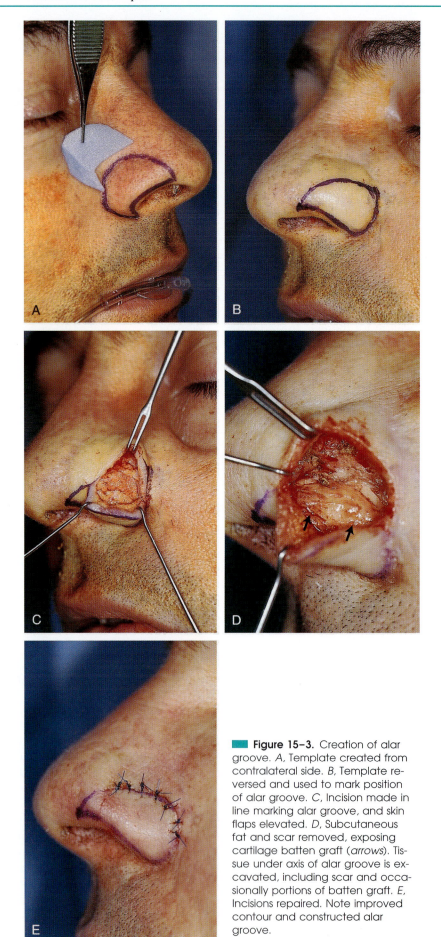

Figure 15–3. Creation of alar groove. *A*, Template created from contralateral side. *B*, Template reversed and used to mark position of alar groove. *C*, Incision made in line marking alar groove, and skin flaps elevated. *D*, Subcutaneous fat and scar removed, exposing cartilage batten graft (*arrows*). Tissue under axis of alar groove is excavated, including scar and occasionally portions of batten graft. *E*, Incisions repaired. Note improved contour and constructed alar groove.

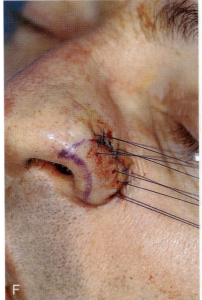
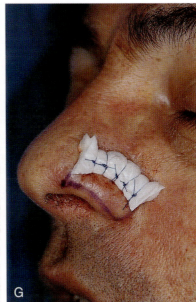

Figure 15-3 *Continued. F* and *G,* Full-thickness bolster sutures straddling constructed alar groove secure dressing that extends length of groove.

fast-absorbing gut suture placed in a vertical mattress fashion.

Correction of Alar Notching

Alar notching or retraction may occur following alar reconstruction in spite of cartilage batten grafts being used for the alar framework. This occurs most frequently when a portion of the distal covering or lining flap has undergone necrosis. Minor notching can sometimes be corrected during construction of the alar groove. Cartilage trimmed during construction of the groove is used to correct the notch (see Chapters 13 and 20). The skin overlying the notched area is undermined from above through the access incision used for the contouring procedure. A subcutaneous pocket is created in the area of the notch to accommodate a cartilage graft of an appropriate size to efface the notch. Care is taken not to penetrate the skin during dissection. In the event of penetration, it is carefully repaired before the cartilage graft is placed. If possible, the superior edge of the graft is secured to the inferior border of any pre-existing cartilage with figure-of-eight 5-0 absorbable sutures. If this is not possible, the cartilage graft is stabilized by a transnasal mattress suture

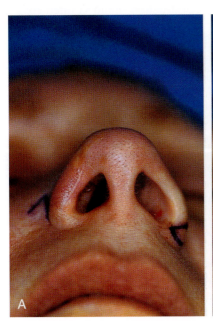
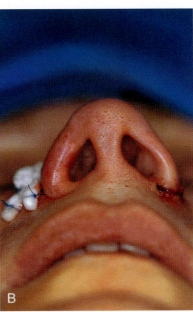

Figure 15-4. Unilateral alar base reduction. *A,* Reconstruction of right ala has resulted in slight reduction in nostril size. Left alar base is marked for reduction. *B,* Left alar base is reduced to improve discrepancy in size. Z-plasty (under bolster dressing) of scar in right alar groove is performed concomitantly.

that straddles the skin of the alar margin on both sides of the graft. More severe notching or greater alar retraction is corrected by complete mobilization of the skin in the affected area and insertion of a cartilage graft to maintain caudal displacement of the mobilized skin (see Chapter 16).

Contour Grafting

Contour depressions are unusual following nasal reconstruction. However, there are instances when contour irregularities occur under skin grafts and flaps used for repair of nasal defects. This is usually the result of too much soft tissue having been removed during a contouring procedure. To correct this problem, it is necessary to undermine the skin covering the involved area and insert a soft-tissue graft consisting of fat, dermis, or fascia. Alloplastic grafts placed subcutaneously may also be used to elevate a depressed area.

Hair Removal

Several options exist for removal of unwanted hair on flaps used for nasal reconstruction. Interpolated cheek flaps in men and interpolated paramedian forehead flaps with extensions to the hair-bearing scalp are the two most common situations involving transfer of a large number of viable hair follicles to the nose. In the paramedian forehead flap, the majority of hair follicles may be removed or destroyed at the time of initial flap transfer. Forehead flaps used as covering flaps are usually thinned to the level of the subcutaneous fat, exposing hair follicles. Using a fine-point tip electrocautery at low setting, each hair follicle is individually cauterized under magnification. It is important to avoid aggressive cautery of a large number of hair follicles in the distal flap, especially in smokers. It may be beneficial to place the epidermal surface of the flap over a sponge moistened with iced saline to reduce thermal damage to the more superficial tissues.

In contrast to the forehead flap, most of the hair follicles transferred to the nose with a cheek flap cannot be obliterated during the initial transfer of the flap. To ensure the vascularity of the flap, a greater amount of subcutaneous fat is maintained on the undersurface, compared with a forehead flap. This prevents exposure of most hair follicles. Although limited depilation can take place during flap transfer and subsequent inset, a second surgical depilation is usually necessary. This is performed during the contouring procedure. One or two procedures to depilate the flap are usually success-

ful in eliminating all hair growth. In contrast to the cheek flap, hair growth on the nose transferred there by a forehead flap is considerably more recalcitrant to treatment. This is because the hair growing in the scalp has three growth phases. One of these is a dormant phase in which the follicles may not be visible in the subcutaneous tissues. Hair on the face is not subject to a dormant phase; all hair follicles transferred with a cheek flap are visible to the surgeon during surgical depilation, thus making it less likely to require additional depilation procedures.

Electrolysis is another option for removal of a limited number of unwanted hairs. The success of this procedure is operator-dependant. A thin wire electrode is passed along the shaft of the hair, and a small flow of current initiates a number of thermal and chemical reactions that destroy the follicle.

Depilatory creams are the most useful for multiple fine vellus hairs not easily addressed with surgery or electrolysis. These are available over the counter and may be used by the patient as needed.

Laser hair reduction is achieved by selective photothermolysis of hair follicles by absorption of light energy through intact skin. A number of laser hair removal systems are available, employing a variety of wavelengths of light. The ideal candidate for this technique is an individual with fair skin and dark hair so that the majority of the light energy is absorbed by the hair follicle, and little thermal damage is incurred to the epidermal layer.

Concurrent Rhinoplasty

Depending on the size and location of a nasal defect and the method of reconstruction, there is often excellent exposure offered to the nasal framework. This exposure may enable concurrent aesthetic modification of the nasal framework or functional procedures to improve an obstructed nasal airway.

Certain cutaneous defects of the dorsum may be repaired primarily if an underlying convexity of the nasal bridge is reduced. Reduction facilitates closure by reducing the skeletal volume of the nose, thus increasing the redundancy of the nasal skin. This may at times allow primary closure of a defect that may have otherwise required a flap or a skin graft for repair. If primary closure is feasible, the remaining nasal skin and soft tissues are widely undermined in the subfascial plane through the access offered by the defect. This is the same plane used for skin elevation in open rhinoplasty and for nasal cutaneous flaps. If the defect does not extend to the nasal skeleton, it is deepened to the level of the subfascial plane by removing soft tissue at its base. Using an angled Aufricht or Converse retractor, dissection is continued in this plane, undermining skin over the entire bony and cartilaginous dorsum, sidewalls, and tip. The cartilaginous convexity is removed sharply with a no. 11 or no. 15 scalpel blade. Osteotomes are used for resection of the bony convexity. Medial and lateral osteotomies may be necessary if dorsal reduction results in a significant bony open roof. A cartilaginous open roof may be repaired with spreader grafts harvested from the septum. Primary closure of the wound is then achieved if it can be performed in a manner that does not create excessive wound closure tension or distortion of free margins of the nose. Depending on skin mobility, proximity of the defect to the tip, and the desired amount of cephalic rotation, wound closure is planned either horizontally or vertically.

Aesthetic or functional rhinoplasty may also be performed subsequent to nasal reconstruction. The reconstruction may involve any combination of surgical procedures and usually does not preclude an aesthetic rhinoplasty. The author recommends postponing aesthetic rhinoplasty for 1 year following nasal reconstruction in which a nasal cutaneous flap or interpolated cheek or forehead flap is used for repair. An open approach is most frequently advised, with standard marginal and transcolumellar incisions. Dissecting the skin from the reconstructed area of the nose is difficult secondary to scarring but can be performed safely. Once the nasal skin has been elevated from the nasal framework, modification of the framework is accomplished in a fashion identical to techniques used in standard rhinoplasty (Fig. 15–5).

Modifications of the bony pyramid may take the form of dorsal reduction and narrowing of an excessively broad bony pyramid. A significant profile reduction of the bony dorsum results in an open roof, requiring osteotomies to mobilize and medialize the bony sidewalls. The medial osteotomy begins at the superolateral portion of the open roof, extending to the junction of the nasal bone with the ascending process of the maxilla at the level of the medial canthus. We perform this osteotomy using a straight guarded osteotome. Perforating lateral osteotomies are performed with a 2-mm chisel, either percutaneously or directly over the periosteum. Digital pressure is used to create the desired infracture.

Narrowing of an excessively wide bony vault may be performed without dorsal reduction. The technique involves a bilateral or unilateral (if asymmetry is present) paramedian ostectomy performed immediately lateral to the bony septum. Removal of a segment of bone 2 to 3 mm in width creates an open roof without a significant reduction in dorsal projection. Osteotomies and infracture will then close the open roof and narrow the bony vault.

The middle vault includes the upper lateral cartilages and the dorsal cartilaginous septum. At the caudal aspect of the middle vault is the internal nasal valve. Narrowing of the angle between the septum and the upper lateral cartilages may result in nasal airway obstruction. The internal valve may be resected by ablative surgery necessary to remove a malignancy. In certain patients with weak upper lateral cartilages, the valve may be compromised by contracture of the overlying skin and soft tissue following reconstruction of nasal cutaneous defects. Spreader grafts are long rectangular grafts of septal or auricular cartilage placed between the dorsal margin of the upper lateral cartilages and the dorsal margin of the septum. Sheen and Sheen[1] described their use of the endonasal approach,

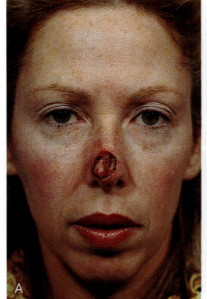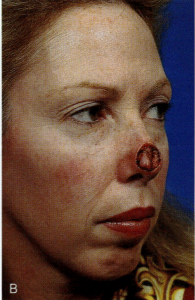

Figure 15–5. Reduction rhinoplasty performed subsequent to nasal reconstruction with paramedian forehead flap A and B, Cutaneous defect of nasal tip.

Illustration continued on following page

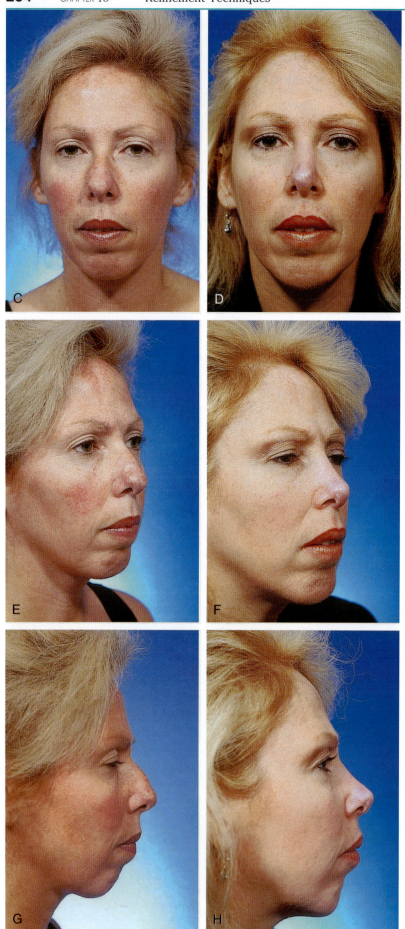

Figure 15–5 *Continued. C–H,* 8 months after paramedian forehead flap repair of nose and 14 months later following aesthetic rhinoplasty and mentoplasty.

and Johnson and Toriumi[2] described their external approach for placement of spreader grafts. When required, we insert spreader grafts through the external approach afforded by the reconstructive procedure. They are utilized to maintain the internal nasal valve or to widen a narrow middle vault (Fig. 15–6). Septal mucoperichondrium is hydrodissected with lidocaine (1% with 1:100,000 concentration of epinephrine). The upper lateral cartilages are detached submucosally from the cartilaginous septum, and mucoperichondrial flaps are elevated on either side of the septal cartilage as described in Chapter 7. Preserving a 1.0- to 1.5-cm dorsal strut of cartilage, sufficient septal cartilage is harvested for grafting. The mucoperichondrial flaps are approximated using a continuous quilting stitch of 3-0 chromic. Grafts are cut with a no. 15 scalpel blade to a

thickness of 1 to 2 mm, width of 4 to 5 mm, and length of 15 to 25 mm. The length depends on the vertical height of the upper lateral cartilages. Thickness depends on the thickness of the septal cartilage and the desired amount of lateralization of the upper lateral cartilages. Grafts are placed on each side and parallel to the dorsal cartilaginous septum. The grafts extend to the junction of the upper lateral cartilages and the nasal bones. We frequently utilize spreader grafts when reducing a markedly overprojected dorsum to prevent pinching of the middle vault. A double-layer spreader graft may occasionally be necessary, either bilaterally or unilaterally, for particularly narrow noses or to correct a longstanding crooked nose. Spreader grafts are held on either side of the septum with Brown-Adson forceps. A 30 gauge needle may be driven through all

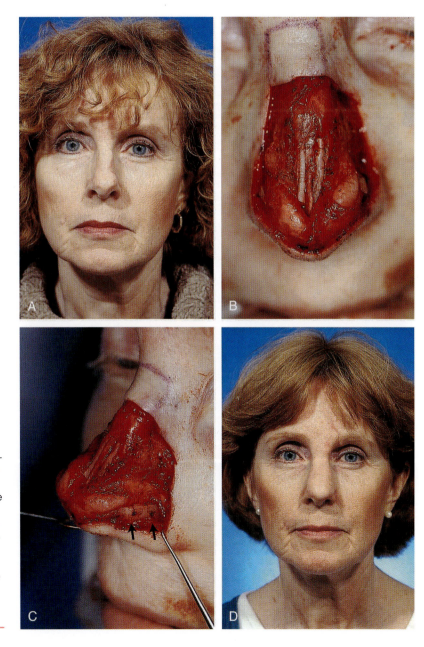

Figure 15–6. Spreader grafts used in reconstructive rhinoplasty. *A*, Preoperative view of patient with basal cell carcinoma of nasal tip and dorsum. Patient experienced nasal obstruction due to constriction of internal nasal valves. Note pinched middle vault. *B*, Following Mohs' surgery. Skin defect facilitated placement of bilateral spreader grafts, used to open apex of middle vault. *C*, Defect extended toward left ala, and a batten graft was secured inferior to left alar cartilage (*arrows*). *D*, 6 months following reconstruction with paramedian forehead flap. Spreader grafts have widened dorsum of middle vault.

three structures to temporarily stabilize them during suture placement. The upper lateral cartilages are retracted laterally. Several horizontal mattress sutures of 5-0 polydioxanone or polypropylene are then passed through both grafts and the intervening septum (see Chapter 5). The upper lateral cartilages are then secured to the spreader grafts and septum using similar sutures (see Fig. 15–6).

Modification of the nasal tip is performed with adherence to principles of cartilage preservation. The nasal framework must withstand the forces of scar contraction as a result of the reconstructive procedures used to repair the nasal skin defect. If the rhinoplasty is performed after the reconstructive procedure, the nasal cartilage must withstand the additional scarring that will result from the rhinoplasty. For this reason, techniques

that may significantly weaken the lower lateral cartilages and tip support are not used.

Volume reduction of the tip may be accomplished by trimming cephalic portions of the lateral crura during primary reconstruction or during a secondary contouring procedure. Before trimming, the intrinsic strength of the cartilages should be assessed to determine whether they will withstand the forces of scar contraction following nasal reconstruction and tip modification. Occasionally, a combination of cartilage trimming and suture contouring is necessary for refinement of the tip (Fig. 15–7). However, volume reduction of the lobule is usually accomplished only by suture contouring of the domes.[3] This may take the form of dome, interdomal, and lateral crural spanning sutures. Dome spanning sutures are used to narrow the individual domes. A mat-

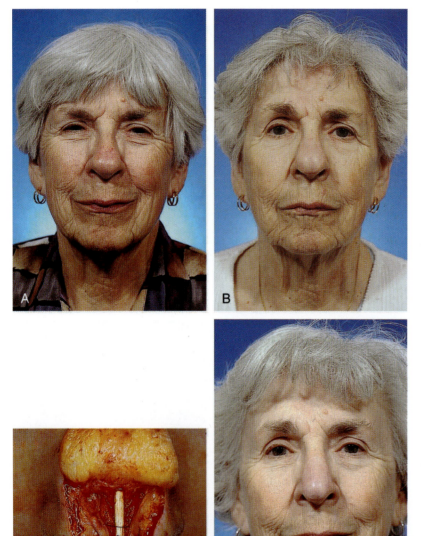

Figure 15–7. Suture narrowing of domes. *A,* Preoperative view of patient with basal cell carcinoma of nasal tip. Note broad tip. *B,* 5 months following paramedian forehead flap repair of tip. *C,* During contouring procedure, cephalic portion of lateral crura trimmed. In addition, dome-spanning sutures and lateral crural-spanning sutures (indicated by wooden applicator) used to narrow dome and supratip. *D,* 10 months following contouring procedure and modification of alar cartilages. Nasal tip and supratip have been narrowed.

tress suture of 5-0 polydioxanone or polypropylene is passed from the intermediate to lateral crus beneath the tip-defining point of the dome complex. Bilateral placement serves to narrow each dome. Depending on the placement of the spanning sutures, greater or lesser portions of the intermediate or lateral crura are recruited into the domal complex. Recruitment of cartilage into the dome region in this manner has the effect of increasing the intrinsic projection of the tip. Whereas dome spanning sutures narrow the domes individually, an interdomal suture has the effect of medializing each dome, narrowing the overall width of the tip.

Columellar struts, fashioned from septal or auricular cartilage, are placed between the medial crura to aid in tip projection and support. A pocket is dissected bluntly between the medial crura remaining above the nasal spine. A 1.5- to 2.0-mm-thick cartilage graft measuring 3 to 4 mm in width and 15 to 20 mm in length is sculpted and placed inside the pocket. The medial crura are secured to the graft with multiple mattress sutures of 5-0 polypropylene (see Chapter 5). Hydrodissection and elevation of the vestibular skin from the lateral aspect of the medial crura facilitate suture placement. Alternatively, percutaneous mattress sutures of 5-0 chromic gut may be placed through all three structures.

In addition to suture contouring, tip grafts may be used to modify the lobule during reconstructive procedures. A full discussion of tip grafting techniques is beyond the scope of this chapter. Grafts of multiple sizes and shapes may be sculpted from autologous septal or auricular cartilage. These grafts are used to enhance projection or modify contour of the nasal tip beyond what is possible using suture techniques and support grafts. Cartilage grafts are secured to the domes using 5-0 polypropylene or polydioxanone sutures. Grafts may be layered for more pronounced changes or crushed for more subtle alterations of tip contour in patients with thin nasal skin.

Scar Revision

Surgical revision of nasal scars may be performed to improve the appearance of depressed or widened scars and trapdoor deformities. Depressed scars may result from inadequate undermining of nasal skin or poor wound approximation during reconstruction of the nose. If the scar is favorably aligned, simple fusiform excision, undermining of the adjacent skin, and layered closure will often improve the appearance. The scar itself is excised superficially, leaving the deeper subdermal scar in situ. This maintains tissue bulk and prevents depression of the new scar. Skin adjacent to the excision is undermined in the subfascial plane, and the wound edges are advanced over the residual scar left

in situ. The wound is repaired in layers using buried absorbable sutures. The skin is approximated with 5-0 or 6-0 nonabsorbable suture.

Trapdoor deformity is often the result of a small hematoma occurring beneath the flap. It may also occur from inadequate undermining of the skin surrounding the periphery of the defect and in some flaps that have a curvilinear configuration. This type of deformity is not corrected with a resurfacing procedure such as dermabrasion and usually requires wide undermining of skin in the involved area and removal of underlying scar tissue. When the scar between flap and nasal skin is curvilinear, it may also be helpful to integrate flap and nasal skin using multiple small Z-plasties. The scar bordering the portion of the flap exhibiting the trapdoor deformity is excised, and undermining is performed in the subcutaneous plane 1.5 to 2 cm on both sides of the scar. Multiple Z-plasties are designed along the length of the scar (Fig. 15–8). Each triangular flap of the Z-plasty measures 5 mm in length and has a 30- to 40-degree angle. The flaps are transposed and secured at each apex with deep buried sutures of 5-0 polydioxanone. A small cutting needle with a half curve configuration is ideal for this purpose. The skin is approximated with interrupted simple or vertical mattress 5-0 or 6-0 polypropylene suture. The wound is cared for in the standard manner and sutures are removed in 5 to 7 days following the procedure. Dermabrasion of the scar and adjacent nasal skin may be performed in 6 to 8 weeks following scar revision.

Dermabrasion

Dermabrasion is one of the oldest resurfacing procedures aimed at improving the appearance of skin. It relies on the fact that there are epithelial elements of follicular and eccrine units located deep within the reticular dermis that are capable of re-epithelializing the denuded skin. As with other resurfacing procedures, dermabrasion results in production of a new epidermal layer as well as new collagen deposition. It can improve surface irregularities of scars bordering a flap or graft and may also improve pigmentary discrepancies between skin of the nose and that of flaps or grafts. The procedure is usually performed 6 to 8 weeks following nasal repair with a nasal cutaneous flap or full-thickness skin graft. When reconstructing the nose with interpolated cheek and forehead flaps, dermabrasion is delayed until all contouring procedures have been completed.

Dermabrasion is performed in the office or clinic procedure room with local anesthesia with or without oral sedation using diazepam. Appropriate photographs are taken prior to performing the procedure. We mark the

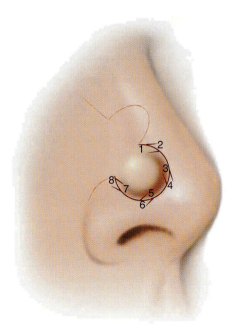
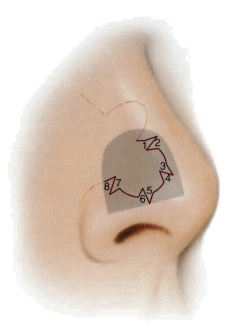

Figure 15–8. Trapdoor deformity corrected with undermining of flap and adjacent nasal skin (*shaded area*) and use of multiple Z-plasties

scars and any elevation or surface irregularity within the flap or graft with a surgical marker. Before infiltration with local anesthesia, the entire aesthetic unit or units involved with the reconstructive procedure are also marked for dermabrasion. For instance, when a small full-thickness skin graft is used to repair a defect of the tip, the entire tip is dermabraded. When a bilobe flap is used for reconstruction, we usually dermabrade the entire nose, sparing alar margins, columella, facets, and the most cephalic portion of the bridge and sidewalls.

The procedure is performed with the patient supine and the head of the bed elevated to reduce bleeding. Nerve blocks are performed in the periphery of the nose using lidocaine (1% with 1 : 100,000 concentration of epinephrine), and several minutes are allowed for the block to take effect. Additional local anesthetic is infiltrated within and just beyond the skin marked for treatment. Anesthetic is infiltrated in the skin as superficially as possible and in the immediate subdermal plane. Intradermal infiltration blocks the numerous sensory branches that terminate in the dermis of the skin.

Our preferred method of dermabrasion involves the use of an electric powered rotary wheel having a speed of 10,000 to 15,000 rpm. Diamond-studded fraises are available in a number of shapes and sizes (Fig. 15–9). The fraises we use most often are wheel-shaped, pear-shaped, or spherical. Steel-wire brush wheels are occasionally used but are more difficult to clean. For smaller areas, spot dermabrasion may be performed with a 5 × 5 cm piece of coarse-grade drywall sandpaper wrapped around a 3-mL syringe for easier handling (Fig. 15–10). This offers the advantage of minimal equipment, no need for cleaning or resterilization of

fraises, and avoids the potential for aerosol spread of blood-borne pathogens.

Powered dermabrasion is performed with the surgeon outfitted in a surgical gown, mask, and a face shield to protect against aerosolized blood and débris. The patient is covered with surgical drapes, and moistened eye pads are placed over both eyes to protect against overhead lighting and debris. Countertraction is applied to tighten the area being dermabraded. Marked scars and areas of contour irregularities are first addressed. Disappearance of the ink marking serves as a rough guide to the required depth of dermabrasion. Dermabrasion is to the level of the upper to mid-reticular dermis along the borders of scars. Elsewhere, the depth

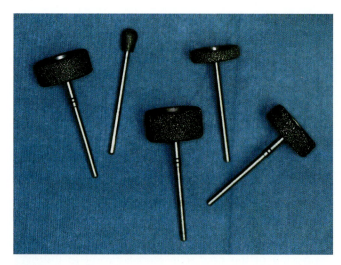

Figure 15–9. Assortment of diamond-studded fraises used for dermabrasion.

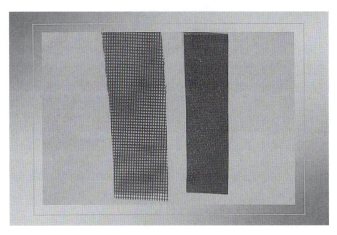

Figure 15–10. Spot dermabrasion may be performed with coarse-grade drywall sandpaper

of dermabrasion is extended to the level of punctate bleeding corresponding to midpapillary dermis. Digital palpation of the flap surface and scars is performed, and projecting areas are further abraded. Hemostasis is achieved by placing a 4 × 4 gauze soaked in hydrogen peroxide over the raw surface of the wound for approximately 5 minutes. The wound is dressed with a thick coat of petroleum-based ointment and covered with a nonadherent dressing. Patients are instructed to keep a generous amount of the ointment on the wound until epithelialization is complete. For the first few nights, the wound may be covered with a piece of household cellophane wrapping to avoid desiccation. Any buildup or crusting is cleaned after adequate soaking with a moistened washcloth or 4 × 4 gauze. The wound is then covered with additional ointment. Makeup may be worn after epithelialization is complete, usually in 7 to 10 days. A green-based concealer is helpful in camouflaging redness that may persist for 8 to 12 weeks. Sun avoidance and daily use of sunscreen are advised for the initial 6 months following the procedure. Irritation, superficial flaking, and itching of the new regenerated skin is common and may be treated twice daily with topical 1% hydrocortisone cream.

Eyebrow Repositioning

The interpolated paramedian forehead flap has the potential of causing residual lowering of the medial aspect of the ipsilateral eyebrow if the proximal pedicle is not carefully returned to the proper position at the time of detachment (see Chapter 14). Should this occur, one technique for elevation of the ptotic brow is a modified direct brow lift. A curvilinear incision is made superior to the medial half of the eyebrow. The incision is bev-

eled, paralleling the hair shafts of the eyebrow. A 2-cm-wide skin flap is dissected superiorly in the subcutaneous plane above the level of the orbicularis oculi and the frontalis muscles. The medial eyebrow is also dissected in the same plane of dissection. It is repositioned superiorly with multiple sutures of 4-0 polypropylene securing the eyebrow to the frontalis and periosteum. Care is taken to avoid placement of sutures in the region of the supraorbital neurovascular corridor. The eyebrow is positioned at a level that is approximately 2 to 3 mm higher that the opposite eyebrow to allow for a small amount of descent during healing. Redundant forehead skin is excised with a counterbevel incision in such a manner that the forehead skin approximates the skin of the eyebrow without traction being applied to the skin. The deep portion of the wound is repaired with 5-0 absorbable suture and the skin with a simple continuous 5-0 polypropylene suture.

When only the extreme medial aspect of the eyebrow is lower than its counterpart, it may be elevated by a Z-plasty. The medial eyebrow is incorporated in the inferior flap of the Z-plasty, and a superior flap is designed with the width necessary to ensure adequate eyebrow elevation following transposition of the two flaps. The medial eyebrow flap is elevated in a plane sufficiently deep to the hair follicles so as not to injure them. The flaps are transposed, and the wound is repaired in the same manner as discussed for scar revision.

Correcting Facial Asymmetry

Tissue transfer from the medial cheek to the nose via the interpolated cheek flap may result in a variable degree of asymmetry between the two melolabial folds. Older patients with redundant melolabial folds will often have an improved appearance on the operated side where skin and subcutaneous tissue were removed as part of the flap. In these instances, direct excision of a portion of the contralateral melolabial fold helps establish symmetry. Excision is planned in such a way that the resulting scar lies within the melolabial sulcus between the cheek and lips. This scar is generally quite acceptable (Fig. 15–11)

Correcting Contour Deformity

Occasionally, there may be persistent contour irregularity on the surface of the nose following repair with nasal cutaneous flaps or skin grafts. Most such deformities significantly improve with time and use of a resurfacing procedure such as dermabrasion. Should a de-

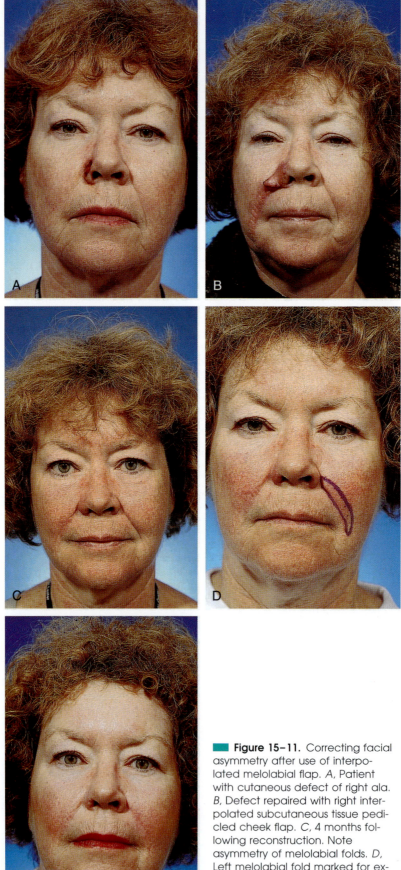

■ **Figure 15–11.** Correcting facial asymmetry after use of interpolated melolabial flap. *A,* Patient with cutaneous defect of right ala. *B,* Defect repaired with right interpolated subcutaneous tissue pedicled cheek flap. *C,* 4 months following reconstruction. Note asymmetry of melolabial folds. *D,* Left melolabial fold marked for excision. *E,* 5 months following excision of left melolabial fold. Note improvement of facial asymmetry.

pressed contour persist following transfer of a flap or a full-thickness skin graft to the nose, it may be improved using dermal allografts. An incision is made at the border of the flap or graft, and small Metzenbaum scissors are used to create a subcutaneous pocket under the area of depression. Sheets of the allograft, which are approximately 1 mm in thickness, are placed inside the pocket and stacked on top of each other to produce the desired contour elevation. The elevation should be slightly overcorrected to allow for some absorption of the grafting material. Preoperative antistaphylococcal antibiotic therapy and a 1-week postoperative course are indicated when using such implants.

References

1. Sheen JH, Sheen A: Aesthetic Rhinoplasty, 2nd ed. St. Louis, Quality Medical Publishing, 1987.

2. Johnson CJ, Toriumi DM: Open Structure Rhinoplasty, Philadelphia, WB Saunders, 1990.

3. Baker SR: Suture contouring of the nasal tip. Arch Facial Plast Surg 2:34, 2000.

16

Complications

Sam Naficy

Complications of nasal reconstruction may occur early or late in the postoperative course. Early complications include bleeding, infection, and flap necrosis. Scarring, nasal airway obstruction, cutaneous pigmentary abnormalities, and vascular abnormalities are late complications.

Hemorrhage

The most common risk factors for perioperative bleeding are hypertension, use of platelet-inhibiting medications such as nonsteroidal anti-inflammatory drugs, and excessive physical activity. High blood pressure, if present, is controlled with medication. Bleeding is most commonly from the undersurface of cutaneous flaps or raw edges of mucosal lining flaps. Preoperative use of topical vasoconstrictive nasal sprays may help reduce mucosal bleeding. When bleeding from the undersurface of forehead flaps is problematic, we apply topical thrombin to the bleeding surface before suturing the flap in place.

External bleeding may ensue from the exposed borders of interpolated flaps. Cauterizing the margins of the pedicle at the time of flap transfer is helpful in retarding postoperative bleeding; however, the pedicle usually oozes blood intermittently for 12 hours following flap transfer. Persistent bleeding beyond this period may be controlled with localized compression or by cautery.

Bleeding beneath a flap may jeopardize blood flow and survival of the flap. Bleeding is prevented by meticulous hemostasis and by judicious use of compression dressings. If blood accumulates beneath a flap and it is recognized, the hematoma is evacuated. One or two sutures are removed, and the blood is expressed manually. Rapid reaccumulation of blood necessitates wide exposure of all wound surfaces to control hemorrhage. Expanding hematomas cause distention of a flap and are easily recognized. These are evacuated immediately. If hematomas are not recognized and evacuated, the subsequent process of clot organization and fibrosis results in contracture of the flap base and development of a trapdoor deformity. The use of oral antistaphylococcal antibiotic therapy reduces the risk of an infected hematoma and is indicated when cartilage or bone grafting is performed. Seroma formation may occur as hematomas resolve. Management of seromas requires multiple needle aspirations 5 to 7 days apart.

Epistaxis may follow use of mucoperichondrial flaps to repair nasal lining defects. The initial step is application of vasoconstrictive nasal sprays such as oxymetazoline hydrochloride. Elevated blood pressure, if present, is reduced. The head is elevated, and appropriate medications are given to reduce anxiety and pain. If these measures fail to control bleeding, the nasal cavity is carefully examined with a 0 or 30 degree rigid fiberoptic nasal endoscope following application of topical anesthetic and vasoconstrictive agents. The topical application of cocaine (4% solution) or a mixture of topical 4% lidocaine and oxymetazoline hydrochloride is useful for this purpose. After anesthetizing the nose, suction cautery is used to control bleeding. Depending on the location of bleeding within the nasal cavity, the area may be compressed with petroleum gauze or an absorbable packing material. If nasal packing is used, the patient is placed on antistaphylococcal antibiotic therapy to reduce the risk of toxic shock syndrome.

Infection

The blood supply of the nasal soft tissue and that of lining and external flaps used for nasal reconstruction is usually abundant. As a result, wound infections following nasal reconstruction are quite uncommon. However, infection may occasionally involve cartilage or bone grafts used for structural support. Severe infections may result in resorption of these grafts.

Our prophylactic regimen involves a single preoperative intravenous dose of an antistaphylococcal antibiotic, such as cephazolin, in all procedures involving skin, cartilage, or bone grafts. We also use perioperative antibiotics if the procedure will expose bone or cartilage grafts used in an earlier reconstructive stage. Patients are continued on a 5-day course of an oral antibiotic such as cephalexin. We do not use antibiotic prophylaxis in cases limited to transfer of local or regional cutaneous flaps.

Typically, infections are minor and manifest as redness, swelling, tenderness, and drainage (Fig. 16–1). Systemic signs, if present, may include fever and malaise. Cellulitis is the most common form of postoperative infection. Should an abscess form, treatment consists of drainage and systemic antibiotic therapy. Sufficient exposure of the infected area is necessary to drain the infected fluid and maintain a path of drain-

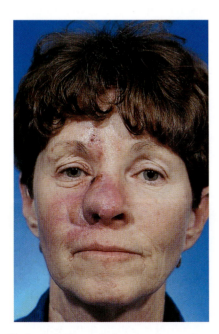

■ **Figure 16–1.** Cellulitis and abscess of nose 2 weeks following detachment of interpolated paramedian forehead flap.

age. Following drainage, the wound is irrigated with an antibiotic solution such as bacitracin or gentamicin. Cultures of the abscess are obtained to ensure proper antibiotic therapy. Empiric systemic antibiotic therapy with coverage for staphylococcus and pseudomonas is initiated.

In less severe cases, aspiration of the infected fluid with an 18 gauge needle and copious irrigation of the wound bed with antibiotic solution through an 18 gauge angiocatheter, together with systemic antibiotic therapy, may prove adequate. Aggressive management of these rare complications may avoid loss of cartilage and bone grafts.

Partial-Thickness Flap Necrosis

There are varying degrees of necrosis of a flap. Superficial necrosis will manifest as epidermal loss that usually heals with little consequence. This is termed epidermolysis and is characterized by superficial crusting and eventual re-epithelialization (Fig. 16–2). The healing epidermis is covered with a moist petroleum-based ointment. Débridement is not necessary, and there is no need for antibiotic therapy. If epidermolysis occurs in an interpolated flap, detachment is delayed until healing is complete.

Full-Thickness Flap Necrosis

Necrosis of a flap may be full-thickness, involving the dermis and subcutaneous tissue. This always involves the most distal aspect of a flap. Initial manifestation of necrosis may be pallor or vascular congestion, followed by mottling and eventually gangrenous necrosis. Flaps with an area of full-thickness necrosis may be managed conservatively, if the involved area is small or is in a region where secondary healing will not result in distortion of free margins. Necrosis of an interpolated flap in a more critical area such as the alar margin may require complete mobilization of the flap, trimming of the necrotic portion, and advancement of the remaining flap to repair the defect (Fig. 16–3). Additional cartilage grafting may also be necessary. After reattachment of the flap, the pedicle is maintained for an additional 3 to 5 weeks to allow for complete healing.

Exposure of native or grafted cartilage and bone may occur as a consequence of full-thickness necrosis of internal lining or external covering flaps. In the case of covering flaps, small (less than 0.5 cm^2) areas of necrosis may be excised, and the wound is closed primarily after undermining adjacent skin. Healing by secondary intention may also result in an acceptable outcome

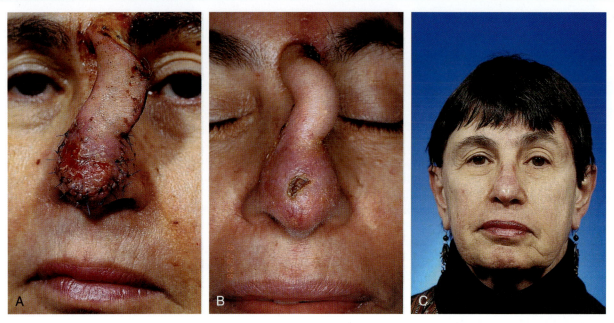

■ **Figure 16–2.** *A,* Epidermolysis of paramedian forehead flap. *B,* Detachment delayed until flap was healed. Partial-thickness necrosis of central flap is present. *C,* 6 months following pedicle detachment. Revision surgery was not required.

over concave areas of the nasal sidewall and alar groove. When necrosis of lining flaps occurs, the involved area is débrided, and exposed cartilage and bone are covered with petroleum-based topical antibiotic ointment. This facilitates granulation tissue formation. The patient is also treated with oral antibiotics. This complication is of minimum consequence when the involved area is small and removed from the nostril margin. However, it may result in notching and deformity if it occurs near the alar margin.

Necrosis of a large portion of a cutaneous flap is very rare and is more likely to occur in heavy smokers. It may also be caused by obstruction of vascular inflow or outflow secondary to a twisted or excessively narrow pedicle. This complication requires a salvage operation to prevent loss of the underlying grafts or contracture of the underlying lining tissue. The necrotic flap is excised, the edges of the defect are freshened, and a second cutaneous flap is designed to provide cover. When 1 cm² or greater exposure of a cartilage graft occurs, the graft will absorb or die unless another covering flap is used in a timely fashion. The cartilage graft will remain viable as long as the underside of the graft is nourished by vascularized lining tissue. Prior to covering the cartilage graft with a second flap, a thin layer of cartilage may be shaved from the exposed surface of the graft. The salvage flap should be designed with a wider pedicle than usual, and initial thinning should be minimized. In patients who use tobacco products, it may be prudent, when possible, to delay the covering flap for 10 days before flap transfer.

Skin Graft Necrosis

Skin or composite grafts undergoing partial necrosis are best kept dry and allowed to form an eschar of the necrotic segment. The eschar remains as a biological dressing. As the surrounding and underlying tissues heal around the eschar, the edges of the eschar will separate from the wound and may be trimmed. The entire eschar is removed when epithelialization is complete beneath it.

Complete full-thickness loss of skin grafts may be due to heavy tobacco use, infection, an excessively thick graft, or an inadequate bolster dressing. The necrotic graft is allowed to form an eschar, and the wound bed heals by secondary intention, sometimes with satisfactory results. Dermabrasion usually improves the appearance of the scar (Fig. 16–4).

Alar Retraction

Alar retraction or notching is the most common complication of reconstructing full-thickness alar defects. It is usually due to necrosis of the lining or covering flap. This exposes the alar batten graft, which subsequently absorbs, resulting in retraction or notching of the nostril (Fig. 16–5). Minor notching of the nostril is corrected

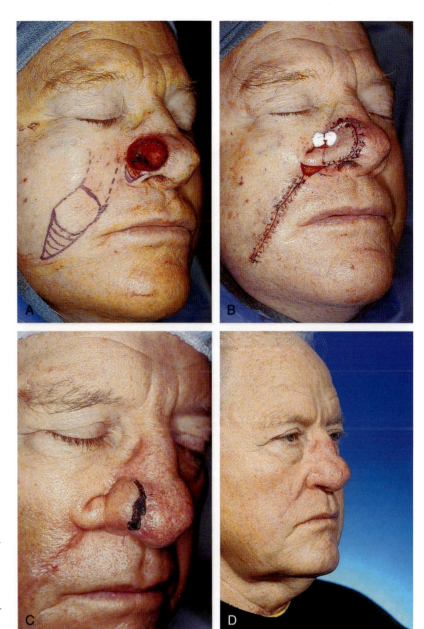

■ **Figure 16–3.** *A*, Cutaneous defect of ala. Remaining skin of ala marked for excision. Interpolated cutaneous pedicled melolabial flap designed for cover. *B*, Flap transferred. *C*, Full-thickness necrosis of distal portion of flap. This was managed by detachment of flap from nose, excision of necrotic portion, and reattachment of flap. Three weeks later the pedicle of flap was divided and flap inset. *D*, 1 year following reconstruction.

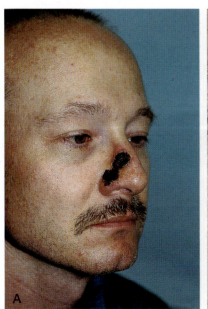

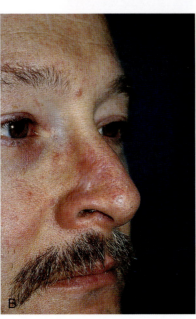

■ **Figure 16–4.** *A*, Necrosis of full-thickness skin graft. *B*, Appearance 6 months following secondary healing and subsequent dermabrasion.

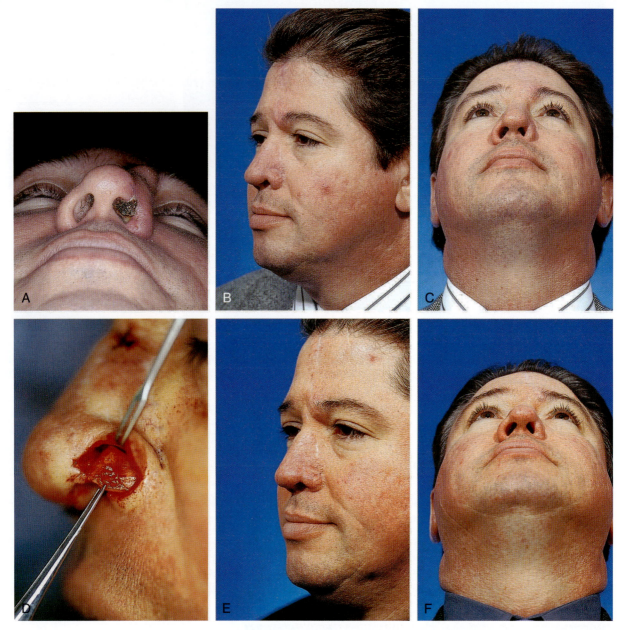

■ **Figure 16-5.** *A*, Full-thickness alar defect reconstructed with septal mucoperichondrial hinge flap, auricular cartilage alar batten graft, and paramedian forehead flap. Necrosis of portion of lining flap is noted. *B* and *C*, Necrosis resulted in notching of nostril margin. *D*, Skin and nasal lining in area of notch mobilized to accommodate auricular cartilage graft held by forceps. *E* and *F*, 1 year following correction of nostril notching.

by subcutaneous undermining in the area of the notch to mobilize the skin caudally to a normal position. The mobilized skin is fixed in place with a cartilage graft positioned caudal to the lateral crus. This prevents cephalic migration of the skin during the healing process. Marked retraction of the nostril may require composite grafting or a three-layer reconstruction using lining, support, and external cover.

■ Nasal Obstruction

Some amount of nasal obstruction is common during the initial 2 or 3 months after an interpolated flap has been used to resurface a defect of the ala or tip. This usually improves with time as the bed of scar tissue beneath the flap softens and matures. In the case of alar reconstuction, nasal obstruction usually persists until a contouring procedure is performed to restore the alar groove. The alar groove is the surface manifestation of the internal nasal valve. Removal of excess subcutaneous tissue during the process of constructing the groove relieves the obstruction. Persistent nasal obstruction may follow reconstruction of any defect involving the ala or nasal sidewall, even when native cartilage has not been removed. This occurs most frequently when two or more nasal aesthetic units are resurfaced in patients with narrow middle vaults and weak upper or lower lateral cartilages. In these cases, nasal obstruction results from constriction of the nasal passage by scar tissue, particularly in the region of the internal nasal valve. The internal nasal valve is at the junction of the caudal aspect of the upper lateral cartilage and the dorsal aspect of the septum. This region represents the narrowest cross-sectional area of the nasal passage and is therefore the most prone to symptomatic airway obstruction.

Identification of patients at risk for postoperative nasal obstruction and taking the necessary preventive steps of using structural reinforcement through the use of spreader and alar batten grafts help avoid this complication. Alar batten grafts are positioned beneath the lateral crura between the crura and vestibular skin. Grafts are of sufficient length to extend from the midportion of the lateral crus to the alar base (see Chapter 5). The batten graft is sutured to the lateral crus in such a manner to cause the ala to flare slightly outward. This is accomplished by medial advancement of the lateral crus on the batten and fixation with permanent mattress sutures. Displacement of the ala laterally also displaces the lateral crus and upper lateral cartilage laterally. This movement has the effect of increasing the aperture of the external and internal nasal valves. Placement of a spreader graft of septal or auricular cartilage between the dorsal septum and upper lateral cartilage also widen the angle of the internal valve and improve the airway. Often, alar batten grafts and spreader grafts are used together.

A defect of cartilage or nasal lining is not a prerequisite for development of internal nasal valve obstruction. Contracture of scar beneath a covering flap may be sufficient to displace the intact upper lateral cartilage, constricting the valve medially. In these instances, prophylactic strengthening of the upper lateral cartilages with an alar batten graft of septal or auricular cartilage, as described in Chapter 5, reduces the risk of persistent postoperative nasal obstruction.

Repair of full-thickness defects of the ala with lining flaps, auricular cartilage grafts, and interpolated cheek or forehead flaps will sometimes result in an excessively bulky ala compromising the nostril aperture. Thinning of the ala may be accomplished through an external approach with subcutaneous undermining to the nostril margin and appropriate contouring of soft tissue and cartilage. If the thickening is from the inter-

nal lining flap, it may be thinned intranasally in a similar fashion through an incision made at the nostril margin. The alar margin may also be thinned directly by elliptical excision of skin and soft tissue at the nostril margin.

Excessive Scarring

There are instances in which the scars resulting from reconstructive surgery may be unsightly or excessive. Complications of wound healing such as infection, hematoma, and partial- or full-thickness necrosis are often contributing factors. A hematoma can produce subcutaneous fibrosis and contracture resulting in a trapdoor deformity of the flap. Younger patients have less skin laxity and may heal with suboptimal scars. Another category of patients who exhibit poor scarring are those with excessively thick and sebaceous skin. These patients are generally poor candidates for skin grafting but are also prone to developing depressed scars from the use of nasal cutaneous flaps (Fig. 16–6). Individuals with thick nasal skin also have a higher rate of skin necrosis and a higher incidence of developing postoperative trapdoor deformities when using nasal cutaneous flaps to repair defects of the nose (Fig. 16–7).

Cutaneous Changes

A number of changes can occur in the skin of flaps and grafts that are used to reconstruct the nose. The most common and, fortunately, most easily managed change is the development of contact dermatitis. This is characterized by pruritis and the development of erythema, occasionally accompanied by vesicles or exudate. Contact dermatitis usually develops 3 to 7 days following the application of antibiotic ointments to the wound (Fig. 16–8). It may also occur from tape or bandages applied to the nose. Contact dermatitis is readily treated by discontinuing the offending agent. The area of dermatitis is treated by cleaning with soap and water and the application of 1% or 2% hydrocortisone cream for a few days. If pruritis is severe, diphenhydramine or hydroxyzine may be prescribed as an oral medication.

Flap and graft erythema is the result of hypervascularity at the capillary level. Erythema is common in the early stages of flap transfer or skin grafting as well as during the dermal remodeling phase following dermabrasion. Persistent flap erythema may, however, compromise the overall aesthetic outcome (Fig. 16–9). A

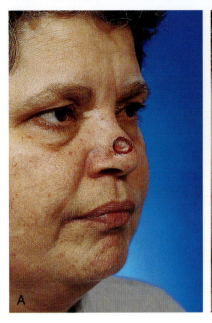
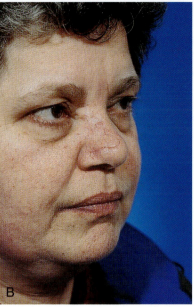

■ **Figure 16–6.** *A,* Cutaneous defect of nasal tip in patient with thick sebaceous skin. *B,* Defect repaired with bilobe nasal cutaneous flap. Note depressed scar outlining borders of the flap.

significant disparity of skin color between the flap and adjacent nasal skin, despite good contour and texture match, will highlight the flap against the native nasal skin. Erythema may be reduced by sun avoidance and use of sunscreen creams. Treatment of the erythematous flap with a pulsed dye laser (577 or 585 nm wavelength) or intense pulsed light (515 to 1200 nm wavelength) may dramatically reduce erythema. The laser energy targets the hemoglobin in the blood vessels and results in selective photothermolysis of the fine capil-

laries, thus reducing erythema. More than one treatment is usually necessary.

Larger, more visible, dilations of arterioles and venules may be visible on the surface of covering flaps or skin grafts (see Fig. 16–9). Telangiectasias may be as large as 2 mm in diameter; if sufficiently superficial, they may be treated with a hyfrecator using a fine-needle electrode inserted into the vessel. Enough thermal energy is delivered to coagulate the vessel. The pulsed dye laser or intense pulsed light treatments may also be used to treat telangiectasias. There may be a moderate amount of temporary bruising and ecchymosis associated with rupture of these vessels following laser treatment.

Flap or graft hyperpigmentation is usually seen in

■ **Figure 16–7.** Trapdoor deformity occurring following partial necrosis of bilobe nasal cutaneous flap.

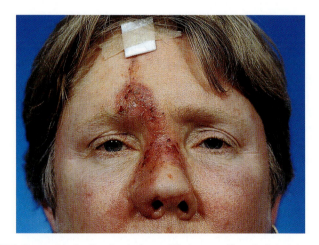

■ **Figure 16–8.** Contact dermatitis from antibacterial ointment applied to suture line.

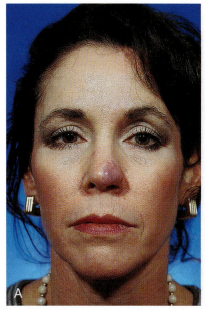
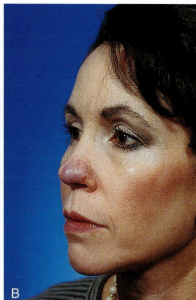

■ **Figure 16–9.** *A* and *B*, 1 year following repair of nasal tip skin defect with interpolated paramedian forehead flap. Note persistent erythema and telangiectasias that cause marked discrepancy between color of flap skin and color of native nasal skin.

patients with Fitzpatrick's skin type III or darker but may even occur in lighter-skinned individuals. Hyperpigmentation is more commonly observed with skin grafts compared with flaps (Fig. 16–10). Postinflammatory hyperpigmentation is a very common occurrence in darker-skinned individuals and usually resolves with time and sun avoidance. In rare instances, the pigmentary changes may persist beyond the initial few months following reconstruction. Fortunately, few of these individuals require nasal reconstruction because of the rare

incidence of cutaneous malignancies in dark-skinned individuals. Hydroquinine (4% concentration) is a topical bleaching agent that may improve hyperpigmentation. The medication is available in cream preparations with or without sunscreen. Sun avoidance and use of sunscreen are key to preventing hyperpigmentation. Lasers with wavelengths aimed at melanin or dermabrasion are also likely to be helpful in reducing persistent hyperpigmentation.

Unlike hyperpigmentation, which usually resolves

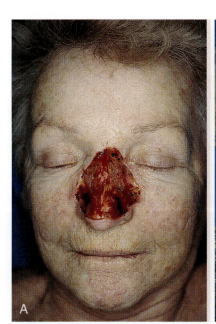
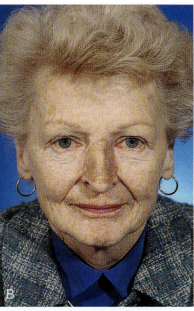
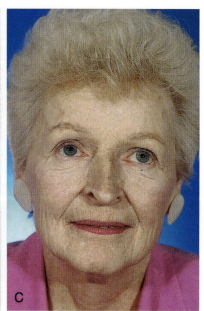

■ **Figure 16–10.** *A,* Large cutaneous defect of nose repaired with full-thickness skin graft. *B,* 2 months following skin grafting. Note postinflammatory hyperpigmentation of skin graft. *C,* 6 months later. Hyperpigmentation has improved, but is still visually distracting. This could likely be improved with dermabrasion.

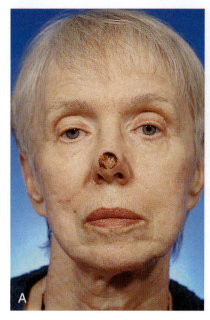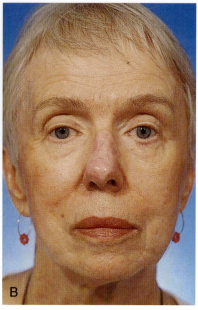

Figure 16–11. *A,* Cutaneous nasal tip defect repaired with bilobe nasal cutaneous flap followed by dermabrasion of flap. *B,* Persistent hypopigmentation from dermabrasion is noted 1½ years following reconstruction.

with time, hypopigmentation is a permanent change. It is important to differentiate between the two types of hypopigmentation. Most resurfacing procedures, such as laser, dermabrasion, or chemical peels, result in some amount of relative hypopigmentation in the treated as compared with the untreated areas (Fig. 16–11). This merely represents improvement of preexisting pigmentary dyschromias and return of the skin to its natural color. This effect can be made less noticeable by resurfacing an entire aesthetic region. Absolute hypopigmentation occurs when there is reduction in the pigment and/or melanocyte count compared with that of the native skin. This can occasionally occur in a flap of skin transferred from one site to another (Fig. 16–12).

Hypopigmentation following dermabrasion may lead to a marked discrepancy in skin color between the abraded area and the adjacent nontreated skin (see Fig. 16–11). This has been a particular problem with forehead skin, which seems to lighten in color more markedly than the remaining facial skin. For this reason we have abandoned the practice of dermabrading forehead donor site scars resulting from transfer of a paramedian forehead flap to the nose. Likewise, we only occasionally dermabrade forehead flaps transferred to the nose unless there are depressed scars or marked skin texture differences between the flap and the adjacent nasal skin.

On occasion we have observed hypopigmentation oc-

Figure 16–12. *A* and *B,* Interpolated paramedian forehead flap used to repair cutaneous defect of nose. Flap was not dermabraded, but it displays marked hypopigmentation 3 months postoperatively.

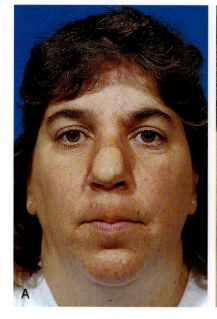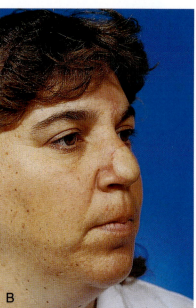

curring in a forehead flap that has been transferred to the nose and not treated with dermabrasion (see Fig. 16–12). Concomitant with these pigmentary changes has been the reversal of solar skin damage such as actinic keratoses and solar lentigenes observed on the forehead skin prior to transfer of the flap. The cause of these cutaneous changes of forehead skin following flap transfer to the nose is unknown. Presumably, the surgical manipulation of dissecting, thinning, and transfer of the forehead skin causes a permanent biological change in the epidermis of the flap. In these instances, hypopigmentation may be improved by camouflaging methods. Micropigmentation (cosmetic tattooing) of the flap may be performed to darken the color. Dermabrasion of the nose in an effort to lighten the native nasal skin surrounding the flap may also be performed. An initial period of postinflammatory hyperpigmentation may temporarily accentuate the disparity in color between flap and native nasal skin. Bleaching creams such as hydroquinone or kojic acid may be used to lighten the native skin. Lasers may also be used in an attempt to reduce pigment in the skin adjacent to the hypopigmented flap.

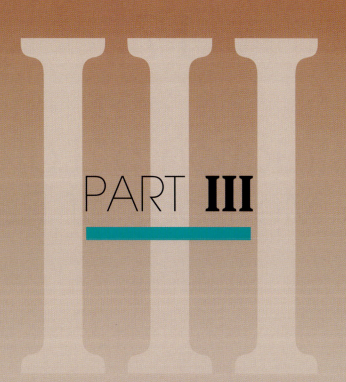

PART **III**

Representative
Cases

17

Reconstruction of Lateral Tip: Two Methods of Repair

Shan R. Baker

Presented are two individuals with similar cutaneous defects involving the lateral tip repaired by two methods. Each approach was selected based on a number of factors.

First Case

The first case was that of a 75-year-old woman treated with Mohs' surgery for basal cell carcinoma of the left lateral nasal tip. She was in good health, lived by herself, and did not use tobacco products. Following surgery, she presented with a 2 × 2 cm skin defect of the lateral tip. The lateral crus of the alar cartilage remained intact (Fig. 17–1). The patient had a large nose, and the defect encompassed only one-third of the surface area of the tip. The circular skin defect was converted to a rectangle by creating corners to the defect, but the remaining skin of the aesthetic unit was not removed (Fig. 17–2). An auricular cartilage graft was placed along the nostril margin spanning the width of the defect. This graft served to reinforce the nostril and was positioned caudal to the lateral crus. It was secured to the lateral crus with 5-0 polyglactin sutures placed in a figure-of-eight fashion to prevent the graft from overlapping the alar cartilage. The skin defect was resurfaced with an interpolated subcutaneous tissue pedicled melolabial flap using techniques described in Chapter 13 (Fig. 17–3). One week later, the distal portion of the flap appeared cyanotic from venous engorgement; however, capillary refill was brisk (Fig. 17–4). Three weeks following flap transfer, the pedicle was detached, and the flap was inset (Fig. 17–5). The distal flap had been thinned to the level of the superficial subcutaneous plane at the initial transfer. The remaining portion of the flap was thinned of excess subcutaneous fat at the time of pedicle detachment and flap inset. A bolster dressing consisting of 4-0 polypropylene sutures passed through the nose and tied over a dental roll compressed the cephalic aspect of the flap and maintained the alar groove. The patient did not require a contouring procedure because the defect did not extend cephalad to the alar groove (Fig. 17–6).

Second Case

The second case was that of a 50-year-old man with a similarly located defect of the nasal skin following surgical resection of a melanoma with a Breslow depth of 1.36 mm. He was in excellent health, had retired, and did not use tobacco products. Like the prior first case, the nasal defect involved the skin of the lateral tip but was slightly larger than the first case, measuring 2.5 × 2.0 cm. Unlike the first case, he had a relatively small nose, and the defect encompassed a portion of the right ala and involved the nostril margin and a small amount of vestibular skin. The lateral crus of the alar cartilage was intact. The patient had a high anterior hairline from male pattern baldness and a youthful face (Fig. 17–7).

It was elected to remove the remaining skin of the ala and hemitip for two reasons. The skin defect was positioned slightly more lateral than the first case so that nearly half of the alar skin was missing. In general, when half or more of the surface area of the alar aesthetic unit is absent, we resurface the entire unit. The second impetus for additional skin removal was the type of tumor resected. Although the surgical margins were shown to be free of tumor by the referring dermatological surgeon, removing additional skin around the resected melanoma provided greater security concerning control of peripheral spread. It was elected not to remove the skin of the entire tip or the sidewall because of their limited involvement by the defect. However, the remaining skin of the hemitip was excised.

A bipedicle vestibular skin advancement flap, described in Chapter 4 and 11, was used to replace the missing lining along the nostril margin. To develop the flap, an extended intercartilaginous incision was made, and the vestibular skin was completely freed from the lateral crus. The flap was mobilized sufficiently so that it could easily be advanced to the nostril margin. An auricular cartilage alar batten graft, described in Chapters 7 and 13, was positioned along the nostril margin extending from the alar base to the nasal facet (Fig. 17–8). Similar to the first case, the graft was nestled between the caudal border of the lateral crus of the alar cartilage and the margin of the nostril. The graft was secured to the bipedicle vestibular skin advancement flap with a few 5-0 polyglactin mattress sutures.

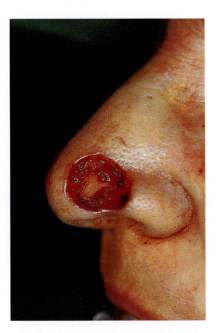

Figure 17–1. 2 × 2 cm skin defect of lateral tip.

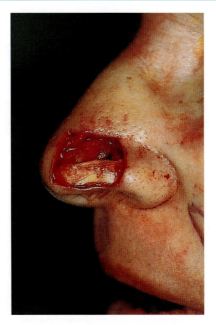

■ **Figure 17–2.** Circular defect is converted to rectangle. Auricular cartilage graft is positioned inferior to intact lateral crus.

A template representing the configuration of the new skin defect that would follow the removal of the remaining skin of the ala and hemitip was used to design a right interpolated paramedian forehead flap. The flap was dissected and transferred to the nose as described in Chapter 14 after removal of the nasal skin. The entire flap covering the defect was thinned to the level of the superficial subcutaneous plane at the initial transfer. The caudal border of the flap was sutured to the caudal border of the bipedicle lining flap (Fig. 17–9). The donor forehead wound was closed primarily by advancing the remaining forehead skin and muscle on either side of the wound. The standing cutaneous deformity that arises in the scalp as a result of repair of the forehead donor wound was excised. It was non–hair-bearing skin and was thinned of its subcutaneous fat and used as a full-thickness skin graft to repair the intranasal donor wound resulting from the bipedicle vestibular skin advancement flap.

The pedicle of the forehead flap was detached 3 weeks later. Although the entire flap attached to the nose had been thinned at the time of transfer, the flap extended cephalad to the alar groove and obliterated it (Fig. 17–10). As a consequence, it was necessary to perform a contouring procedure 3 months following pedicle detachment. An alar groove was constructed using techniques described in Chapter 13, and a bolster dressing was applied. Figure 17–11 shows the results of the three-stage reconstruction 4 months following the contouring procedure. There is asymmetry of nostril size; however, he did not suffer any restriction of the nasal airway.

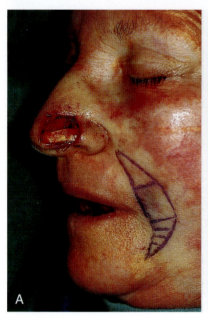
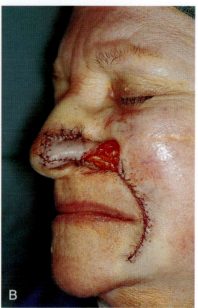

■ **Figure 17–3.** *A,* Interpolated subcutaneous tissue pedicled melolabial flap is designed. *B,* Cheek flap in position. Distal half of flap was thinned to level of superficial subcutaneous plane.

Discussion

A cutaneous defect of the nasal tip is most commonly reconstructed with a bilobe flap, if the flap is sufficiently small, or with an interpolated paramedian forehead flap for defects that have a maximum dimension of 2.0 cm or greater. Laterally located defects of the tip may also be resurfaced with interpolated cheek flaps. This flap can be developed with sufficient length to

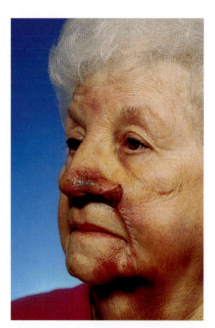

■ **Figure 17–4.** 1 week following flap transfer. Note cyanosis of distal portion.

reach the midline of the tip, but it cannot resurface an entire nasal tip without jeopardizing the vascularity of the flap. In large noses, extending the cheek flap to the lateral tip may occasionally stress the capability of the pedicle to support the distal flap. Such was the reason for the distal flap developing cyanosis in the first case (see Fig. 17–4).

When repairing nasal cutaneous defects of the tip, we reserve the use of the interpolated subcutaneous tissue pedicled cheek flap to small (2.0 cm or less) laterally located skin defects in older patients who have cheek skin laxity. Such a flap was selected in the first case because of the size and location of the patient's defect and the laxity of cheek skin. The patient was elderly and lived by herself. Caring for a paramedian forehead flap during the 3 weeks that the pedicle remains attached to the forehead would have been problematic. She also had a relatively low anterior hairline, with the likelihood of having to transfer hair to the nose if a paramedian forehead flap were selected. All these factors suggested the cheek as the preferred source for a covering flap.

Like the first case, a number of factors influence the selection of an interpolated paramedian forehead flap to resurface the nasal defect of the second case. The defect was enlarged to increase surgical margins around the tumor and to allow the resurfacing of the entire alar aesthetic unit and the hemitip. The overall size of the new defect encouraged the selection of a forehead flap for cover. In addition, the patient had a receding hairline that provided an ample supply of non–hair-bearing skin for the covering flap. He had a youthful face having minimal cheek skin laxity and typical male pattern facial hair. A cheek flap would have transferred hair to the nose and may have caused a

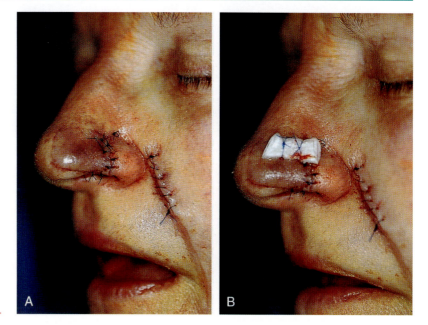

■ **Figure 17–5.** *A,* Pedicle detached and flap inset. Proximal half of flap was thinned before inset. *B,* Bolster dressing used to maintain alar groove.

more noticeable scar, compared with the scar typically observed from use of a paramedian forehead flap. He was retired and could easily avoid social engagements for the 3 weeks between the first and second surgical stage.

Two nasal cutaneous defects of similar location and size were repaired with two different covering flaps. The method of reconstruction was based on a host of factors that determined the selection of the flap. Often the surgeon is confronted with a relatively small nasal cutaneous defect that may be repaired using more than

one technique. Foremost in the selection of a surgical approach is the priority of restoring normal nasal function and contour. When these requirements can be met using more than one technique, other factors are considered before deciding on the method of repair. Defect size and location were similar in these two cases; however, age, gender, pattern of scalp and facial hair growth, and living arrangements were all dissimilar. Other factors that may come into play when selecting the cheek or forehead as the source for a covering flap is the patient's occupation and whether tobacco prod-

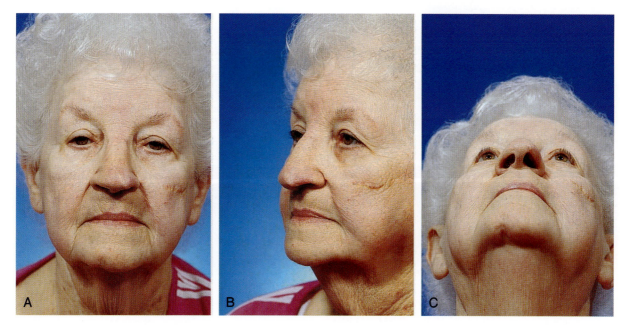

■ **Figure 17–6.** *A* to *C,* 8 months postoperative. Contouring procedure was not necessary.

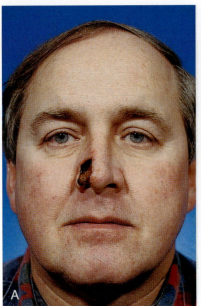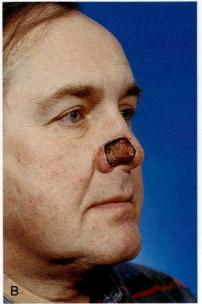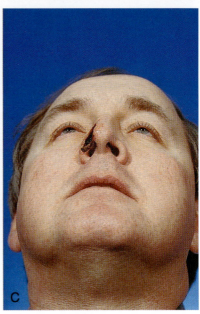

Figure 17–7. *A* to *C*, 2.0 × 2.5 cm skin defect of lateral tip.

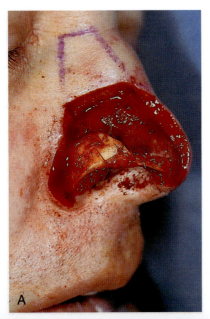

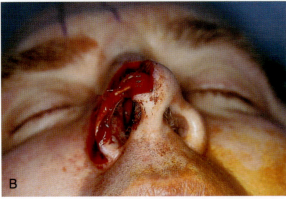

Figure 17–8. *A,* Defect enlarged by removing skin of ala and hemitip. Auricular cartilage batten graft in place. *B,* Bipedicle vestibular skin advancement flap provided lining to nostril margin.

ucts are habitually used. When either an interpolated forehead or cheek flap may be equally effective in repairing a nasal defect, a cheek flap is usually selected in patients who express a desire to continue to work at their employment between the first and second stage of reconstruction. While the pedicle of a forehead flap is attached, it is difficult to properly wear eye and safety glasses and to cover the flap with a bandage without obstructing the vision. In contrast, while the pedicle of a cheek flap remains attached, the flap may easily be covered with a bandage, keeping it from the sight of coworkers. The cheek donor site wound is more problematic because of its inferior extent, but it may also be covered with a bandage if desired. Cheek flaps do not impair the use of eyeglasses. In patients who use tobacco products, cheek flaps are more likely to suffer necrosis of the distal portion compared with paramedian forehead flaps. This is because cheek flaps have a more random vascularity than the well-developed axial vascular pattern of the paramedian forehead flap. For this reason we are inclined to select the forehead as the preferred donor site for reconstruction of alar or tip defects in patients who use tobacco products.

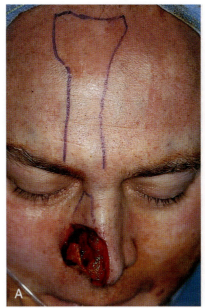
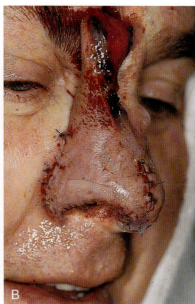

Figure 17–9. *A*, Interpolated paramedian forehead flap designed for external cover. *B*, Entire flap covering defect was thinned and caudal border sutured to vestibular skin advancement flap along nostril margin.

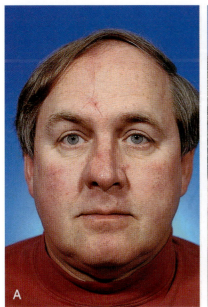
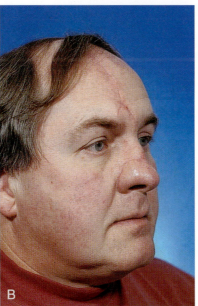

Figure 17–10. *A* and *B*, 3 months following detachment of forehead flap. Flap is bulky, and alar groove is absent, necessitating contouring procedure.

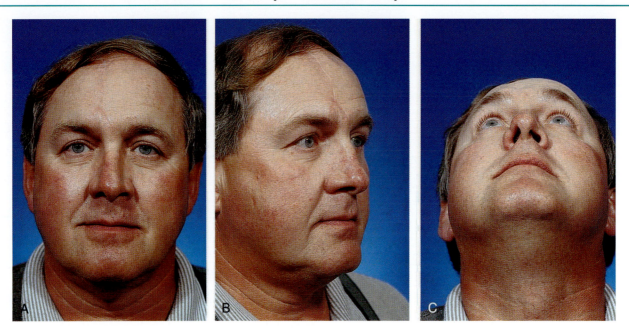

Figure 17–11. *A* to *C*, 4 months following contouring procedure.

18

Reconstruction of Central Tip: Three Methods of Repair

Shan R. Baker

Presented are three individuals with cutaneous defects of the central portion of the nasal tip. Each defect was repaired with a different surgical approach. Selection of the method of repair was based on a number of factors.

First Case

The first case was that of a 56-year-old woman who presented with a 5 mm nodular basal cell carcinoma of the nasal tip. The tumor was treated with Mohs' surgery, following which she presented with a 2 × 2 cm skin defect predominantly involving the right hemitip (Fig. 18–1). The defect was at the upper size limit for repair with a bilobe nasal cutaneous flap. However, her relatively large nose and the amount of laxity of skin covering the dorsum and sidewalls encouraged the selection of a bilobe flap. Another factor influencing that decision was the location of the defect. It was cephalic to the tip-defining points and away from the free margin of the nostril by more than 1 cm. The skin defect was repaired with a laterally based bilobe flap using techniques described in Chapter 10 (Fig. 18–2). The flap and adjacent nasal skin were dermabraded 5 months following reconstruction. Figure 18–3 shows the result of surgery a year later. There is a very subtle contour

depression over the right side of the caudal portion of the dorsum.

Second Case

The second case was that of a 67-year-old woman who was seen for recurrent basal cell carcinoma of the nasal tip. The tumor had been present for a number of years before she sought medical attention. Examination showed a scaly lesion involving most of the skin of the nasal tip. Mohs' surgery was performed to remove the tumor. This necessitated removal of all of the skin of the tip. The 3 × 3 cm skin defect extended to the nostril margin and involved a full-thickness loss of a small portion of the facet. The size of the defect precluded reconstruction with a nasal cutaneous flap. The full-thickness loss of a portion of the nostril margin prevented the use of a full-thickness skin graft for repair. A graft would likely contract sufficiently to cause retraction of the nostril margin. In addition, a skin graft could not replace the missing soft-tissue loss in the area of the facet. An interpolated paramedian forehead flap was the obvious choice for reconstruction.

The internal lining for the facet was provided by developing a vestibular skin advancement flap. The cephalic borders of the lateral crura were trimmed to refine the tip. The excised segments of alar cartilage were approximated with fine sutures to create a double

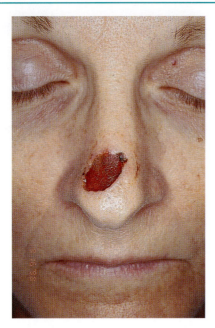

■ Figure 18–1. *2 × 2 cm skin defect of nasal tip.*

layer cartilage graft that served as a framework for the facet. The graft spanned the angle between the intermediate and lateral crura and was secured to the caudal border of the alar cartilage with figure-of-eight 5-0 polyglactin sutures. The vestibular skin advanced for lining was secured to the graft with mattress sutures of similar material.

The remaining skin of the tip was removed, and the surrounding nasal skin was widely undermined in the

subfascial plane using techniques described in Chapter 14. An interpolated paramedian forehead flap was used to cover the tip and left facet (Fig. 18–4). Three weeks later, the pedicle of the forehead flap was divided and the flap inset. No additional surgical procedures were necessary (Fig. 18–5).

Third Case

The third case was that of a 65-year-old woman who presented with two independent basal cell carcinomas. One was on the left aspect of the tip, and the other was on the caudal aspect of the right sidewall. Seven years earlier, she had a basal cell carcinoma removed from the nasal tip, and the wound was left to heal by secondary intention. Examination showed two 2-mm areas of erythema from the biopsy sites used to confirm the presence of the neoplasms. No obvious tumor was palpable or visible. There was moderate skin laxity over the dorsum and sidewalls of the nose. The anterior hairline was low, necessitating transfer of hair-bearing skin to the nose, should a paramedian forehead flap be required for repair. Alternative methods of reconstruction following Mohs' surgery were discussed with the patient. A bilobe nasal cutaneous flap was anticipated as the most likely choice for repair.

Following Mohs' surgery for the two tumors, the patient was examined. A very superficial 3.0 × 1.5 cm skin defect of the tip was observed. The defect was too large to repair with a bilobe nasal cutaneous flap. A

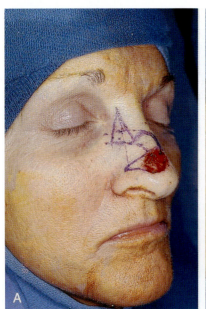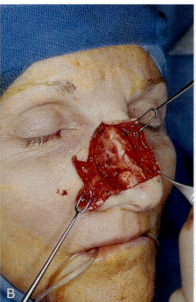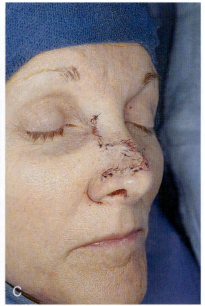

■ Figure 18–2. *A*, Lateral-based bilobe nasal cutaneous flap designed for repair. *B*, Skin flap and adjacent nasal skin widely undermined in subfascial plane. *C*, Standing cutaneous deformity resulting from pivoting flap is excised in alar groove.

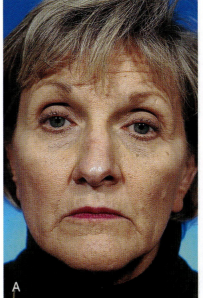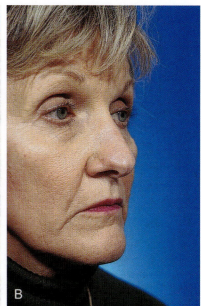

Figure 18–3. *A* and *B*, 1 year postoperative. Subtle contour depression is noted over right side of caudal dorsum.

paramedian forehead flap was recommended, but the patient was reluctant to undergo such surgery. Because of the superficial depth of the wound, a full-thickness skin graft offered a reasonable alternative. The defect was repaired with a graft harvested from the supraclavicular area. The graft was secured in place with a bolster dressing as described in Chapter 9. The graft survived completely and was dermabraded 3 months later. Because of the limited depth of the nasal defect, the patient healed without a depressed contour in the area of the skin graft. Dermabrasion assisted in reduc-

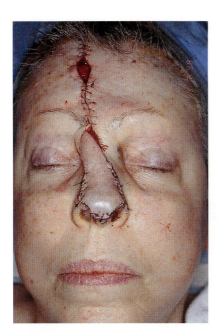

Figure 18–4. Interpolated paramedian forehead flap used to repair skin defect of tip and left nasal facet.

ing discrepancies in color match between the graft and adjacent nasal skin (Fig. 18–6).

Discussion

In alar reconstruction, surgical approaches are limited because the ala contributes to the caudal free margin of the nose and entrance to the nasal airway. Use of nasal cutaneous flaps distorts the ala, and skin grafts may cause constriction of the external nasal valve. In contrast, when reconstructing skin defects of the nasal tip the surgeon has a greater number of options. Skin defects measuring up to 2.5 cm, centrally located on the tip and remaining at least 0.5 cm from the margin of the nostril, are best repaired with nasal cutaneous flaps (see Chapter 10). The preferred nasal cutaneous flap for repairing skin defects of the central tip is the bilobe flap. The flap is ideally suited for a skin defect less than 1.5 cm in maximum dimension, located on the central or lateral tip without extension to the ala. The larger the nose and the older the patient, the greater the ease of repairing a cutaneous defect of the tip with a bilobe flap. Relative to overall nasal size, the surface area of a given defect is smaller for a large nose compared with a small nose. Larger cutaneous flaps can be developed in larger noses, which translates to less wound closure tension. In the case of age, elderly individuals tend to have greater laxity of skin covering the nasal sidewalls and dorsum. Greater skin laxity means there is more tissue available for construction of the flap and less wound closure tension.

The first case represents a skin defect that was at the upper limit in size for repair with a bilobe flap. How-

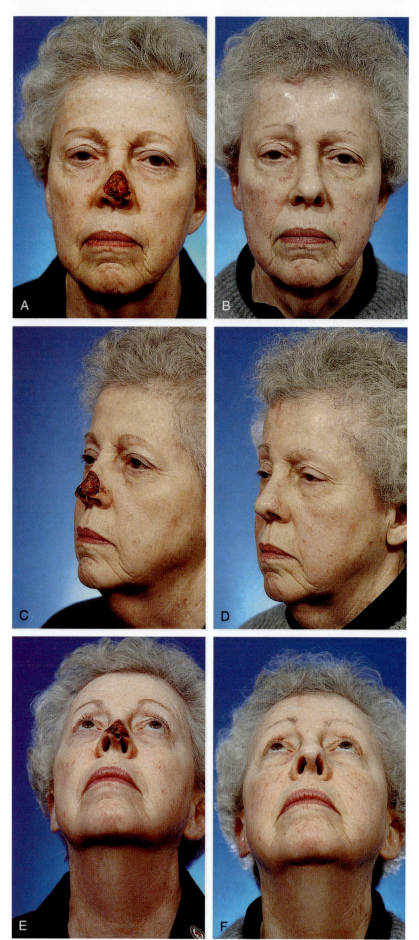

Figure 18–5. *A* to *F*, Preoperative and 3 months postoperative. A contouring procedure was not necessary.

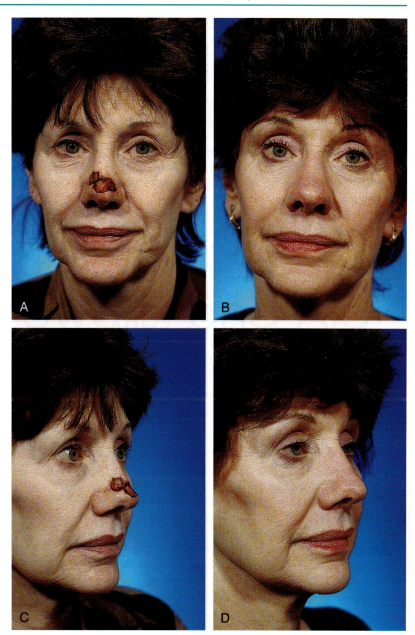

Figure 18–6. *A* to *D,* Preoperative and 6 months postoperative. Wound was repaired with full-thickness skin graft from supraclavicular area. Graft was dermabraded 3 months following grafting.

ever, the defect was small relative to the overall size of the nose. This fact, along with modest laxity of the nasal skin, convinced us that a bilobe flap was the preferred method of repair. The patient was left with a slight contour depression on the right side of the lower dorsum. Abnormal contour and distortion of the tip or margin of the nostril are the most common problems encountered when using a bilobe flap for nasal reconstruction (see Chapter 10). When the defect is small (maximum dimension 1 cm or less) and located cephalic to the apex of the domes, distortions and contour irregularities do not occur. However, larger skin defects repaired with a bilobe flap result in greater wound closure tension, which may lead to distortion of the topography of the nose. In addition, larger defects require greater quantities of skin transfer from the dor-

sum and sidewalls. This skin typically is thinner than the skin of the tip and may lead to subtle contour discrepancies as observed in this case. In Chapter 10 we discuss some of the techniques that may be used in an attempt to avoid contour deformities.

The second case represents the opposite end of the spectrum from case one. The patient's nose was small, and she had a recurrent basal cell carcinoma of the nasal tip for several years. Recurrent basal cell carcinomas typically are larger than primary tumors. Because of this, preparation for a paramedian forehead flap was made when the patient was interviewed at the initial consultation. As anticipated, the skin defect following Mohs' surgery was too large for repair with a nasal cutaneous flap. A skin graft would have left the patient with a noticeable notching and likely retraction of the

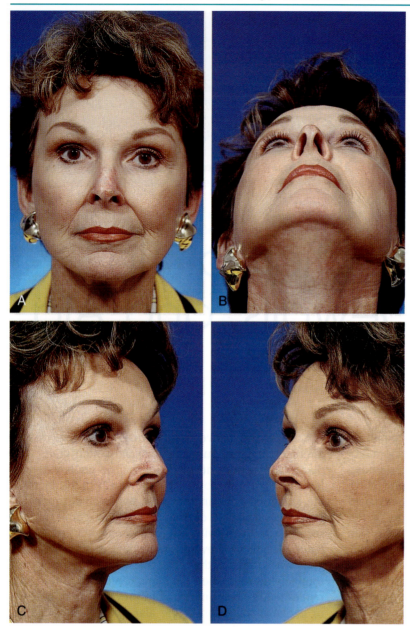

■ **Figure 19–1.** A–D. Patient with basal cell carcinoma of nose. Clinically, tumor appeared to involve tip and caudal aspect of dorsum and sidewalls.

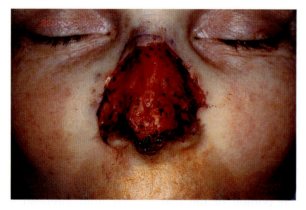

■ **Figure 19–2.** Nasal defect following Mohs' surgery. Skin defect involved entire tip, dorsum, right ala, both nasal facets, sidewalls, and entire margin of right nostril. All native nasal cartilage remained intact.

scalp skin prevented an axial pattern blood flow to the hair-bearing portion of the flap (Fig. 19–4). In spite of this, epidermolysis of the most distal hair-bearing portion of the flap occurred. This is a very superficial partial-thickness necrosis of the skin that results from vascular insufficiency. Fortunately, epidermolysis rarely leads to a visible scar. The width of the flap measured 6 cm; the size prevented complete primary closure of the donor wound. The portion of the wound not closed primarily was kept moist with petroleum ointment and left to heal by secondary intention.

Three weeks following transfer of the forehead flap, the pedicle was detached, and the flap was inset. The native skin of the nasion and cephalic sidewalls was preserved. Before inset, the flap was thinned by removing muscle and some of the subcutaneous fat on the

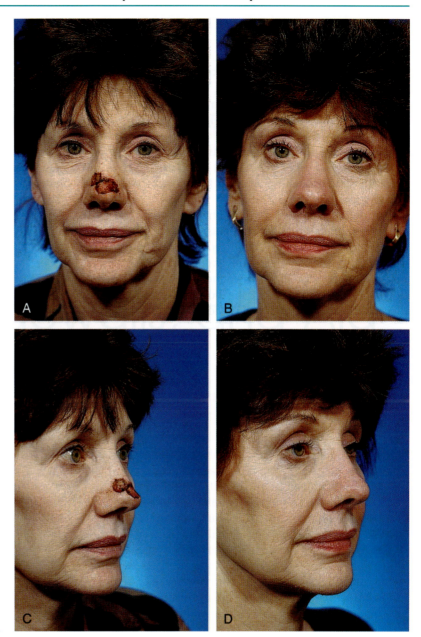

■ **Figure 18-6.** *A to D,* Preoperative and 6 months postoperative. Wound was repaired with full-thickness skin graft from supraclavicular area. Graft was dermabraded 3 months following grafting.

ever, the defect was small relative to the overall size of the nose. This fact, along with modest laxity of the nasal skin, convinced us that a bilobe flap was the preferred method of repair. The patient was left with a slight contour depression on the right side of the lower dorsum. Abnormal contour and distortion of the tip or margin of the nostril are the most common problems encountered when using a bilobe flap for nasal reconstruction (see Chapter 10). When the defect is small (maximum dimension 1 cm or less) and located cephalic to the apex of the domes, distortions and contour irregularities do not occur. However, larger skin defects repaired with a bilobe flap result in greater wound closure tension, which may lead to distortion of the topography of the nose. In addition, larger defects require greater quantities of skin transfer from the dor-

sum and sidewalls. This skin typically is thinner than the skin of the tip and may lead to subtle contour discrepancies as observed in this case. In Chapter 10 we discuss some of the techniques that may be used in an attempt to avoid contour deformities.

The second case represents the opposite end of the spectrum from case one. The patient's nose was small, and she had a recurrent basal cell carcinoma of the nasal tip for several years. Recurrent basal cell carcinomas typically are larger than primary tumors. Because of this, preparation for a paramedian forehead flap was made when the patient was interviewed at the initial consultation. As anticipated, the skin defect following Mohs' surgery was too large for repair with a nasal cutaneous flap. A skin graft would have left the patient with a noticeable notching and likely retraction of the

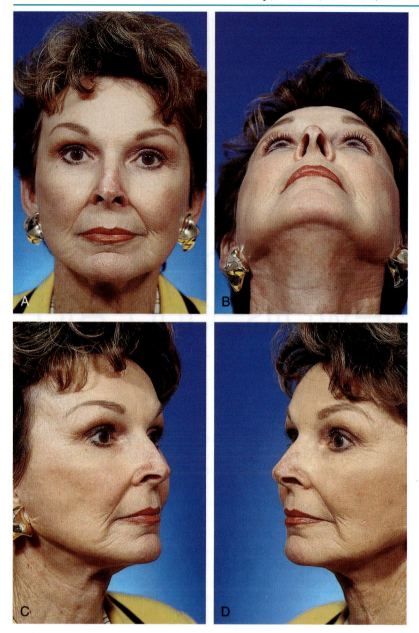

Figure 19-1. A–D. Patient with basal cell carcinoma of nose. Clinically, tumor appeared to involve tip and caudal aspect of dorsum and sidewalls.

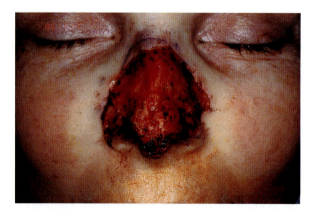

Figure 19-2. Nasal defect following Mohs' surgery. Skin defect involved entire tip, dorsum, right ala, both nasal facets, sidewalls, and entire margin of right nostril. All native nasal cartilage remained intact.

scalp skin prevented an axial pattern blood flow to the hair-bearing portion of the flap (Fig. 19–4). In spite of this, epidermolysis of the most distal hair-bearing portion of the flap occurred. This is a very superficial partial-thickness necrosis of the skin that results from vascular insufficiency. Fortunately, epidermolysis rarely leads to a visible scar. The width of the flap measured 6 cm; the size prevented complete primary closure of the donor wound. The portion of the wound not closed primarily was kept moist with petroleum ointment and left to heal by secondary intention.

Three weeks following transfer of the forehead flap, the pedicle was detached, and the flap was inset. The native skin of the nasion and cephalic sidewalls was preserved. Before inset, the flap was thinned by removing muscle and some of the subcutaneous fat on the

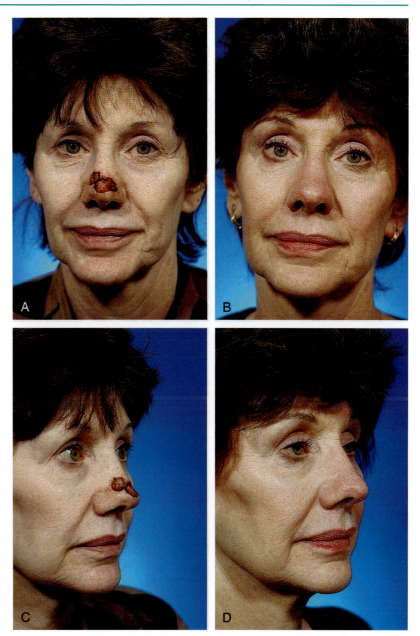

Figure 18–6. *A* to *D*, Preoperative and 6 months postoperative. Wound was repaired with full-thickness skin graft from supraclavicular area. Graft was dermabraded 3 months following grafting.

ever, the defect was small relative to the overall size of the nose. This fact, along with modest laxity of the nasal skin, convinced us that a bilobe flap was the preferred method of repair. The patient was left with a slight contour depression on the right side of the lower dorsum. Abnormal contour and distortion of the tip or margin of the nostril are the most common problems encountered when using a bilobe flap for nasal reconstruction (see Chapter 10). When the defect is small (maximum dimension 1 cm or less) and located cephalic to the apex of the domes, distortions and contour irregularities do not occur. However, larger skin defects repaired with a bilobe flap result in greater wound closure tension, which may lead to distortion of the topography of the nose. In addition, larger defects require greater quantities of skin transfer from the dor-

sum and sidewalls. This skin typically is thinner than the skin of the tip and may lead to subtle contour discrepancies as observed in this case. In Chapter 10 we discuss some of the techniques that may be used in an attempt to avoid contour deformities.

The second case represents the opposite end of the spectrum from case one. The patient's nose was small, and she had a recurrent basal cell carcinoma of the nasal tip for several years. Recurrent basal cell carcinomas typically are larger than primary tumors. Because of this, preparation for a paramedian forehead flap was made when the patient was interviewed at the initial consultation. As anticipated, the skin defect following Mohs' surgery was too large for repair with a nasal cutaneous flap. A skin graft would have left the patient with a noticeable notching and likely retraction of the

nostril. A paramedian forehead flap enabled resurfacing of the entire aesthetic unit of the tip and covered the framework graft used for support of the facet.

The third case is somewhere between the first and second case in complexity. The patient had a large nose and moderate nasal skin laxity. The defect was confined to the central tip, and its borders were well removed from the margin of the nostril. These factors would have led to the use of a nasal cutaneous flap for repair; however, the skin defect measured 3 cm in greatest dimension. The size of the defect prevented use of such a flap.

The defect extended through the skin only. The underlying subcutaneous fat and muscle remained, which could provide a well vascularized recipient site for a skin graft. A full-thickness skin graft of moderate thickness could fill the shallow wound, preventing a step-down contour deformity at the border of the graft. All these factors supported the choice of a full-thickness skin graft as the preferred method of repair. Had the depth of the defect extended to the level of the alar cartilages as observed in the first two cases, the choice of a skin graft for repair would have been less attractive because a contour depression and visible transition between graft and nasal skin would have been likely.

Pre- and postauricular and supraclavicular skin are preferred sources of full-thickness skin grafts used to cover defects of the nose. We prefer the preauricular area because skin color and solar aging more closely match those of the nasal skin. However, the quantity of skin available from the preauricular area is limited to approximately 3 cm^2. Larger grafts prevent primary closure of the donor wound. In contrast, supraclavicular skin is abundant. This site can provide sufficient skin to cover the entire nose while closing the donor wound primarily. Supraclavicular skin has a color similar to that of nasal skin and frequently has a similar amount of changes from solar aging.

19

Reconstruction of Tip, Dorsum, Sidewalls, and Ala

Shan R. Baker

The patient was a 62-year-old woman in consultation for basal cell carcinoma of the nose. Ten years earlier, she had undergone a pretrichial forehead lift and cervicofacial rhytidectomy. Physical examination revealed extremely thin nasal skin showing the outline of her delicate alar cartilages. A scaly lesion involved the skin covering the tip and a portion of the left nasal sidewall. The tumor extended inferiorly to the junction of the tip and columella and appeared to involve most of the skin of the right ala (Fig. 19–1). The patient had a relatively high forehead and a pretrichial scar that extended through the full width of the anterior hairline.

The tumor was excised using Mohs' surgery. Tumor ablation required removal of skin from the entire tip, both nasal facets, right ala, approximately half of both sidewalls, and the majority of the dorsum. The skin defect involved the entire margin of the right nostril (Fig. 19–2). An interpolated paramedian forehead flap was the preferred method of reconstructing the nose. However, the patient's pretrichial scar raised concern for the possibility of vascular compromise of the distal portion of the flap. For this reason, the flap was designed with an oblique angle near the hairline to limit extension of the flap distal to the scar (Fig. 19–3). In spite of the oblique design and extending the pedicle slightly into the eyebrow, the flap encompassed approximately 8 cm^2 of hair-bearing scalp distal to the pretrichial scar. This was necessary because nearly the entire nose, except for the left ala, and cephalic portion of the sidewalls required resurfacing.

Although no native nasal cartilage was removed by tumor extirpation, auricular cartilage batten grafts were placed along both nostril margins. The grafts extended from the alar base to the medial aspect of the facets at the junction of the intermediate and medial crura. The grafts were placed caudal to the alar cartilages and secured to them with 5-0 polyglactin sutures placed figure-of-eight to prevent overlapping of their edges. A graft was used on the right because batten grafts are routinely utilized when the ala is resurfaced. Such grafts reinforce the nostril margin and prevent partial collapse or cephalic migration of the alar margin. Although the left ala was not resurfaced, a batten graft was placed along the margin of the left nostril to serve as a safeguard against retraction of the nostril margin at the junction of the tip and ala and because of concern that the patient's delicate alar cartilages did not have sufficient intrinsic rigidity to resist the forces of wound contraction. Each of the batten grafts also served as a scaffold for the facets.

The defect extended to the left medial cheek. Cheek skin was advanced to the nasal facial sulcus and secured to the periosteum of the nasal process of the maxilla. A left interpolated paramedian forehead flap was used to resurface the nasal defect. To limit the amount of hair-bearing scalp included in the flap, the pedicle was incised through the medial eyebrow. The distal portion of the flap derived from forehead skin was thinned by removing the galea and frontalis muscle. The hair-bearing portion of the flap was not thinned because the scar separating forehead from

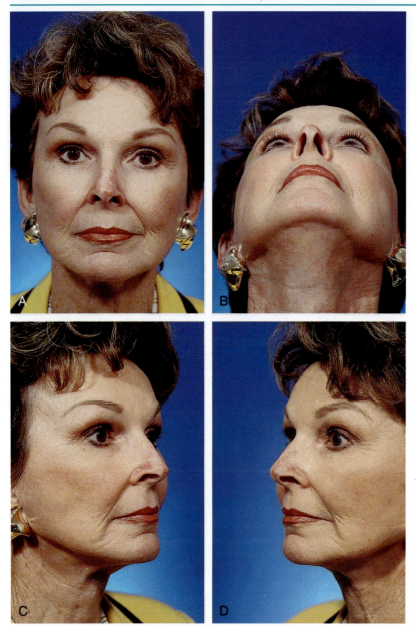

Figure 19–1. A–D. Patient with basal cell carcinoma of nose. Clinically, tumor appeared to involve tip and caudal aspect of dorsum and sidewalls.

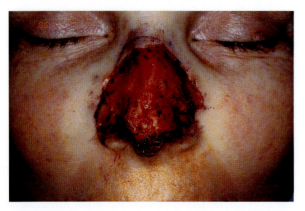

Figure 19–2. Nasal defect following Mohs' surgery. Skin defect involved entire tip, dorsum, right ala, both nasal facets, sidewalls, and entire margin of right nostril. All native nasal cartilage remained intact.

scalp skin prevented an axial pattern blood flow to the hair-bearing portion of the flap (Fig. 19–4). In spite of this, epidermolysis of the most distal hair-bearing portion of the flap occurred. This is a very superficial partial-thickness necrosis of the skin that results from vascular insufficiency. Fortunately, epidermolysis rarely leads to a visible scar. The width of the flap measured 6 cm; the size prevented complete primary closure of the donor wound. The portion of the wound not closed primarily was kept moist with petroleum ointment and left to heal by secondary intention.

Three weeks following transfer of the forehead flap, the pedicle was detached, and the flap was inset. The native skin of the nasion and cephalic sidewalls was preserved. Before inset, the flap was thinned by removing muscle and some of the subcutaneous fat on the

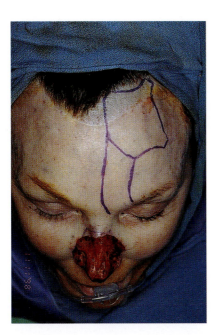

Figure 19–3. Oblique angled paramedian forehead flap designed to limit extension of flap beyond pretrichial scar.

undersurface of the flap. The inferior aspect of the donor wound was open, and the area between the eyebrows was widely undermined to release wound contracture and free the medial aspect of the left eyebrow. The proximal pedicle was converted to a small triangular skin flap that was advanced superiorly to restore the original position of the left eyebrow. It was necessary to excise a Burow triangle immediately above the medial aspect of the eyebrow as described in Chapter 14 (Fig. 19–5).

Four months following inset of the forehead flap (Fig. 19–6), a contouring procedure and a 2-cm-long revision of the inferior donor site scar were performed. The scar revision consisted of a simple elliptical excision of redundant skin in the glabella and reapproximation in layers of the wound edges. The flap was contoured by incising along the entire inferior border of the flap and elevating the entire flap in a superficial subcutaneous plane, exposing all hair follicles (Fig. 19–7). Using magnification, the hair follicles were individually cauterized and mechanically removed. Subcutaneous fat and scar deposition were sharply dissected from the underlying alar cartilages. The incision was repaired with 5-0 vertical mattress cutaneous sutures. A nasal cast served as a compression bandage.

Four months after the contouring procedure, the patient complained of bilateral partial nasal obstruction. Examination of the nose revealed mild constriction of the internal nasal valves. This occurred presumably from generalized contraction of scarring encompassing nearly the entire surface of the nasal framework. Although auricular cartilage alar batten grafts had served their purpose in preventing retraction or constriction of the nostril, the more cephalically located internal valves were compressed by overlying scar tissue.

Bilateral incisions were made along the inferior border of the flap at the margin of the nostrils. The flap was elevated on the left for a distance of 1.5 cm to expose some persistent hair follicles. These were cauterized individually. The marginal incisions exposed the previously placed auricular cartilage grafts that were removed by blunt and sharp dissection. These grafts had served their purpose in providing structural support to the alae; however, they appeared to be contributing to the bulk of soft tissue and scar surrounding the region of the internal nasal valves. The nasal obstruction was rectified by first harvesting septal cartilage through a Killian septal incision. The septal cartilage was cut in two strips, each 5 mm wide and 3 cm long. These strips serving as alar batten grafts were inserted in a pocket created in the alar base and were tunneled under the lateral crura where they were sutured to the crura in such a fashion that the cartilage grafts caused the nostrils to flare outward. The marginal incisions were repaired with 5-0 interrupted cutaneous sutures. Additional sutures were passed full-thickness through the nose and tied over a bolster to compress the flap on the left side.

In addition to nasal obstruction, careful inspection of the topography of the reconstructed nose had revealed persistent fullness in the cephalic portion of the flap and a noticeable transition between the skin of the flap and nasion. To improve contour, the cephalic third of the flap was thinned by incising the scar at the superior border of the flap. To lessen the abrupt transition between the skin of the flap and nasion, two Z-plasties were performed in the scar. The patient has remained free of recurrent skin cancer and has an improved nasal airway, although she still complains of minor nasal stuffiness on the right side. The transition between forehead and nasal skin at the nasion improved as a result of the Z-plasties (Fig. 19–8).

Discussion

This case is informative in a number of ways. One lesson that it demonstrates is that nasal obstruction may occur after the majority of the nose is resurfaced with a cutaneous flap even when native cartilage has not been removed. Obstruction may occur in spite of cartilage grafts in the form of battens used to supplement the native nasal framework. This phenomenon occurs most frequently when two or more nasal aesthetic units are resurfaced in patients with fragile or flaccid upper and lower lateral cartilages. Both of these predisposing factors were exhibited in this case.

It is not uncommon for patients to complain of some

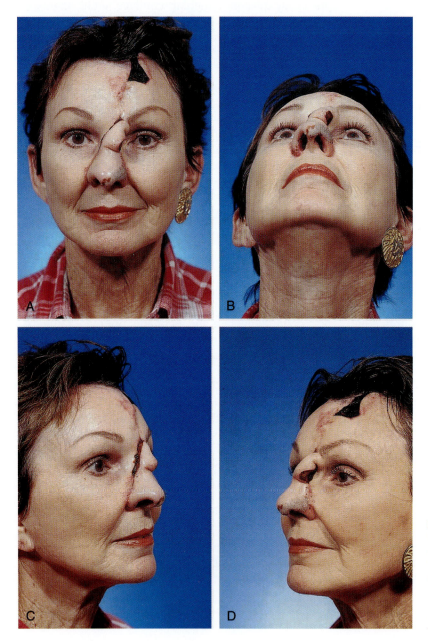

Figure 19–4. *A* to *D,* 3 weeks following flap transfer. Donor wound partially closed. Distal portion of flap derived from scalp is growing hair. This portion was not depilated at time of flap transfer. Superficial necrosis (epidermolysis) of skin covering tip has occurred as noted by darkened skin. This represents most distal portion of hair-bearing component of flap.

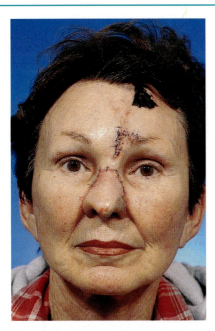

Figure 19-5. 1 day following flap detachment. A Burrow triangle was removed from above medial aspect of left eyebrow to restore proper positioning.

nasal stuffiness or obstruction for the first few months following resurfacing of the tip or ala with a paramedian forehead flap. This is because scar tissue between the flap and underlying nasal framework reaches maximal induration within the first 2 to 3 months following flap transfer. Nasal obstruction usually improves with time as the sheet of scar beneath the flap softens and matures. In the case of alar reconstruction, nasal obstruction on the side of reconstruction is common until a contouring procedure is performed that relieves the

obstruction by removing excessive tissue in the area of the internal nasal valve during the process of constructing an alar groove. Those cases that do not improve with time or after a contouring procedure are usually from persistent compression by scar tissue of the nasal passage, particularly in the critical area of the internal nasal valve. The problem is best addressed by inserting alar batten grafts through marginal incisions. The grafts are positioned deep to the lateral crura, between them and the vestibular skin. They should be of sufficient length to extend from the crura to the alar bases and are sutured to the lateral crura in such a manner that they cause the ala to slightly flare outward. This is accomplished by medial advancement of the lateral crus on the batten. Batten grafts expand the lumen of the nasal airway, displacing the alar and upper lateral cartilages laterally, which has the effect of widening the internal valves. Spreader grafts may also be helpful, but by themselves they are usually insufficient to improve the airway. This is because scar tissue typically causes compression of the entire cartilaginous skeleton supporting the sidewall and lateral tip. The scar constricts the internal valve along its entire perimeter from the attachment of the upper lateral cartilage to the septum medially to the bony piriform aperture laterally. Spreader grafts expand the angle between the septum and upper lateral cartilage but have no influence on the lateral aspect of the internal valve. Batten grafts have the capacity of lateral displacement of the entire upper lateral cartilage, which expands the cross-sectional area of the internal valve medially near the septum as well as laterally at the bony piriform aperture. If alar batten grafts have been used, they may sometimes be exposed, freed from surrounding tissue and readjusted to create greater alar flare. Other times, as in this

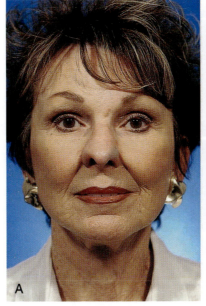
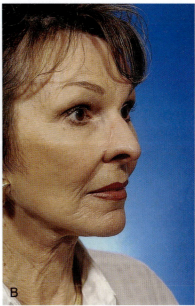

Figure 19-6. *A* and *B*, 4 months following pedicle detachment and before contouring procedure. Note general bulkiness of flap and lack of alar grooves.

A

B

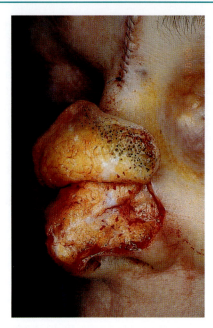

■ **Figure 19-7.** Contouring was accomplished by incising inferior border of flap and elevating entire flap in superficial subcutaneous plane exposing all hair follicles. Follicles were individually cauterized and resected.

case, it may be more expedient to replace them with new grafts.

The need to perform two depilation procedures to free the flap from hair growth is typical of most forehead flaps that transfer hair to the nose. This was true in this case in spite of meticulous exposure, cautery, and excision of all visible hair follicles during the initial contouring procedure. In addition to persistent hair growth, another disadvantage of transferring hair-bearing skin of the scalp with a forehead flap is the occasional poor texture and color match with native nasal skin. Scalp skin, particularly if hair-bearing, differs in texture and color from skin of the forehead. It is also thicker, less flexible, and has subcutaneous fat that is more adherent to the dermis. Transferring a forehead flap to the nose where both forehead and scalp skin will remain as part of the reconstructed nose may cause mild discrepancies in the nature of the skin covering the nose.

We attempt to limit the amount of scalp skin in-

cluded in a paramedian forehead flap for the reasons discussed. We often recruit skin in the temporal recession adjacent to the axis of the paramedian flap in instances where necessary flap length would require extending the flap to hair-bearing scalp. In such instances, the forehead flap is angled obliquely beneath the anterior hairline extending laterally toward the temporal recession (see discussion of oblique forehead flap in Chapter 14). This modification in flap design sometimes circumvents the need to include hair-bearing skin in the flap. Other times, as in the case presented, the design reduces the surface area of scalp that must be included.

This patient did not have the fine vellus hair typically observed at the anterior hairline because it was removed at the time of her forehead lift. Typically, however, this fine hair is transferred with a forehead flap that extends to the hair-bearing scalp. Vellus hair cannot be removed by exposing and removing the follicles (see discussion of this in Chapter 14). It is best managed with electrolysis or depilatory creams.

When using a paramedian forehead flap for repair of the nose, we have found the transition between forehead and nasal skin is often most noticeable in the area of the medial canthus, rhinion, and nasion, depending on how cephalically the flap extends. The thickness of skin in these regions is different from that of forehead skin. In the case of the extreme cephalic portion of the dorsum, there is a rapid tapering of skin thickness from the nasion to the rhinion, which is difficult to replicate with forehead skin. For this reason, we avoid replacing skin over the rhinion even when the remaining caudal portion of the dorsum is resurfaced with a forehead flap. In situations like this case where the defect involves the skin over the rhinion, we thin the forehead flap covering this portion of the nose to the level of the dermis. As in this case, we often use Z-plasties along the cephalic border of the flap to interface the skin of the flap with that of the nasion. This technique has the effect of interdigitating flap skin with nasal skin, making the transition between the two less visible. We often preserve the native skin of the cephalic third of the sidewalls when possible. The skin in this region is thin and devoid of subcutaneous fat. It is often difficult to replicate the thinness of this skin using forehead skin.

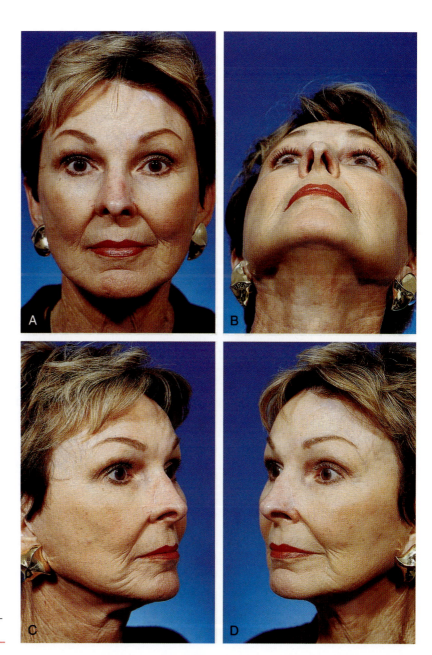

■ **Figure 19–8.** *A* to *D*, 1½ years following contouring procedure.

Sequential Paramedian Forehead Flaps

Shan R. Baker

The patient was a 44-year-old woman who had Mohs' surgery for treatment of a basal cell carcinoma of the right ala. Examination of her nasal defect following surgery revealed a 2.0 × 2.5 cm skin defect of the ala and tip (Fig. 20–1). A portion of the alar margin was missing. An interpolated paramedian forehead flap was used for repair of the nose. This flap was selected because of the patient's youthful face and lack of cheek skin laxity. The lining of the nostril margin was supplied by advancement of vestibular skin. The vestibular skin was dissected from the entire lateral crus of the alar cartilage and mobilized inferiorly to the level of the alar margin. The remaining skin of the alar aesthetic unit was removed, and an auricular cartilage alar batten graft described in Chapters 7 and 13 was secured along the nostril margin. The height of the graft extended from the nostril margin to the caudal border of the lateral crus of the alar cartilage. It was secured to the advanced vestibular skin with two 5-0 polyglactin mattress sutures. The graft was also sutured to the lateral crus, with similar sutures placed in a figure-of-eight fashion to prevent overlapping of the graft with the crus (Fig. 20–2).

A right interpolated paramedian forehead flap was used to cover the graft and resurface the skin defect (see Fig. 20–2). The forehead donor wound was repaired primarily by advancement. The caudal border of the forehead flap was sutured to the caudal border of the advanced vestibular skin. Three weeks later the pedicle of the forehead flap was detached. Three

months following pedicle detachment, a contouring procedure was performed to restore the alar groove. The patient did not return for examination following the contouring procedure.

Three years later, she was seen in consultation for another basal cell carcinoma located on the opposite side of the nose. Examination of the nose showed a reasonable restoration of the right ala except for a mild retraction of the nostril margin. A 1 × 1 cm yellowish ulcerating skin lesion involved the left nasal sidewall and left aspect of the tip. The forehead donor site scar was as expected, and there was slight inferior displacement of the medial aspect of the right eyebrow (Fig. 20–3).

Mohs' surgery was again used to excise the second cutaneous malignancy of her nose. The procedure left the patient with a large skin defect encompassing the nasal tip, portions of the dorsum, and left ala and sidewall (Fig. 20–4). Because the defect involved the rhinion, the remaining skin of the dorsal aesthetic unit was removed in conjunction with the remaining skin of the tip. The patient had a broad tip caused by marked convexity of the alar cartilages in both vertical and horizontal axes, giving the tip a bulbous appearance. She was agreeable to modification of her nasal tip contour. Exposed alar cartilages were modified with a dome-spanning suture to narrow the tip and reduce convexity of the lateral crura. An auricular cartilage alar batten graft was positioned along the nostril margin to provide a framework for the left ala. A left interpolated paramedian forehead flap was used to cover the

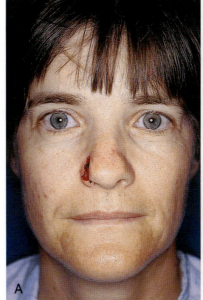
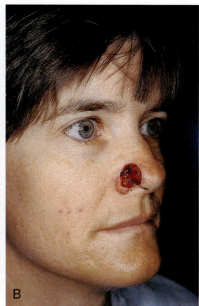

■ **Figure 20–1.** *A* and *B*, 2.0 × 2.5 cm skin defect of right ala and lateral tip. Small amount of lining is missing on inner aspect of nostril margin.

tip, dorsum, and left ala. This flap was designed so that the medial border of the entire flap was positioned along the donor scar of the previous paramedian forehead flap (Fig. 20–5). The left forehead flap measured 4.2 cm at the widest point, and it was necessary to incorporate hair-bearing scalp in the distal portion. The inferior portion of the donor forehead wound was closed in the scar line resulting from her first flap. However, complete wound approximation superiorly was not possible, and the defect was allowed to heal by secondary intention.

Similar to the first forehead flap, the second one was detached 3 weeks following transfer. Three months later, a contouring procedure was performed to construct an alar groove and depilate persistent hair follicles. This was accomplished by incising the entire inferior border of the flap and elevating it in the subdermal plane. Under magnification, all exposed hair follicles were cauterized and then mechanically removed. The left alar groove was constructed by sculpturing the exposed soft tissue. A bolster dressing as described in Chapter 13 was used to maintain the constructed groove.

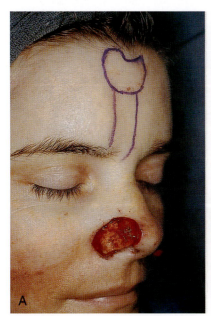
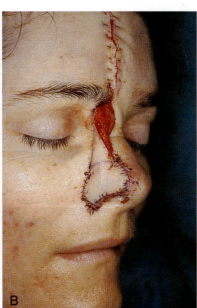
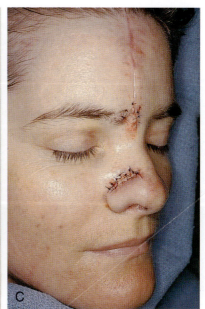

■ **Figure 20–2.** *A,* Remaining skin of alar unit removed. Auricular cartilage batten graft in place. Vestibular skin freed from lateral crus and stretched inferiorly to replace lining deficit. *B,* Right paramedian forehead flap used to resurface defect. *C,* Flap detached from forehead 3 weeks following transfer.

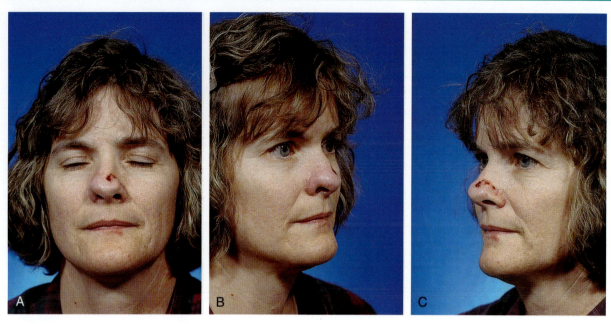

■ **Figure 20–3.** *A to C,* 3-year postoperative result of reconstruction. Patient has retraction of right nostril margin. She has developed second skin cancer on left side of nose.

Revision of the forehead donor site scar was also performed. Revision consisted of opening the inferior portion of the scar and excising a triangle-shaped section of forehead skin just above the medial aspect of the left eyebrow as described in Chapter 14. The medial eyebrow was undermined and mobilized superiorly, elevating it to the level of the opposite eyebrow. The wound was repaired in a V-to-Y configuration.

Eight months later, a second depilation of the flap was performed with the same approach as for the contouring procedure. In addition, an incision was made in the scar separating the reconstructed right ala and native skin of the right nasal sidewall. A flap was elevated by dissecting inferiorly in the subcutaneous plane to the level of the nostril margin. In the vicinity of the

retracted nostril margin, an auricular cartilage graft was positioned inferior to the previously placed alar batten graft. This second graft improved the retraction by lowering the level of the nostril (Fig. 20–6).

Discussion

The lining defect of the right ala was only 3 mm in vertical height, and the mobilized vestibular skin appeared to easily reach the inferior border of the nostril without tension. However, the nostril retracted subsequent to reconstruction of the ala in spite of using an

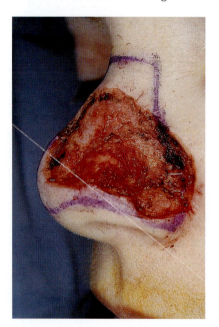

■ **Figure 20–4.** Skin defect following removal of second cutaneous malignancy.

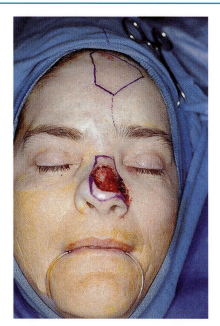

Figure 20–5. Left paramedian forehead flap designed to resurface nasal defect. Medial border of flap is positioned in donor site scar of first forehead flap.

alar batten graft. The error was in not releasing the vestibular skin from its cephalic attachment by performing an intercartilaginous incision. This incision is required for the development of a bipedicle vestibular skin advancement flap (see Chapters 4 and 11). Although an alar batten graft was used, and the patient had sturdy alar cartilages, scar contraction within the vestibule was sufficient to elevate the nostril. Fortunately, we were able to improve this condition somewhat by mobilizing the skin in the area of the retraction and by placing a cartilage graft caudal to the inferior border of the batten graft used in the initial reconstruction of the ala. The lesson taught by this case is that when vestibular skin is advanced inferiorly to line the nostril margin, it should be mobilized as a bipedicle advancement flap of vestibular skin. This is true even when repairing very small lining deficits.

One of the great advantages of designing a forehead flap with a paramedian axis compared with a midline design is that it leaves the patient with the possibility of having a second flap harvested from the contralateral side, should it be necessary at a later time. The second flap is based on the supratrochlear artery contralateral to the one used to supply the first flap. Depending on the size of the flap, typically, there is limited or no laxity of forehead skin following transfer of the first forehead flap. Thus, the donor wound resulting from the second flap usually cannot be completely closed and must heal in part by secondary intention. However, the narrow pedicle width of 1.5 cm required by each flap usually enables sequential primary closure of the inferior portion of the donor wounds. The medial bor-

der of the second flap should be positioned in the paramedian scar resulting from transfer of the first flap. This design and the narrow width of the two pedicles ensure a single unobtrusive scar in the inferior two-thirds of the forehead (Fig. 20–7). Although the superior portion of the donor site typically cannot be closed primarily after the transfer of the second flap, the wound heals without complications, resulting in a wide, somewhat atrophic-appearing flat scar that is acceptable to most patients. Secondary healing in the superior aspect of the central forehead usually results in an acceptable scar. This is due to the convexity of the upper forehead and the relative immobility of skin in this region. Facial wounds that heal by secondary intention on concave and convex surfaces produce less apparent scars when compared with flat surfaces. In addition to topography, skin immobility may play a role in scarring. Less noticeable scars occur in areas of limited skin mobility. In the case of the superior central forehead, the lack of skin mobility is related to the natural midline dehiscence of the frontalis muscle creating a deficiency of muscle in this region.

Alar cartilages are not commonly modified during reconstruction of the nose. Occasionally, a patient will express a desire to reduce the size of the nasal tip. Volume reduction using limited trimming of the alar cartilages may be performed simultaneously with repairing a skin defect of the tip. In the case presented, the alar cartilages were modified because of the patient's desire to have a less broad nasal tip. Alar cartilages may be compressed by the forces of wound contraction constricting the airway (see Chapter 19), and modification for the purpose of aesthetic improvement is performed only in patients with alar cartilages that have sufficient intrinsic strength to resist these forces. In most instances, alar cartilages are contoured using sutures rather than excisional techniques.[1] This approach maintains the structural integrity of the cartilages while modifying the shape of the tip.

This patient presented with her first basal cell carcinoma at a young age relative to most patients who develop skin cancer of the nose. Because the nasal skin had sustained sufficient sun damage to cause one cancer, it is not unreasonable to assume that the nasal skin not removed with resection of the first cancer may have a high potential for developing a second basal cell carcinoma. The younger a person is when developing skin cancer, the more likely that individual will live to see others develop. Surgeons should keep this in mind when planning nasal reconstruction. Depending on the defect, the forehead can usually provide sufficient skin for two independent nasal repairs. Skin of the two cheeks is also available as a source for covering flaps, provided the nasal defect is located laterally.

The potential for developing a second or third cutaneous malignancy of the nose may influence the surgical approach. If the patient has lost considerable nasal skin from removal of a cancer, and the remaining nasal

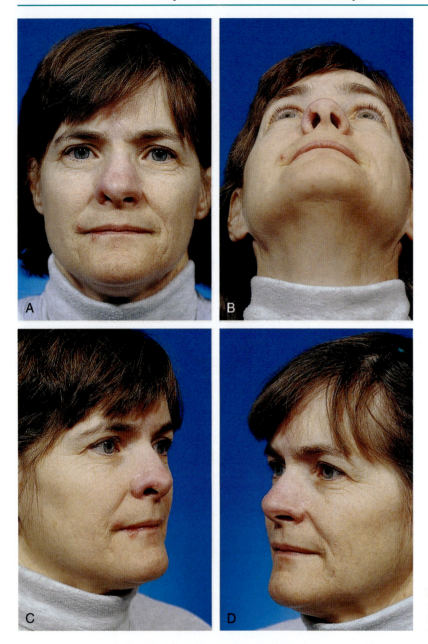

Figure 20–6. *A* to *D*, 2 years postoperative following transfer of second paramedian forehead flap to nose.

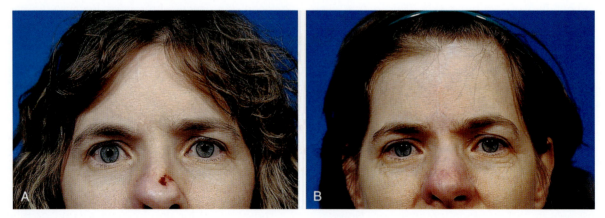

Figure 20–7. *A*, Forehead scar 3 years following transfer of right paramedian forehead flap to nose. *B*, Forehead scar 2 years following transfer of second (left) paramedian forehead flap to nose.

skin has numerous actinic changes, we recommend removal of all remaining skin of the nose. The entire nose is then resurfaced with an interpolated paramedian forehead flap. In some instances we have also resurfaced all or the majority of the nose when a patient has developed three or more nasal cutaneous malignancies at independent locations. This approach markedly reduces but does not eliminate the risk of developing future nasal skin cancers. Forehead skin transferred to the nose, like native nasal skin, has the potential for developing malignancies. Although the entire face is exposed to sunlight, the nasal skin receives a greater amount of ultraviolet radiation than forehead skin because of the position and angle of exposure to the sun. As a result, cancer arising from forehead skin is considerably less common than from nasal skin, particularly skin from the central portion of the forehead.

Reference

1. Baker SR: Suture contouring of the nasal tip. Arch Facial Plast Surg 2:34, 2000.

21

Reconstruction of Nasal Facet

A 50-year-old man presented with a 0.4-cm basal cell carcinoma of the left infratip lobule encroaching on the nostril margin. He had a basal cell carcinoma removed from the right nasal dorsum a year earlier. The dorsum had been repaired with a full-thickness skin graft. He did not use tobacco products.

Following Mohs' surgery, the patient was observed to have a 1.3-cm skin defect of the left infratip lobule and facet. It extended to the margin of the nostril (Fig. 21–1). The defect was repaired with a 1.0 × 1.5 cm auricular composite graft harvested from the preauricular skin and helical crus (see Chapter 9). In spite of postoperative ice compresses and the small size of the graft, it did not survive. Suppuration did not occur, so the graft was left in place to serve as a biological dressing while the wound healed beneath it by secondary intention. Ultimately, the eschar formed by the composite graft was removed, and the patient was left with a significant notching and distortion of the nostril margin (see Fig. 21–7).

Two surgical options were available to repair the defect. A second composite graft or a staged reconstruction could have been performed. A staged reconstruction required replacement of lining, structural support, and external covering. These alternative methods of repair were discussed with the patient. We both selected the staged repair because it was more likely to be successful.

The lining defect measured 0.5 cm in vertical height and 0.3 cm in width. Replacement was provided by a bipedicle vestibular skin advancement flap by means of surgical techniques discussed in Chapter 11 (Fig. 21–2). The advancement flap was sufficient because of the limited height of the lining deficit. An auricular cartilage graft served as framework for the facet. The remaining skin of the left half of the infratip lobule was removed. The adjacent nasal skin was undermined in a plane immediately above the perichondrium of the alar cartilage. The cartilage graft measuring 2.5 × 0.6 cm was sculpted, trimmed, and inset between the intermediate and lateral crura of the left alar cartilage. It was secured to the caudal border of the alar cartilage with figure-of-eight 6-0 polyglactin sutures as described in Chapter 7 (Fig. 21–3). The bipedicle vestibular skin advancement flap was suspended to the graft with a few mattress sutures of similar material (Fig. 21–4).

A template was used to design an interpolated paramedian forehead flap that served as covering for the defect. The flap was dissected and transferred to the nose using techniques discussed in Chapter 14. To prevent the transfer of hair to the nose, the pedicle of the forehead flap was extended below the level of the eyebrow (Fig. 21–5). The entire portion of flap covering the defect was thinned to the level of the superficial subcutaneous plane. The caudal border of the forehead flap was sutured to the caudal border of the lining flap. The forehead donor wound was closed by advancement of adjacent muscle and skin. The donor wound of the lining flap was repaired with a full-thickness skin graft.

Three weeks following transfer, the pedicle of the forehead flap was divided, and the flap was inset. The skin surrounding the medial aspect of the left eyebrow

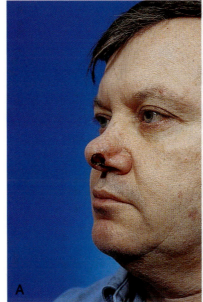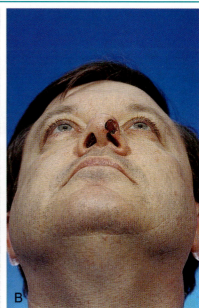

Figure 21-1. A and B, Skin and soft-tissue deficit of nasal facet. Auricular composite graft used to repair this was unsuccessful.

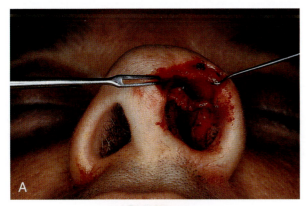

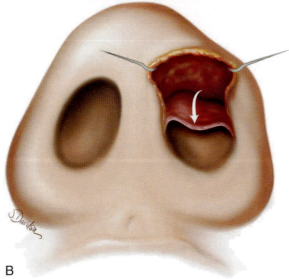

Figure 21-2. A and B, Bipedicle vestibular skin advancement flap used as lining flap.

was widely undermined in the subfascial plane, and the proximal pedicle was inset between the eyebrows. This restored the natural anatomical relationship of the two eyebrows (Fig. 21-6).

The patient did not require a contouring procedure; however, 3 months following reconstruction, he presented with partial extrusion of the auricular cartilage graft. This was causing a point of crusty inflammation on the infratip skin. This was treated in the office by injecting the area with local anesthesia and trimming the protruding cartilage. Reconstruction left him with subtle asymmetry of the nostrils that is only appreciated on the base view of the nose (Fig. 21-7).

Discussion

Limited full-thickness defects of the nostril margin may be successfully reconstructed with a composite graft. This has the advantage of providing in one surgical stage the lining, structural support, and external covering required for proper repair (see Chapter 9). With thoughtful case selection, composite grafts used in primary repair of the nose survive in their entirety in approximately 50% of cases. If grafting is delayed until healing by secondary intention has occurred and the graft is small (1.0 cm or less), it is more likely to survive.

The other alternative for repair of full-thickness defects of the nostril involves a more complex two- or three-stage surgical procedure. This represents a long

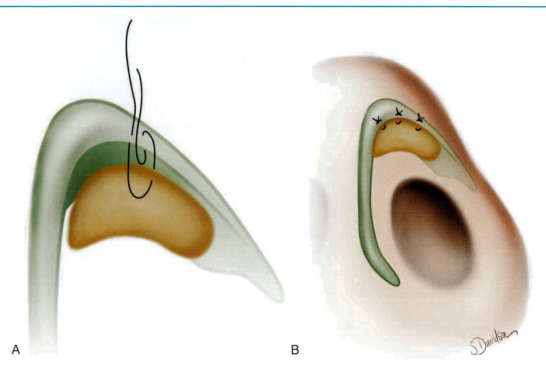

■ **Figure 21–3.** *A* and *B,* Auricular cartilage graft is secured to caudal border of alar cartilage with figure-of-eight sutures.

run for a short slide. That is, it requires the use of multiple flaps and cartilage grafting to successfully transfer a very small quantity of tissue to the margin of the nostril.

This case represented a dilemma that occasionally confronts the surgeon. The dilemma is that a small skin defect of the nose that could easily be repaired with a skin graft or nasal cutaneous flap involves the nostril margin excluding the use of these surgical approaches. The surgeon must decide whether to perform a staged reconstruction or attempt a composite graft, which has considerably greater risk of failure. Patients may sometimes have difficulty accepting a complex surgical procedure when the defect is so small. However, even minor irregularities of the nostril margin are apparent to the casual observer. Patients presenting with full-thick-

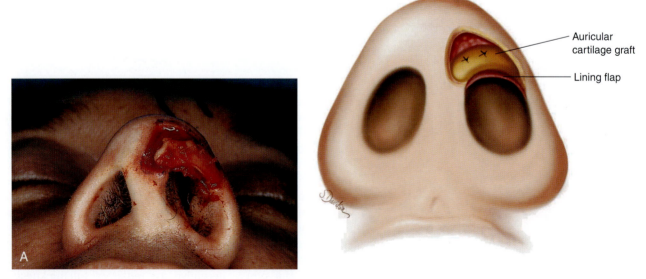

■ **Figure 21–4.** *A* and *B,* Auricular cartilage graft served as framework for repair. Lining flap was suspended to inner aspect of cartilage graft (note sutures through cartilage). Unencumbered caudal border of lining flap extends beyond framework graft.

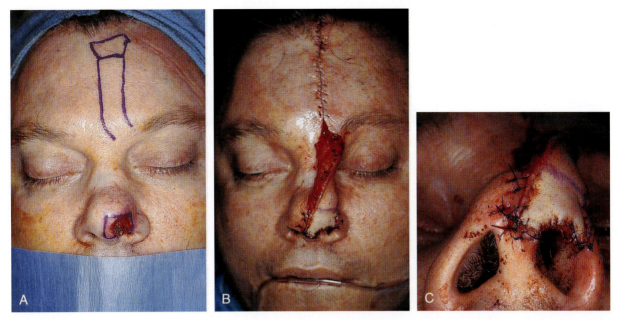

■ **Figure 21–5.** *A*, Skin of left half of infratip is marked for excision. Interpolated paramedian forehead flap is designed as covering flap. *B* and *C*, Forehead flap in position. Caudal border is sutured to distal border of lining flap.

ness defects of the nostril are instructed that simpler methods of repair, such as full-thickness skin grafts, will ultimately result in distortion, notching, or retraction of the nostril. Composite grafts are offered as an alternative to a staged reconstruction in persons with small defects who do not use tobacco or who have peripheral vascular disease. They are informed of the limited success of composite grafts and the possible need for subsequent, more elaborate, surgical procedures, should the graft not survive. Patients who are not candidates for composite grafts are instructed on the critical location of their defect. They are told that a staged

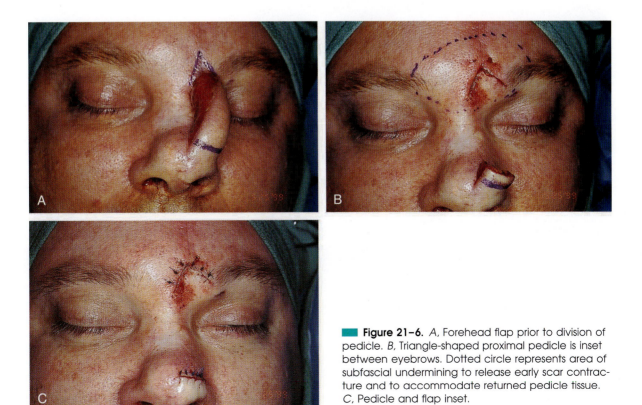

■ **Figure 21–6.** *A*, Forehead flap prior to division of pedicle. *B*, Triangle-shaped proximal pedicle is inset between eyebrows. Dotted circle represents area of subfascial undermining to release early scar contracture and to accommodate returned pedicle tissue. *C*, Pedicle and flap inset.

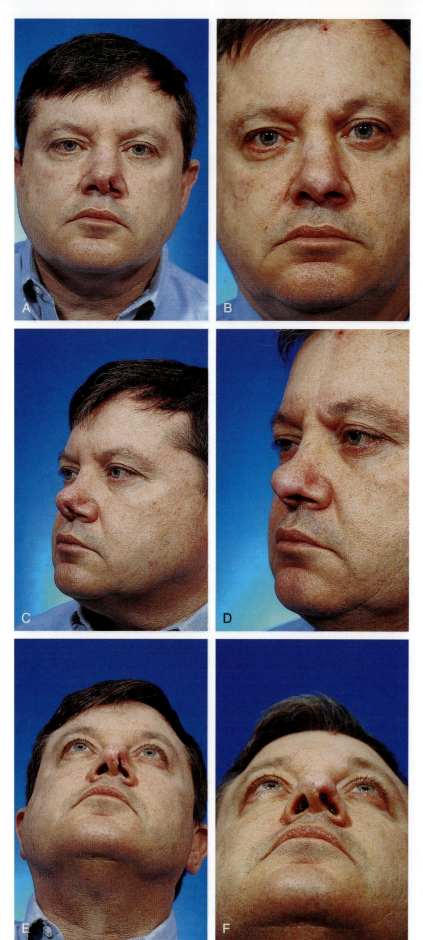

Figure 21–7. *A to F,* Full-thickness defect of nasal facet after failure of auricular composite graft and 1 year postoperative results using two-stage surgical repair.

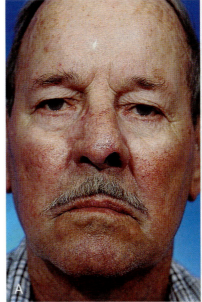
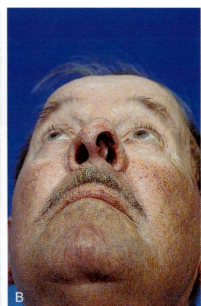

■ **Figure 21-8.** *A* and *B,* 1.0 × 1.5 cm full-thickness defect of nasal facet. Height of lining defect is too great to repair with bipedicle vestibular skin advancement flap.

surgical procedure is necessary in spite of the limited size of the defect to prevent the development of an unsightly notch of the nostril.

The forehead rather than the cheek was selected as the donor site for the covering flap in this case. The choice of a paramedian forehead flap provided greater confidence that the covering flap would survive because forehead flaps have a greater vascular supply compared with interpolated cheek flaps (see Chapters 13 and 14). This is especially true when a cheek flap

must be of sufficient length to reach the midline of the tip. The first surgical procedure used to repair the nose had failed. To maintain the confidence of the patient, it was important to select a covering flap that was most likely to survive and provide a successful reconstruction.

The vertical height of the lining defect in this case was 0.5 cm. Full-thickness defects of the nasal facet that have a greater vertical height cannot be repaired with a bipedicle vestibular skin advancement flap because there is insufficient skin remaining in the nasal vesti-

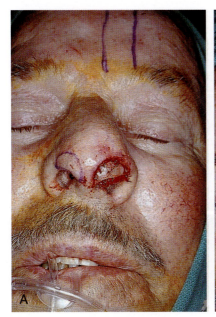
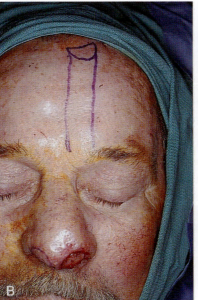
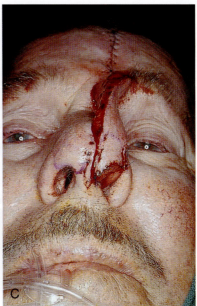

■ **Figure 21-9.** *A,* Lining of defect was provided by ipsilateral septal mucoperichondrial hinge flap. Septal cartilage served as framework and flap was suspended to cartilage graft (note sutures through cartilage). Unencumbered caudal border of lining flap extends beyond framework graft. *B,* Interpolated paramedian forehead flap designed as covering. *C,* Forehead flap in position. Caudal border was sutured to distal border of lining flap.

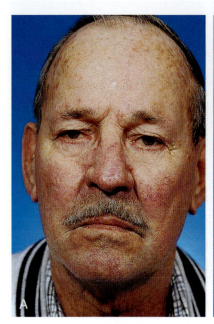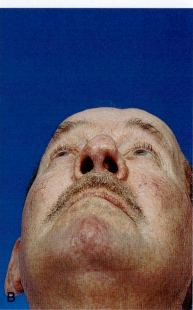

Figure 21–10. *A* and *B*, 6 months following pedicle detachment of covering and lining flaps. Contouring procedure was not required.

bule to line the defect. In these instances, an ipsilateral septal mucoperichondrial hinge flap (see Chapters 4 and 11) is required for lining.

The full-thickness defect shown in Fig. 21–8 is an example of a defect of the nasal facet that cannot be lined with a bipedicle vestibular skin advancement flap because of its size. The patient was a 76-year-old man who smoked a pack or more of cigarettes a day for most of his life. After Mohs' surgery for a basal cell carcinoma, he presented with a 1.0 × 1.5 cm full-thickness defect of the nasal facet. A septal mucoperichondrial flap hinged on the caudal septum (see Chapters 4 and 11) was used to line the defect. Septal cartilage exposed by transferring the flap to the facet was removed and used as a framework graft positioned caudal to the alar cartilage. The cartilage graft was covered with an interpolated paramedian forehead flap. The caudal border of the forehead flap was sutured to the caudal border of the lining flap (Fig. 21–9).

The distal portion of the lining flap became necrotic, exposing the overlying cartilage graft. Three weeks postoperatively, the flap was débrided. The pedicle of the flap was dissected more caudally to give length to the flap so that it could be reattached to the caudal border of the forehead flap. Detachment of the forehead flap was delayed. The distal end of the lining flap necrosed again; however, granulation tissue was noted to be

present on the inner aspect of the septal cartilage graft. Two weeks following reattachment of the lining flap, it was débrided, and the pedicle was detached from the septum. The pedicle of the forehead flap was also divided, and the forehead flap was inset in the nose. The interior aspect of the reconstructed facet eventually healed by secondary intention without stenosis of the apex of the nasal dome. No additional surgical procedures were required.

The lining flap was a complete failure in this case. However, together with the forehead flap and adjacent nasal tissue, it may have contributed sufficient vascularity to enable the interior of the reconstructed facet to heal by secondary intention. Probably, the rich vascular supply of the forehead flap provided sufficient nourishment to the cartilage graft to enable the graft to survive. It also provided a vascular supply to the margins of the defect, which facilitated the growth of granulation tissue on the deep surface of the cartilage graft. The granulation tissue in turn enabled healing without loss of the graft and without notching of the nostril margin (Fig. 21–10). Although septal mucoperichondrial hinge flaps have a rich vascular supply, they are subject to necrosis, particularly in smokers. When this occurs, reattachment is unlikely to be successful as noted in this example. Fortunately, in this case the patient healed without excessive scarring or deformity.

22

Reconstruction of Ala and Lateral Tip

Shan R. Baker

A 44-year-old woman developed melanoma of the left alar groove. This was resected by her referring dermatological surgeon, and the patient was referred for wider surgical margins. She was in excellent health and did not have other cutaneous malignancies. Examination of the nose revealed a 0.8-cm ulcer in the anterior portion of the alar groove where the wound had been left open following her resection. A chest radiograph revealed no evidence of metastases. Pathological examination of the excised specimen showed a melanoma of a Breslow level of 2.13 mm. The recommended treatment was full-thickness resection of the tumor with a 1.5-cm wide soft-tissue margin (Fig. 22–1).[1] The tumor was excised by removing the entire ala, lateral tip, and caudal portion of the sidewall to the level of the base of the piriform aperture. The lateral crus and upper lateral cartilage was included in the specimen. Resection left a 3.0 × 2.75 cm full-thickness defect of the left nose (Fig. 22–2).

Reconstruction required replacing missing tissue with like tissue in three layers: lining, framework, and external cover. Internal lining was provided by an ipsilateral septal mucoperichondrial hinge flap described in Chapters 4 and 11. The flap measured 5 × 3 cm and was incised through the defect by an angled scalpel blade. The flap, hinged on the caudal septum, was dissected from the bony perpendicular ethmoid plate and cartilaginous septum (Fig. 22–3). The exposed septal cartilage was removed as a single piece for grafting purposes. This was accomplished by incising the cartilage with a scalpel while preserving the contralateral mucoperichondrium. The borders of the incised mucosa along the perimeter of the remaining intact septum were cauterized to prevent postoperative hemorrhage.

The hinge flap was reflected laterally to provide internal lining to the defect. The borders of the flap were sutured to the margins of the mucosal defect with interrupted 5-0 polyglactin sutures. The proximal margins of the flap were sutured to each other to develop a closed cul-de-sac that separated the nasal passage from the exterior wound (see Fig. 22–3). The caudal border of the flap was left unencumbered to serve as lining for the nostril margin. The cartilage removed from the septum was thinned with a scalpel and trimmed to precisely replace the missing upper lateral cartilage and lateral crus. The specimen was tailored to the defect and secured by suturing the edges of the cartilage to the surrounding periosteum laterally, septum medially, and lateral aspect of the dome cartilage inferiorly. The caudal aspect of the cartilage graft was scored to create a convex contour simulating the topography of the lateral crus. This provided sufficient convexity to the re-

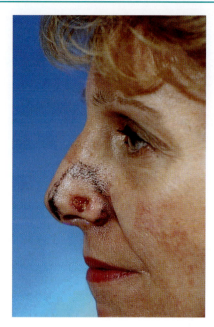

■ **Figure 22-1.** Open wound following resection of melanoma of alar groove. Black marking indicates margins for planned full-thickness resection.

gion of the lateral tip so that a separate piece of cartilage to replace the lateral crus was not necessary. The mucoperichondrial hinge flap was suspended to the undersurface of the cartilage graft using 5-0 polyglactin mattress sutures that passed full-thickness through the cartilage and partial-thickness through the lining flap (see Chapter 11).

A 3.0 × 1.5 cm auricular cartilage graft was removed from the right ear with techniques described in Chapter 7. The purpose of this graft was to provide structure for the ala. After sculpturing, the graft was scored to en-

hance its convexity, better simulating contour of the ala. One end of the graft was inserted into a soft-tissue pocket created at the alar base. The other end was tapered to fit in the nasal facet (Fig. 22–4). The graft that slightly overlapped the caudal aspect of the septal cartilage graft was sutured to the septal cartilage and medial crus with mattress 5-0 polydioxanone sutures. These sutures served to stabilize the two grafts with respect to each other, providing a more solidified framework. The caudal aspect of the septal mucoperichondrial hinge flap was suspended to the alar batten graft with a single mattress suture.

A template of the surface defect was made before resection. The template represented the precise pattern of the nasal skin removed. It was used to design a left interpolated paramedian forehead flap measuring 10 cm in length and 3 cm in width. The flap extended to the hair-bearing scalp. It was elevated from the frontal bone, and the distal two-thirds covering the defect was thinned as described in Chapter 14. Interrupted vertical mattress 5-0 polypropylene sutures were used to approximate the flap to the adjacent nasal skin. The caudal border of the forehead flap was sutured to the caudal border of the mucoperichondrial hinge flap with a continuous 5-0 polyglactin suture. The donor forehead wound was repaired primarily by advancement of wound margins (Fig. 22–5).

Three weeks following the first stage of reconstruction, the pedicle of the interpolated paramedian forehead flap was detached. The portion of the flap not thinned at the initial transfer was thinned of its muscle, and most of the subcutaneous tissue and the flap were inset. The septal mucoperichondrial hinge flap was also detached from the septum by incising through the pedicle and removing redundant mucosa. This restored the patency of the nasal passage.

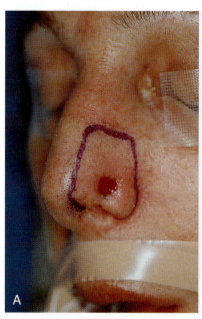
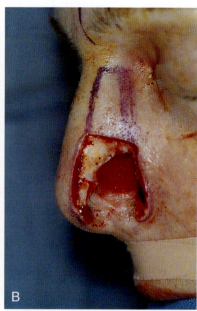

■ **Figure 22-2.** *A,* Marking indicates planned resection margin. *B,* Full-thickness resection of ala, caudal sidewall, and hemitip. Upper lateral cartilage exposed in wound was resected to level of septum and nasal bone before reconstruction.

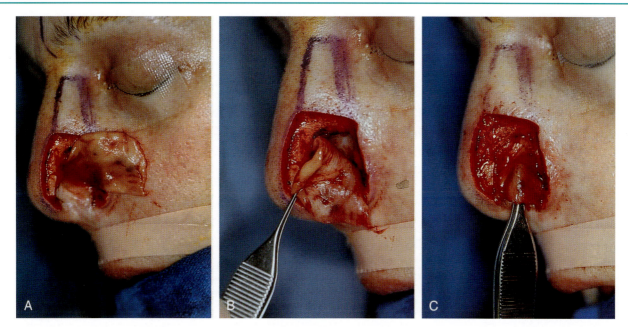

■ **Figure 22–3.** *A,* Septal mucoperichondrial flap reflected laterally. *B,* Lining flap hinged on caudal septum is folded on itself. *C,* Blind cul-de-sac lined by mucosa is created by suturing borders of flap to margins of lining defect. End of forcept is within cul-de-sac.

Ten weeks later, a contouring procedure was performed to restore the alar groove. A template of the contralateral ala was fashioned, reversed, and used to outline the alar groove on the reconstructed side. A 3-cm incision was made through the middle of the flap along this line. Skin flaps were elevated on either side of the incision. Subcutaneous fat, scar deposition, and some cartilage (alar batten) were removed as described in Chapter 13 to construct the groove. Persistent hair follicles surviving the depilation efforts administered at the time of the initial flap transfer were individually cauterized using magnification. The constructed alar groove was maintained with compression by using a bolster dressing consisting of 4-0 polypropylene sutures passed full-thickness through the ala and tied loosely over a dental roll. The patient had developed a syn-

echia between the septum and the interior of the reconstructed nostril. This was resected with a scalpel. A silastic splint was positioned alongside the septum and secured with a single trans-septal suture. The bolster was removed 5 days later and the splint 10 days following surgery.

At the initial consultation, the patient had expressed interest in reducing the overall size of her nose and the convexity of her nasal bridge. Aesthetic procedures on the nose were postponed until reconstruction was complete. Three months following the contouring procedure, a reduction rhinoplasty was performed. This was accomplished through an open approach using transcolumellar and marginal incisions. The skin was dissected from the native nasal cartilaginous and bony framework as well as from the cartilage grafts used for

■ **Figure 22–4.** *A* and *B,* Septal cartilage graft used to replace missing upper lateral cartilage and lateral crus. Caudal portion of graft scored to create convex surface, simulating contour of lateral crus. Auricular cartilage alar batten graft positioned along nostril margin and slightly overlaps septal cartilage. Forceps retract caudal border of lining flap.

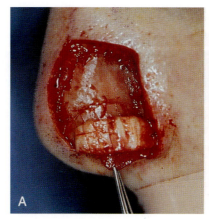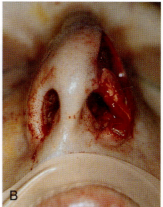

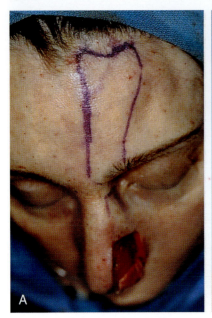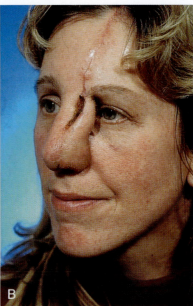

Figure 22–5. *A,* Interpolated paramedian forehead flap designed for external flap. Flap extends to hair-bearing scalp. *B,* 3 weeks following transfer of forehead flap.

reconstruction of the nose. The right upper lateral cartilage was detached from the septum. The remaining dorsal septum was 1 cm wide, enabling a 3 mm trim of the cartilaginous dorsum. The bony dorsum was lowered a similar degree with an osteotome. The right upper lateral cartilage and left septal cartilage graft were also trimmed to accommodate the lowered nasal bridge. Bone wedges 1 mm thick were removed from the bony vault on either side of the bony septum. This increased the open roof deformity without the need for further lowering of the bony dorsum. Medial and lateral osteotomies were performed, and the nasal bones were infractured to narrow the bony vault. A columella strut was fashioned from cartilage trimmed from the septum. This was secured to the medial crura with 5-0 polypropylene sutures. The crura were advanced on the strut to increase tip projection.

The septal mucoperichondrial hinge flap used to line the reconstructed ala and tip was thick, thus causing mild compromise of the internal nasal valve on the left side. The flap was thinned through the marginal incision by dissecting rostrally in the submucosal plane of the flap. Contouring the interior of the nostril was accomplished by removing submucosal tissue and scar deposition. A bolster dressing consisting of 4-0 polypropylene sutures that passed from the nasal skin through the mucoperichondrial flap and back again and tied over a dental roll compressed the flap and eliminated dead space. Skin incisions were repaired, and a nasal cast was applied as with standard rhinoplasty. The cast and bolster were removed 1 week later. The patient has remained free of recurrent tumor. She has a pleasant nasal appearance (Fig. 22–6).

Discussion

Loss of the upper lateral cartilage and lateral crus of the alar cartilage seen with full-thickness nasal defects of the sidewall and lateral tip can frequently be replaced with a single piece of septal cartilage as in this case. The caudal portion of the graft is thinned more severely and scored to increase its convexity. This in turn causes the cartilage to bend outward, assuming the contour of the lateral crus. This technique may not always restore a natural contour to the lateral tip. In such instances, a second cartilage graft is sculptured in the shape of the lateral crus and placed over the first graft in a position corresponding to that of the missing lateral crus. In all instances of full-thickness defects of the lateral nose involving the ala, an alar batten graft is included in the construction of the framework. The batten is made 1.5 cm wide, which corresponds to the approximate vertical height of the ala. This width ensures proper contour of the reconstructed ala and provides a continuous sheet of cartilage extending from the nostril margin to the alar cartilage. When the lateral crus of the alar cartilage has been resected, it is replaced with a septal cartilage graft. When the upper lateral cartilage is absent, it is also replaced with a septal cartilage graft. In such instances, a wide (1.5 cm) alar batten graft is made to overlap the caudal portion of the graft replacing the upper lateral cartilage. The batten concomitantly provides a framework for the ala and restores the contour of the missing lateral crus of the alar cartilage without the necessity of replacing the

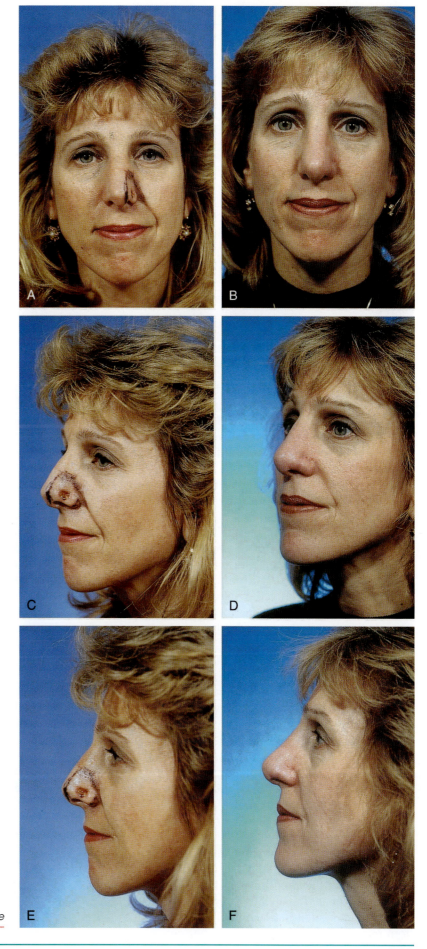

■ **Figure 22–6.** *A* to *H,* Preoperative and 1 year following reconstruction and subsequent conservative reduction rhinoplasty. Black markings on preoperative views indicate margins of subsequent surgical resection.
Illustration continued on following page

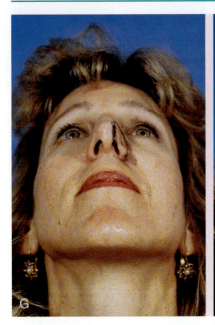
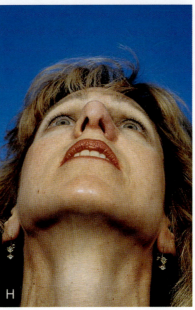

■ **Figure 22–6** *Continued.*

crus with a separate piece of cartilage. When covered with a skin flap, this arrangement of cartilage grafts produces a natural valley between constructed sidewall and ala simulating the alar groove. This groove is enhanced by a subsequent contouring procedure as discussed in Chapter 13.

The internal lining used in the reconstruction of this case was provided by a septal mucoperichondrial flap. The flap is reflected laterally from the septum and is sutured to the margins of the lining defect. To provide the maximum mucosal surface area to the region that requires the greatest quantity of lining material, the flap is often angulated so that a portion of the inferior or superior border is recruited alongside the distal margin to provide the necessary lining for the caudal border of the missing nostril. To facilitate the positioning of the flap, it is sometimes necessary, as in this case, to suture the more proximal borders of the flap together (see Chapter 11). This may cause a mucosally lined cul-de-sac that seals off the nasal passage from the exterior. This in turn separates the framework grafts from the nasal passage, preventing contamination of the grafts. The cul-de-sac is opened by incising through the pedicle of the flap, separating it from the septum. This is accomplished at the same time as detachment of the pedicle of the covering flap. Redundant mucosa is trimmed from the lining flap after dividing the pedicle. This usually restores the patency of the airway without additional surgical procedures. A synechia may occasionally form between septum and constructed nasal sidewall, as occurred in this case. Management consists of resection of the synechia and temporary placement of a septal splint. The splint prevents the synechia from reforming and is left in place until the raw surfaces left from resection of the synechia have healed.

Septal mucoperichondrial flaps used for lining ala and nasal sidewall transfer to these regions erectile tissue located in the submucosa of the posterior septum. This tissue retains its capacity to become engorged with blood after being transferred to the constructed nasal passage. The erectile nature of the mucosa of the lining flap tends to involute with time but may be of sufficient bulkiness to crowd the area of the internal nasal valve. Such was the condition in this case. Management consists of making an incision along the caudal border of the lining flap, dissecting rostrally in a submucosal plane, and removing the erectile tissue that is in the form of redundant submucosal tissue. The lining flap is then coapted to the overlying cartilage framework with a bolster suture.

Aesthetic rhinoplasty is not often requested by patients undergoing nasal reconstruction. As in this case, when such patients do make a request for aesthetic improvement of the nose, these changes are usually delayed until the nose has been completely reconstructed. The exception to this is in patients undergoing a nasal cutaneous flap to repair the nose. In this situation, the rhinoplasty is performed concurrent with repair of the nasal defect. The "open sky" effect of dissecting the nasal cutaneous flap exposes the entire nasal skeleton, facilitating necessary modifications as called for by the rhinoplasty (see Chapter 10). When reduction rhinoplasty is planned, reducing the projection of the dorsum or tip creates a redundancy of skin that often reduces wound closure tension following transfer of the nasal cutaneous flap.

Reference

1. Baker SR: Major Nasal Reconstruction. In Facial Plastic and Reconstructive Surgery, 2nd ed. New York, Thieme, in press.

23

Bilateral Paramedian Forehead Flaps

Shan R. Baker

The patient was a 66-year-old man with type II diabetes mellitus who developed an adenoid cystic carcinoma of the left posterior nasal passage. Computerized axial tomography demonstrated that the epicenter of the tumor was arising from the deep surface of the left nasal bone. The nasal bones and posterior superior bony septum were eroded by the tumor. The cribriform plate appeared intact; however, the tumor extended into the posterior ethmoid cells. The neoplasm was removed by a craniofacial resection through a bicoronal approach. Surgery included an ethmoidectomy, partial medial maxillectomy, and resection of the cribriform plate and posterior superior bony septum. Full-thickness resection of the left bony and cartilaginous nasal sidewall was performed. A portion of the bony dorsum was also removed. The patient refused postoperative radiotherapy because of the small risk of blindness.

Examination following resection of the neoplasm revealed a 3.0 × 4.5 cm full-thickness defect of the nasal sidewall and medial cheek (Fig. 23–1). There was complete absence of the left upper lateral cartilage, nasal bone, and medial maxilla. The superior bony septum was also absent, thus interrupting the branches providing blood supply to the nasal septum from the anterior and posterior ethmoidal and sphenopalatine arteries. The portion of the bony septum contributed by the vomer was present inferiorly. Interruption of the posterior blood supply of the septum gave concern for the use of a contralateral septal mucoperichondrial hinge flap based on the remaining bony dorsum. This is the preferred lining flap for repairing full-thickness defects of the cephalic portion of the sidewall (see Chapters 4 and 11).

A Killian incision near the caudal border of the nasal septum was used to remove the majority of the cartilaginous septum, maintaining a 1.5–cm-wide continuous strip of dorsal and caudal septal cartilage for support of the tip and middle vault. A portion of the vomer was harvested in continuity with the cartilage graft using techniques discussed in Chapter 11. This provided a sizable composite graft of bone and cartilage for use as framework for the nasal sidewall. A large auricular cartilage graft measuring 4.0 × 1.5 cm was obtained from the left ear by techniques discussed in Chapter 5.

The absence of the majority of the dorsal and posterior blood supply to the remaining septum encouraged the use of a forehead flap for lining the nasal defect (Fig. 23–2). A right interpolated paramedian forehead flap measuring 3 cm in width was dissected and transferred to the interior of the nasal passage. The flap was tunneled beneath the intervening skin of the glabella and delivered to the interior of the nose by hinging rather than pivoting the pedicle at the level of the eyebrow (see Chapter 14). The flap was thinned of its muscle and some subcutaneous tissue and sutured to the mucosal borders of the lining defect with the skin of the flap turned toward the nasal passage.

The composite graft of bone and septal cartilage was used for the framework of the repair. The graft was cut to the appropriate size and placed over the exposed surface of the lining flap and secured to the flap with 4-

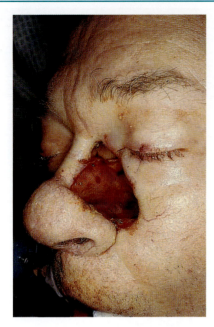

■ **Figure 23–1.** 3.0 × 4.5 cm full-thickness defect of nasal sidewall and medial cheek. There is complete absence of left upper lateral cartilage, nasal bone, and medial maxilla.

0 polyglactin sutures (Fig. 23–3). The graft served as a large batten for the sidewall. The nasal skin was elevated from the remaining nasal bridge, creating a space to accommodate an auricular cartilage graft. A double-layered dorsal onlay graft was fashioned from the cartilage and used to augment the dorsal line of the middle and bony vaults. The graft extended the full length of the two vaults.

The cutaneous component of the defect extended to the medial cheek. Cheek skin was dissected in a subcutaneous plane and advanced to the level of the anticipated nasal facial sulcus. It was secured in position using 4-0 polyglactin sutures that passed from the deep surface of the cheek flap to the exposed raw surface of the lining flap previously attached to the interior of the nasal passage. A template of the nasal skin defect was used to design a left interpolated paramedian forehead flap. The flap was 3 cm wide and was dissected to the level of the left eyebrow. It was pivoted inferiorly to provide external cover. The flap was thinned of muscle and the majority of subcutaneous tissue and was sutured to the periphery of the cutaneous defect with interrupted vertical mattress sutures (Fig. 23–4).

The forehead donor wound was 6 cm wide, and no attempt was made to advance the remaining forehead skin. The open wound was kept moist with petroleum ointment. It was anticipated that the majority of the forehead skin comprising the proximal pedicles of the two flaps would be returned, replacing much of the missing skin from the lower central forehead. Three

weeks following transfer of the paramedian forehead flaps, their pedicles were divided, and the flaps were inset. The pedicle of the internal lining flap was transected inside the nasal passage with an angled scalpel blade inserted through the skin tunnel created to deliver the flap to the interior of the nose. The proximal pedicle beneath the glabellar skin was pulled out of the tunnel and returned to the forehead without trimming. Using the skin tunnel for access, the incised border of the distal flap was sutured to the cephalic border of the mucosal defect with interrupted 5-0 polyglactin sutures. This sealed off the connection between the nasal passage and the exterior. The pedicle of the external flap was divided, and the proximal pedicle was returned to the forehead in its entirety. The portion of the external flap left attached to the nose was inset. A compression dressing was applied over the area. Returning all of the tissue comprising the proximal pedicles of the two flaps restored all of the forehead skin between the eyebrows as well as some skin to the central forehead. The medial aspect of both eyebrows was widely undermined in the subfascial plane and spread apart in order to accommodate return of the two pedicles. This in turn restored a normal anatomical relationship between the two eyebrows.

The patient did not require a contouring procedure. He was monitored closely for possible recurrent tumor by periodic examinations of the nasal passage with a nasal endoscope and yearly magnetic resonance imaging studies. Three years following reconstruction he presented with a complaint of left nasal obstruction. Examination showed medial displacement of the constructed nasal sidewall that appeared to be obstructing the nasal passage in the area of the internal nasal valve. It was apparent that the composite graft used as framework for the sidewall was not providing sufficient rigidity to prevent partial collapse of the soft tissues composing the sidewall.

The loss of the entire medial maxilla accounted for the lack of support to the soft tissues of the cheek and nasal sidewall. This great deficiency of bone made bone grafting a difficult proposition. Restoring continuity of bone from the nasal dorsum to the midportion of the maxilla would have required several split rib or cranial bone grafts. An alternative to bone grafting was selected as the preferred method of lateralizing the nasal sidewall and restoring structural support to the cheek and nose. A 3 × 4 cm titanium mesh was implanted beneath the skin of the nasal sidewall and medial cheek. An incision was made in the left alar groove between the inferior border of the forehead flap used for external cover and the native nasal skin. A large subcutaneous pocket was dissected to accommodate the mesh. The pocket extended to the glabella superiorly, nasal dorsum medially, and residual maxilla laterally. The portion of mesh extending from the nasal

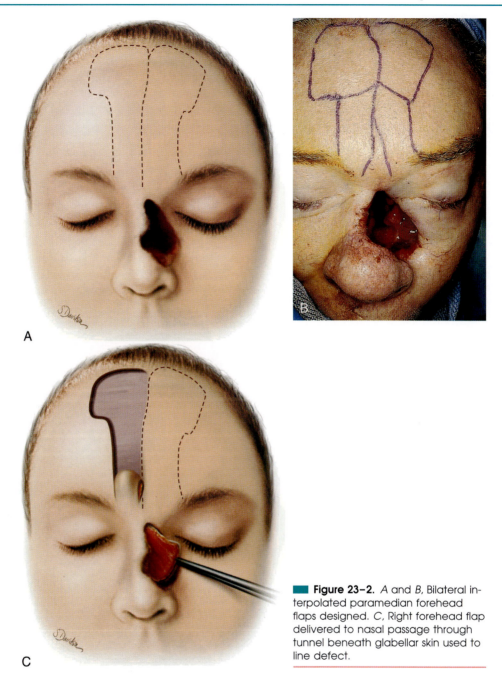

A

B

C

■ **Figure 23–2.** *A* and *B*, Bilateral interpolated paramedian forehead flaps designed. *C*, Right forehead flap delivered to nasal passage through tunnel beneath glabellar skin used to line defect.

dorsum to the nasal facial sulcus was bent outward to create a slight convexity to the contour of the mesh beneath the soft tissues of the nasal sidewall. This maneuver lateralized the sidewall and opened the interior of the left nasal passage. Thus, the mesh served as a large solitary batten spanning the bone deficiency that existed from the nasal dorsum to the central portion of the maxilla. The access incision used for implanting the mesh was closed in layers. The patient has maintained his improved nasal airway to the present time, now 4 years since implantation (Fig. 23–5).

Discussion

When repairing full-thickness defects of the nose, the nasal septum is the preferred source of lining in the form of mucoperichondrial flaps reflected from the septal bone and cartilage (see Chapter 4). In the case presented, the posterior septum was absent, and the blood supply to the remaining anterior septum was impaired. The lining defect was too cephalic to be re-

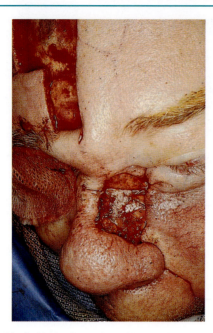

■ **Figure 23-3.** Lining flap sutured to borders of lining defect with skin of flap turned inward. Composite graft of septal cartilage and bone is seen covering raw surface of flap. Graft served as framework batten for repair. Double-layered auricular cartilage onlay graft has been placed beneath nasal skin to augment nasal dorsum.

paired with turbinate mucoperiosteal flaps. In the rare cases where there is insufficient mucosa from the interior of the nose to line a nasal defect, an interpolated paramedian forehead flap provides an alternative to septal flaps. If necessary, a sufficiently large flap may be transferred to line the entire interior of the nasal passage from the anterior nares to the region of the posterior choanae. A forehead flap used for nasal lining may be delivered to the interior of the nasal passage beneath the skin of the glabella or through a nasal cutaneous fistula created at the side of the nose (see Chapters 4 and 11). In the later case, the fistula is closed after dividing the pedicle of the lining flap.

There are disadvantages to using a paramedian forehead flap to line the nose. Forehead flaps are thick compared with septal mucoperichondrial flaps and may have sufficient bulk to crowd the nasal airway. This is especially true if used to line the lower nasal vault. As in this case, forehead flaps works best when used to line the more posterior cephalic portions of the nasal airway. When the septum is absent, there is sufficient space in this region to accommodate the flap without constriction of the nasal passage. Another disadvantage is the lack of a self-cleansing mechanism for ridding the nasal passage of squamous epithelial debris that is continually shed by the skin. If sufficient mucosa remains in the interior of the nose, this debris is moved toward the nasopharynx by the cilia of the remaining mucosa. However, if the surface area of the forehead flap lining

the nose is large, there may not be sufficient mucus produced by the residual mucosa still present in the nose to provide a travel medium for transport of the squamous epithelial debris. In such circumstances, periodic manual cleaning of the nose using saline irrigations may be necessary (see Chapter 11 for discussion of maintaining nasal hygiene).

Following the division of the pedicle of a paramedian forehead flap, the proximal portion is usually converted to a V-shaped flap of tissue that is inset between the eyebrows to restore their natural relationship. Any excess pedicle extending above the level of the eyebrow is excised (see Chapter 14). This approach results in a

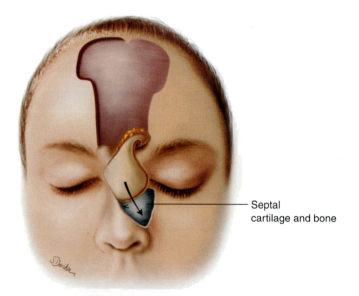

Septal cartilage and bone

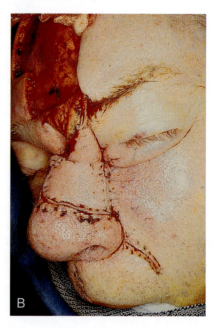

■ **Figure 23-4.** *A* and *B*, Left forehead flap used to cover framework graft and repair cutaneous portion of defect.

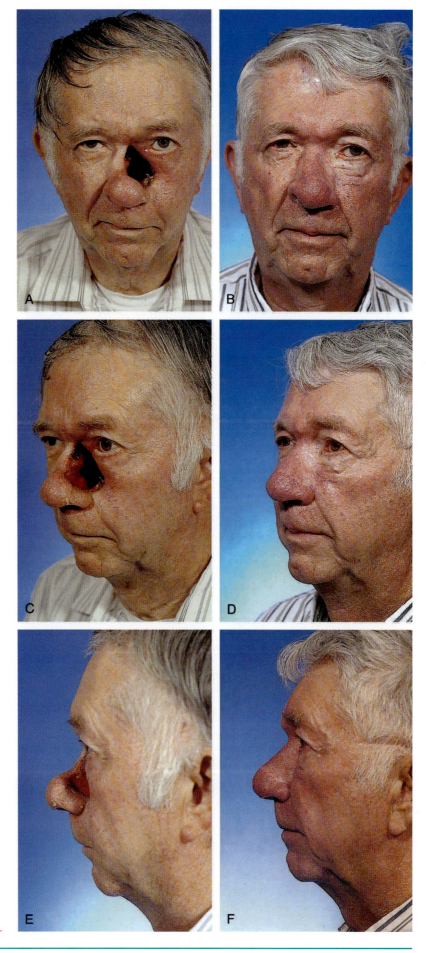

Figure 23–5. *A* to *F*, Preoperative and 4 years postoperative.

single unobtrusive vertical scar in the paramedian position extending from the eyebrow to the hairline. When large forehead flaps are used for nasal reconstruction, the donor wound cannot be completely closed primarily. In these cases, the superior portion of the donor wound is left open to heal by secondary intention. Large flaps are transferred on a narrow pedicle approximately 1.5 cm wide. This design minimizes the quantity of skin removed from the lower two-thirds of the forehead. Thus, even with very large forehead flaps, the lower forehead donor wound can usually be repaired primarily, yielding a narrow vertical scar.

In the case presented, bilateral paramedian forehead flaps were transferred to the nose, removing a strip of skin from the lower forehead approximately 6 cm wide. The wide donor wound could not be closed primarily. Although the superior third of the donor wound healed by secondary intention, the inferior two-thirds of the wound was closed at the time of detachment of the two flaps. Instead of insetting the pedicles between the eyebrows and trimming the excess tissue, all of the tissue of the proximal pedicles were preserved. This enabled the return of all of the skin and muscle previously removed from the lower and central forehead. This approach of managing the forehead donor wound resulted in a near normal appearing forehead. Only the superior portion of the donor scar was apparent because of the necessity for secondary intention wound healing.

The composite bone and cartilage graft used for structural support for the nasal sidewall eventually proved to be inadequate. It stented the nasal sidewall but was not sufficiently large to span the gap between the bony nasal dorsum and the remaining portion of the maxilla. If therefore served strictly as a batten rather than as a framework graft that was continuous from stable nasal bone to stable maxillary bone. The error was in not providing a continuous lamina of support. The loss of the medial buttress of the maxilla accounted for the progressive collapse of the reconstructed region from the weight of the skin and soft tissues composing the medial cheek and lateral nose. The collapse was remedied by providing a rigid framework in the form of a titanium mesh that replaced the structural support normally provided by the nasal bone and ascending process of the maxilla.

24

Reconstruction of Nasal Sidewall and Dorsum

Shan R. Baker

A 56-year-old man presented with progressive swelling over the bridge of the nose during the preceding 3 years. Eighteen years earlier he had an adenoid cystic carcinoma removed from the right nasal passage in the area of the upper lateral cartilage. Examination revealed a 3.0 × 2.5 cm immobile mass in the area of the rhinion (Fig. 24–1). There was no visible mass noted on inspection of the nasal airway. Biopsy of the tumor revealed an adenoid cystic carcinoma. Computerized axial tomography demonstrated only limited erosion of the nasal septum. There was no apparent involvement by tumor of the ethmoid cells or nasal bones. Tumor resection necessitated a partial rhinectomy that included resection of the right upper lateral cartilage, portions of the dorsal nasal septum, and all of the skin covering the upper and middle nasal vaults. The caudal 0.5 cm of the nasal bones was removed. Surgical margins were free of malignancy.

Following surgery, the patient was examined in preparation for reconstruction of his nose (Fig. 24–2). Most of the dorsum of the middle and bony vaults was absent. There was full-thickness loss of the entire right nasal sidewall with extension of the soft-tissue defect to the medial cheek. Although considerable dorsal bony and cartilaginous septum had been resected, the majority of the left upper lateral cartilage and mucosa lining the left middle vault remained intact. The overall dimensions of skin resection measured 5.5 × 5.5 cm. He had advanced male pattern baldness and wore a hairpiece.

It was elected to use a cranial bone graft to provide the framework for the nasal dorsum and a septal cartilage graft as framework for the right sidewall. The ascending process of the maxilla was exposed but remained intact. This provided a bony buttress to anchor the cartilage graft. The remaining portions of both nasal bones were entirely exposed by the loss of skin and soft tissue in the area of the nasion. This bone provided a buttress on which to anchor the cranial bone graft. The bone graft was obtained from the right parietal bone using techniques described in Chapter 8. A drill was used to create a trough measuring 4.5 × 1.4 cm around the bone graft. Angled saws were then used to remove the graft preserving the inner cortex of the cranium.

Working through the open wound on the right side, a septal mucoperichondrial hinge flap was dissected (see Chapters 4 and 11). This was accomplished by making an incision 1 cm below and parallel to the exposed dorsal septal cartilage and bone. A second incision parallel to the first was made along the floor of the nose. The two incisions were connected posteriorly with a vertical incision across the perpendicular plate of the ethmoid bone. The flap was elevated in the subperiosteal and subperichondrial plane to create a flap 4 cm long and 3 cm wide based on the anterior portion of the nasal septum. The exposed septal cartilage was removed as a single piece, preserving a strip of dorsal cartilage 1 cm wide and the contralateral mucoperichondrium. The flap, hinged caudally, was turned anteriorly and laterally to provide lining to the entire right

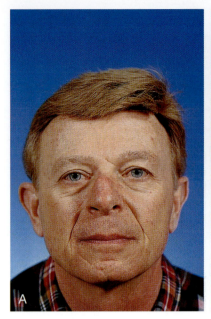
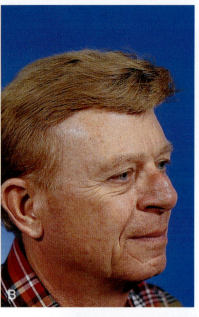

Figure 24–1. *A* and *B*, Presenting complaint was swelling over nasal bridge.

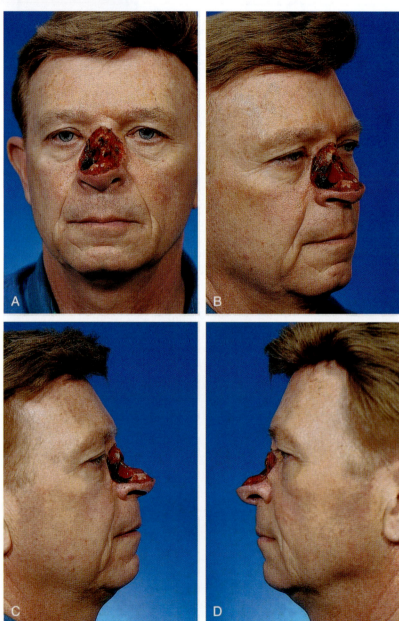

Figure 24–2. *A* to *D*, 5.5 × 5.5 cm nasal defect. There was complete loss of entire right sidewall.

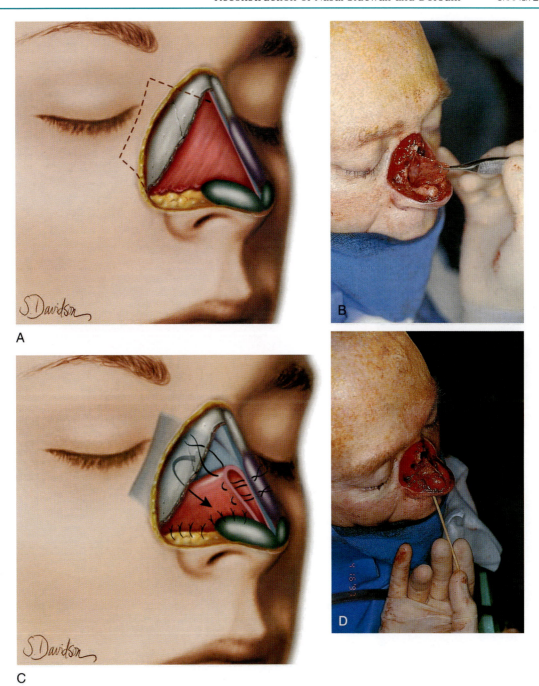

■ **Figure 24–3.** *A,* Dotted line indicates incision made to create septal mucoperichondrial hinge flap. *B,* Lining flap reflected from septum. *C,* Proximal portion of lining flap folded on itself and borders sutured together. *D,* Applicator inserted in nasal passage demonstrates mucosally lined closed cul-de-sac.

nasal passage defect (Fig. 24–3). The mucoperichondrial flap was sutured to the surrounding mucosal borders of the defect with interrupted 5-0 polyglactin sutures. Proximal portions of the flap were folded on itself, and the borders were sutured together to seal off the nasal passage from the exterior. This created a mucosally lined closed cul-de-sac in the superior aspect of the right middle vault (see Chapter 11). The lining defect on the left side of the nose was repaired primarily

by suturing the mucosa along the border of the septum to the remaining mucosa of the middle vault roof.

The bone graft was sculptured with a drill as described in Chapter 8 and secured to the exposed nasal process of the frontal bone with fixation plates using 3- and 4-mm screws, 1.5 mm in diameter (Fig. 24–4). The septal cartilage graft was sculpted with a scalpel, trimmed for a precise fit, and positioned along the right nasal sidewall. It was attached to the underlying lining

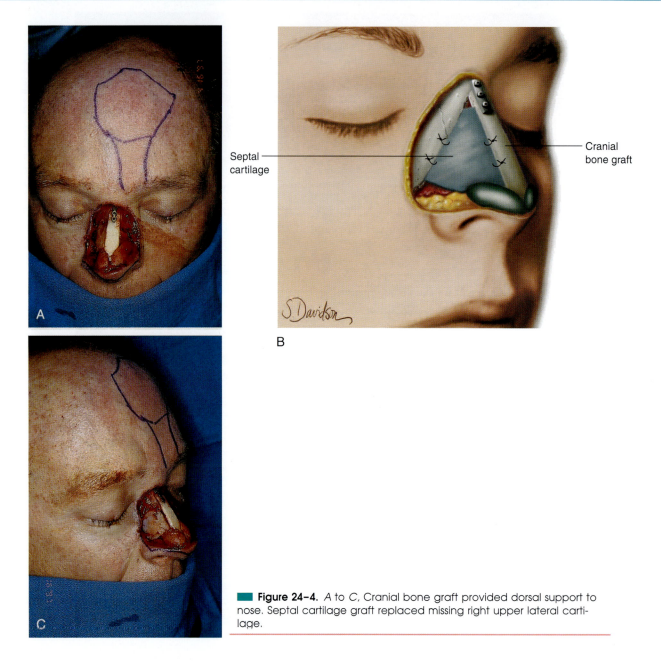

Septal cartilage

Cranial bone graft

Figure 24–4. *A* to *C*, Cranial bone graft provided dorsal support to nose. Septal cartilage graft replaced missing right upper lateral cartilage.

flap with 5-0 polyglactin horizontal mattress sutures that passed from the external surface of the cartilage full-thickness through cartilage and flap and back again. The graft was also attached superiorly to the remaining right nasal bone with sutures that passed through small holes drilled through the bone to accommodate them. Medially the cartilage was attached to the dorsal bone graft using similar techniques. Laterally the graft rested on the medial maxilla.

To repair the cheek component of the defect, adjacent cheek skin was dissected in the subcutaneous plane, and the medial cheek skin was advanced to the lateral border of the nasal sidewall. The skin was secured to the lateral aspect of the cartilage graft with 3-0 polyglactin sutures.

A left interpolated paramedian forehead flap was de-

signed to resurface the entire dorsum, tip, and both sidewalls. It measured 15.0 × 5.5 cm and was dissected and transferred to the nose with techniques described in Chapter 14 (Fig. 24–5). The caudal two-thirds of the portion of flap covering the nose was thinned by removing muscle and the majority of subcutaneous tissue. The flap was secured to the cheek skin laterally and nasal skin caudally with 5-0 polypropylene vertical mattress sutures. The majority of the forehead donor wound was closed by medial advancement of the remaining forehead muscle and skin. The remainder of the wound was allowed open to heal by secondary intention.

Three weeks following the initial reconstructive procedure, the pedicle of the forehead flap was divided and the flap inset in the nose after thinning the proxi-

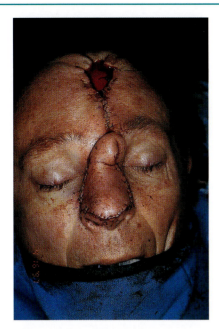

Figure 24–5. Left interpolated paramedian forehead flap served as external cover.

mal portion of the flap not thinned at the time of transfer. The pedicle was trimmed and inset so as to restore the normal anatomical relationship of the medial aspect of the eyebrows. A scalpel was used to transect the pedicle of the septal mucoperichondrial hinge flap, releasing it from the septum. This opened the cul-de-sac created by the lining flap, restoring the nasal airway on the right side. Redundant mucosa from the pedicle was resected, and the incised edges of the mucosa were cauterized with an extended insulated suction cautery device (see Chapter 11).

The patient completed a full course of postoperative external beam irradiation. Additional surgical procedures were not required. The patient has not complained of any nasal obstruction. At the time of writing, he is 4 years postoperative and has not developed recurrent tumor locally (Fig. 24–6).

Discussion

This case demonstrates the principle of replacing missing tissue with like tissue in three layers when reconstructing full-thickness defects of the nose. Missing lining was replaced with mucosa by using a mucoperichondrial flap from the septum. Missing cartilage and bone was replaced with similar tissue to restore the nasal skeleton. External coverage was provided by a skin flap. Ipsilateral septal mucoperichondrial hinge flaps based on the caudal septum are usually employed to line the caudal nasal passage (see Chapter 11). However, in this case, the flap was not dissected caudally to the level of the nasal spine as typically required when using the flap to line the ala or tip. It was dissected only to the caudal-most extent of the lining defect, which was midway between the nostril and the choana. Extending the length of the flap posteriorly to near the level of the posterior choana gave the flap sufficient length to provide lining to the entire mucosal defect of the right bony and middle vaults. Reflecting the lining flap toward the roof and lateral wall of the middle vault required folding the flap on itself in its more proximal portion and suturing the borders to each other. This technique is discussed in Chapter 11. It is an effective method of restoring lining to the roof of the lower or middle vault without placing excessive torsion on the pedicle of the flap. This approach causes a closed cul-de-sac that is lined by mucosa. The cul-de-sac is opened by detaching the pedicle from the nasal septum 3 weeks later. The mucosa reflected laterally to line the lateral wall and roof of the nasal vaults is preserved, and the pedicle spanning between the sidewall and septum is resected. This restores the patency of the nasal passage.

In cases where nasal malignancies are treated with surgery and postoperative radiotherapy, we recommend that irradiation be administered before nasal reconstruction is performed. This prevents delay in completion of multimodality therapy. In the case presented, radiotherapy was delayed until after reconstruction because of the patient's desire to have immediate repair of his nose. Because his malignancy was an adenoid cystic carcinoma, the urgency of administering early postoperative radiotherapy was not critical to the management of his tumor.

The cranium offers an ample source of bone grafts that can be used for nasal reconstruction. Cranial bone is preferred to bone from the rib because it may be thinned to a thickness of 2.0 mm and still maintain sufficient strength to support the soft tissues of the nose. In addition, compared with rib bone, cranial bone is less likely to resorb, and there is considerably less donor site discomfort. We prefer to stabilize cranial bone grafts with a fixation plate system.

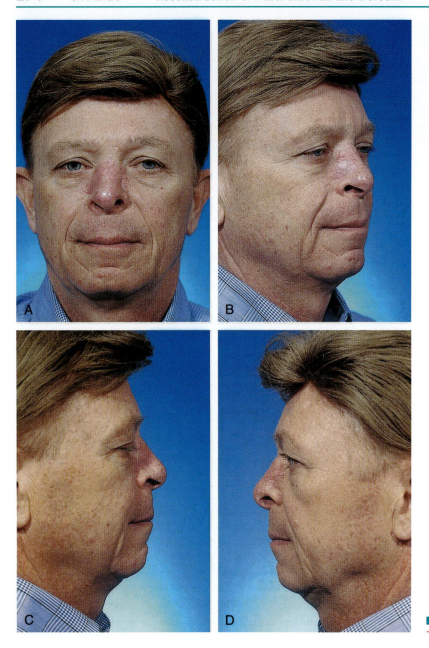

Figure 24-6. *A* to *D*, 1 year postoperative.

25

Near-Total Nasal Reconstruction

Shan R. Baker

The patient was a 61-year-old man who presented with a 2-year history of progressive swelling of the nose. Physical examination showed a mass involving the nasal bridge. The skin was indurated over the entire nasal tip and dorsum to the level of the rhinion (Fig. 25–1). The tumor was fixed to the underlying nasal cartilages and caudal aspect of the nasal bones. It appeared to involve the tip and alae. The neoplasm was not visible intranasally, and the patient did not complain of nasal obstruction. There was no evidence of cervical lymphadenopathy. A biopsy confirmed the presence of a squamous cell carcinoma, probably arising from nasal skin.

A near total rhinectomy was performed. To achieve surgical margins free of tumor involvement, it was necessary to resect the nasal bones, upper and lower lateral nasal cartilages, and the entire nasal tip and columella. The majority of the cartilaginous septum was also removed. Only a small residual segment of alar bases remained in addition to most of the bony septum (Fig. 25–2). The patient received a full course of postoperative external beam irradiation before reconstruction was planned. Three months following radiotherapy, reconstruction was initiated. There was limited septum remaining to line the nose, and there was concern that radiotherapy might have impaired the vascularity of the remaining mucosa within the nasal passage. For these reasons, it was elected to reconstruct the nose using two additional stages beyond that which is typically required for reconstruction of most full-thickness nasal defects.

As with all cases of nasal reconstruction, the goal was to replace the tissue deficiencies with like tissue. This required mucosa for lining, cartilage and bone for framework, and skin for external coverage. The first stage consisted of delaying a composite septal chondromucosal pivotal flap. This was accomplished by making a cut through the remaining cartilagenous and bony septum just below the cribriform plate with Mayo scissors. A right-angled scalpel was then used to continue the incision inferiorly through the thin perpendicular plate of the ethmoid bone. This incision was carried to the level of the floor of the nose. In addition, limited bilateral mucoperichondrial flaps were elevated anteriorly near the nasal spine, and a small wedge of remaining septal cartilage was removed as described in Chapter 11. The purpose of this excision was to provide a space to accommodate the pivoted movement of the flap in the second surgical stage. The two mucoperichondrial flaps were then approximated with nasal packing consisting of petroleum-impregnated gauze.

Three weeks following delay of the composite flap, the nose was reconstructed. The delayed composite septal chondromucosal flap was gently mobilized with a chisel to make a full-thickness inferior septal cut along the floor of the nose to connect with the posterior vertical incision through the perpendicular plate of the ethmoid bone made at the time of the delay. This incision remained 1.5 cm posterior to the caudal margin of the remaining nasal septum to maintain the integrity of the previously dissected mucoperichondrial flaps that served as the pedicles. The flap was gently

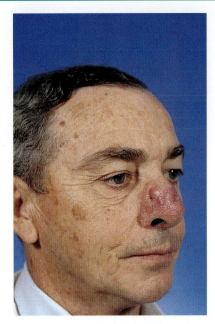

■ **Figure 25-1.** Preoperative view of squamous cell carcinoma of nasal skin.

pivoted anteriorly, pulling it outward from the nasal passage through the open wound. It was mobilized caudally as far as possible so the cartilage of the flap could serve as the framework for the columella and the accompanying mucosa could provide lining for the lower nasal vault as discussed in Chapters 4 and 11. The small amount of septum left intact following resection of the nose limited the size of the composite flap. This in turn limited the amount of caudal extension of the flap. As a consequence, it was not possible to restore an ideal length to the nose. The flap was stabilized in its new position by attaching it to the nasal spine with a 5-0 polypropylene suture placed in a figure-of-eight configuration. The cephalic border of the pivoted flap, which consisted of the perpendicular plate of the ethmoid bone, was connected to the frontal bone with a fixation plate that spanned the distance between the flap and bone (Fig. 25-3). Bilateral mucoperichondrial flaps were reflected laterally away from the most anterior portion of the pivoted composite flap. This provided sufficient mucosa to line the nasal domes but not the more lateral aspects of the nasal vestibules.

The inferior turbinates were small and scarred from adhesions created by irradiation of the nasal passage; however, the middle turbinates were large and not scarred. Bilateral turbinate mucoperiosteal flaps were developed from the two middle turbinates by techniques described in Chapter 11. The flaps were hinged on an anterior attachment to the nasal sidewall (Fig. 25-4). All of the bones of the turbinates were removed and discarded. These flaps provided sufficient mucosa to line the lateral portion of the nasal vestibules that could not be covered by the lining flaps developed from the composite septal pivotal flap (Fig. 25-5). Medially, the turbinate flaps were sutured to the mucosal flaps developed from the composite flap. Laterally, they were sutured to the residual skin of the vestibules near the alar bases. Interrupted 5-0 polyglactin sutures were used for this purpose. The lining flaps reflected from the composite flap together with the turbinate flaps were also sufficient to line the middle nasal vault. The caudal borders of the lining flaps were left unencumbered so they could be sutured to the covering flap.

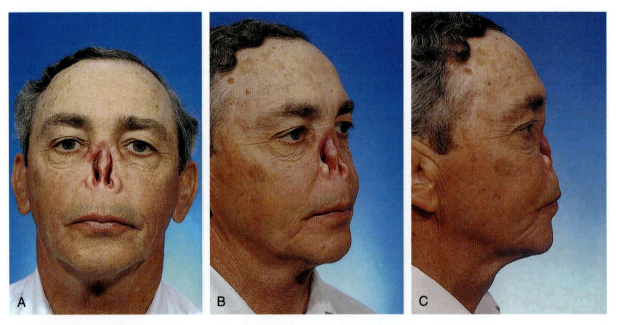

■ **Figure 25-2.** *A* to *C,* Following near-total rhinectomy and postoperative radiotherapy.

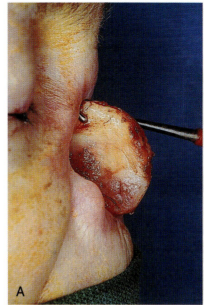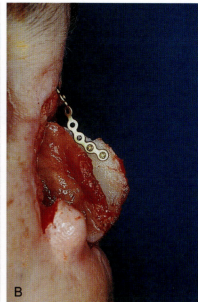

■ **Figure 25–3.** *A,* Composite septal flap pivoted anteriorly from posterior nasal passage. *B,* Position of flap maintained by fixation plate extending from flap to frontal bone. Septal mucoperichondrial flaps have been reflected to assist with nasal lining.

Auricular cartilage grafts were obtained from both ears by techniques discussed in Chapter 7. The concha cavum and concha cymba were removed as a single piece to provide grafts measuring 4.0 × 1.75 cm. These served as framework grafts for the nasal tip and alae.

A cranial bone graft was obtained from the left parietal bone with techniques discussed in Chapter 8. The graft measured 5.0 × 1.5 cm. An oscillating angled saw was used to harvest the graft after it was outlined with a side-cutting bur. The bone graft was cut in half to create two grafts, each 2.5 cm long and 1.5 cm wide (Fig. 25–6). The bone grafts were positioned on either side of the spanning plate used to stabilize the composite septal pivotal flap. They provided the framework for the sidewalls and nasal dorsum. Because there was no septal cartilage available for replacing the upper lateral cartilages, the bone grafts served the purpose of providing structural support for the middle vault. The grafts were attached to each other and to the ascending processes of the maxillae with 1.2 mm titanium fixation plates with 3-mm screws. This provided rigid skeletal support to the upper and middle nasal vaults. The lining flaps were suspended to the bone grafts by 5.0 polyglactin mattress sutures that passed through several 1-mm holes drilled in the bone grafts.

The auricular cartilage grafts were sculpted and tailored using a scalpel. The full length of each graft

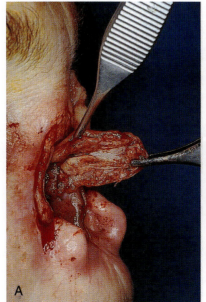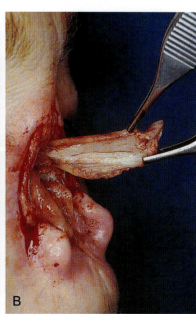

■ **Figure 25–4.** *A* and *B,* Right and left middle turbinate mucoperiosteal flaps hinged on anterior attachments.

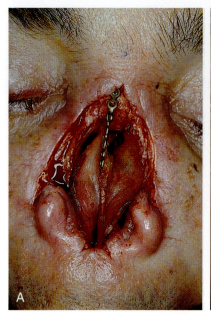
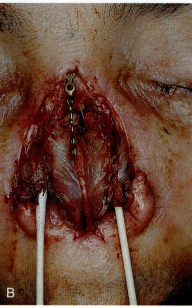

Figure 25–5. *A,* Bilateral mucoperichondrial flaps reflected laterally from composite septal flap. This provided sufficient mucosa to line nasal domes but was insufficient to line lateral aspects of nasal vestibules. *B,* Middle turbinate flaps provided lining for lateral portion of nasal vestibules. Applicators inserted in nasal passage identify suture lines between lining flaps.

was utilized to restore the arc of the nasal domes and provide a framework for the alae. The grafts extended from the cartilage of the composite flap to the alar bases. The lateral aspect of the grafts was secured in soft-tissue pockets created in the remaining alar bases. The medial aspect of the positioned grafts was sculpted and scored to create a contour typical of the intermediate and lateral crura. The cartilage grafts were sutured to the cartilage of the composite flap in the midline and to the caudal end of the bone grafts via drill holes in the bone created for this purpose (Fig. 25–7). The auricular cartilage grafts provided a desirable contour to the tip and alae because of their natural convexity. The length (4 cm), width (1.75 cm), and contour of the grafts were sufficient to replace the intermediate and lateral crura of the alar cartilages and provide a framework for the alae. The caudal border of the cartilage

contained within the composite flap served as a replacement for the medial crura and provided a framework for the columella and support to the nasal tip. The lining flaps were suspended to the cartilage grafts with 5-0 polyglactin mattress sutures that passed from the external surface of the grafts through cartilage and flaps and back again (see Chapters 4 and 11).

A template was fashioned from foam rubber that was carefully tailored to drape the constructed framework. This was accomplished by suturing the template in the position that a covering flap would eventually assume (Fig. 25–8). The template was then detached from the framework and used to design a right interpolated paramedian forehead flap that was 6.5 cm in width (Fig. 25–9). The flap was dissected and transposed to the nose after muscle and the majority of subcutaneous fat were removed from the distal portion by techniques

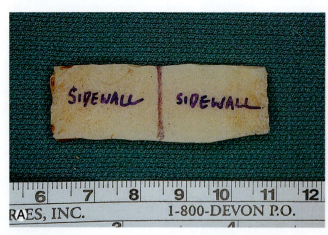
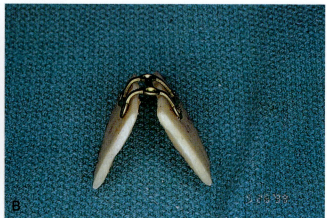

Figure 25–6. *A,* 5.0 × 1.5 cm cranial bone graft. *B,* Graft divided and segments attached by fixation plate. Each segment provided structural support for half of upper and middle nasal vaults.

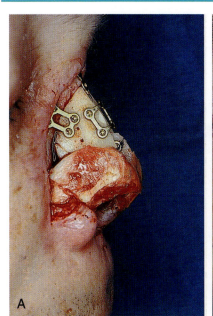 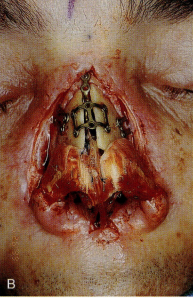 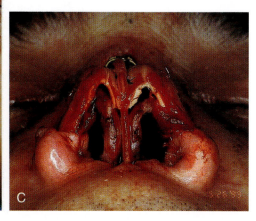

Figure 25-7. *A* and *B*, Auricular cartilage grafts provided framework for lower nasal vault. Grafts overlapped bony framework cephalically, simulating contour of alar grooves. *C*, Lining flaps were suspended to cartilage and bone grafts. Caudal borders left unencumbered.

described in Chapter 14. The forehead flap was secured to the medial cheek skin with vertical mattress 5-0 polypropylene sutures. The caudal border of the lining flaps was sutured to the caudal aspect of the forehead flap. The portion of the forehead flap replacing the columella was sutured to the caudal edges of the mucosa covering the composite flap.

Before detachment, the portion of the forehead flap not thinned of its muscle and subcutaneous fat at the time of flap transfer was contoured. This was done 2

months after flap transfer. Bilateral incisions were made in the scars between flap and cheek skin along the entire length of the sidewalls. The forehead flap was freed from the underlying bone grafts and cephalic portions of the auricular cartilage grafts by dissecting in the superficial subcutaneous plane. This created a bipedicle flap attached to the nasal tip caudally and forehead cephalically. All of the fat and scar deposition left attached to the framework grafts were removed. The skin incisions were repaired, and a compression dress-

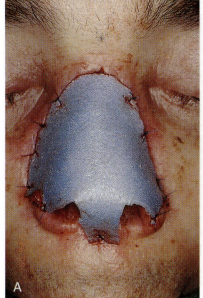 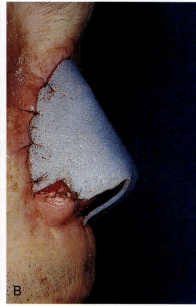

Figure 25-8. *A* and *B*, Template of foam rubber crafted for design of paramedian forehead flap.

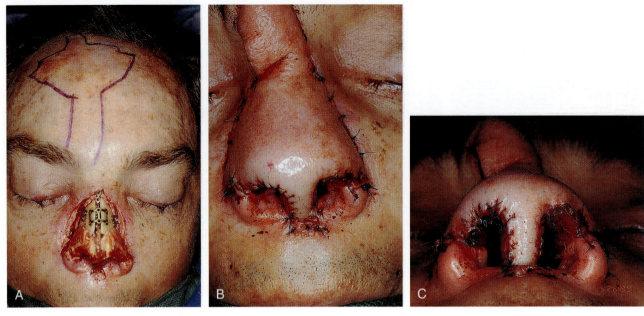

Figure 25–9. *A,* Interpolated paramedian forehead flap designed. *B* and *C,* Caudal aspect of forehead flap was sutured to caudal borders of lining flaps. Portion of forehead flap replacing columella was sutured to borders of mucosa covering composite flap.

ing was applied to the nose. Six weeks later, alar grooves were constructed with techniques described in Chapter 13. Incisions corresponding to the ideal position of the alar grooves were made in the covering flap. The underlying auricular cartilage grafts were exposed, and cartilage was removed along the projected line of the grooves. Bolster dressings secured with transnasal sutures were employed for 5 days to maintain the constructed grooves (Fig. 25–10). Two months later, the pedicle of the forehead flap was divided, and the flap

was inset. The proximal pedicle was trimmed and inset between the medial aspect of the eyebrows as described in Chapter 14.

The patient required one additional surgical procedure to correct a minor notch of the right nostril. This was performed in the office 7 months following pedicle detachment. The notch was improved with a Z-plasty and inserting a small auricular cartilage graft harvested from the helical crus (Figs. 25–11). He has maintained an ample nasal airway (Fig. 25–12).

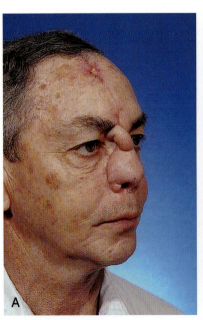
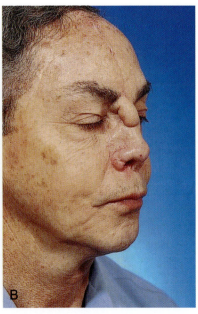

Figure 25–10. *A,* 6 weeks following transfer of paramedian forehead flap. Note edema and general bulkiness of flap. *B,* Result of two contouring procedures before detachment of flap from forehead.

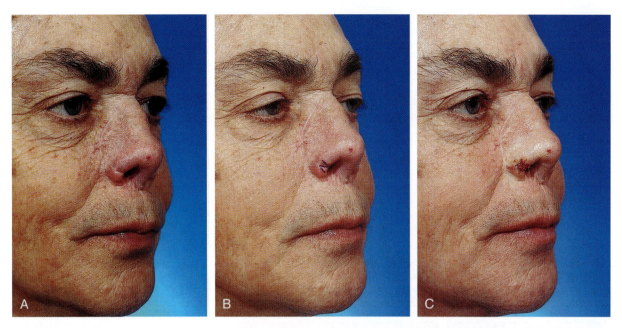

■ **Figure 25–11.** *A*, Minor notch of right nostril margin. *B*, Z-plasty designed for correction. *C*, Completion of Z-plasty supplemented by small auricular cartilage graft placed deep to repair.

Discussion

Total and near total reconstruction of the nose is a formidable challenge, even to an experienced surgeon. The project requires replacing the nose with like tissue whenever possible. The lining of the entire nasal passage must be restored. Missing bone and cartilage are replaced with grafts that are sculpted and tailored to replicate the contour of the natural nasal skeleton. The exterior of the reconstructed nose is restored with an interpolated forehead flap. All flaps must have sufficient blood supply to survive and provide adequate nourishment to grafts they cover. All flaps and grafts must be carefully planned and precisely constructed to achieve the goal of successfully restoring a nose with natural form and function. If any component of the restoration fails, it is unlikely that this goal will be entirely achieved.

Constructing the lining of the nose is the most difficult aspect of nasal reconstruction. If an ample portion of the nasal septum is remaining, the task of reconstructing the nose is considerably simpler and usually more successful because the septum is the primary source for lining flaps. The first step is to mobilize the septum out of the nasal passage in the form of a composite septal pivotal flap based caudally on the floor of the nose. The composite flap provides structural support to the tip and caudal dorsum and serves as a source of mucosa for lining the middle and lower nasal vaults.

In the case presented, all of the remaining septum was utilized as a composite flap for the purpose of providing structual support and lining to the nose. However, the flap was not of sufficient size to provide an ideal length to the nose nor to completely line the nasal passage. The flap was mobilized as far caudally as possible and secured in this position by a fixation plate used to span the gap between flap and frontal bone. The composite flap did not provide adequate mucoperichondrium to completely line the lower nasal vault. Fortunately, the patient had large middle turbinates that provided a second source for lining. Mucoperiosteal flaps were developed from the middle turbinates as described in Chapter 11. These flaps were essential in providing sufficient mucosa to line the nasal passages entirely.

We do not delay composite septal chondromucosal pivotal flaps when the caudal septum remains intact because of the ample blood supply provided to the flap by the septal branches of the superior labial artery (see Chapter 4). However, when the caudal septum has been resected as in the case presented, it is prudent to delay the flap before pivoting it forward out of the nasal passage. The flap is large relative to the pedicle, which consists of two mucoperichondrial flaps located at the anterior floor of the nasal passages. It is also prudent to delay large composite septal chondromucosal flaps for patients who use tobacco products and those who have received previous irradiation of the nasal passages.

The pedicles of interpolated forehead flaps used as covering for the nose are typically divided 3 weeks

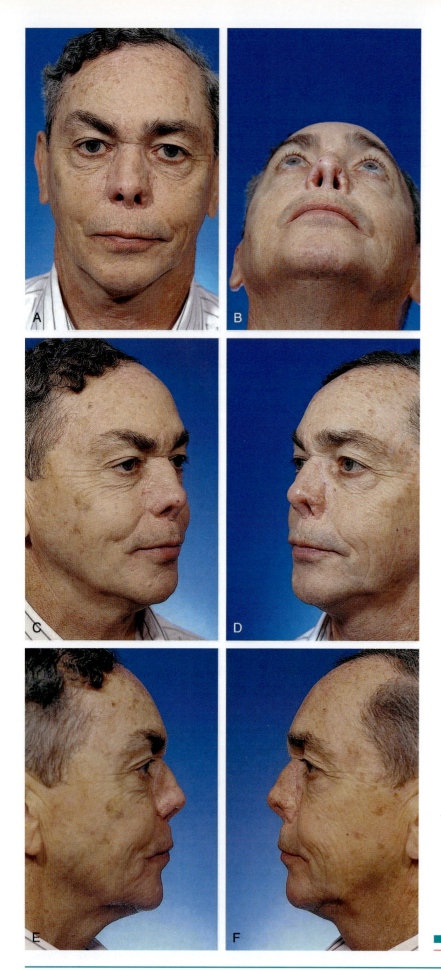

Figure 25–12. *A* to *F*, 1 year postoperative.

following transfer of the flap of the nose. However, when the surgeon is confronted with complete loss of the nose, there is less surface contact between the covering flap and vascularized tissue at the recipient site. As in this case, ingrowth of vessels required to revascularize the covering flap is derived only from scar tissue along the border of the constructed nose and the caudal border of the lining flaps. This limited access for revascularization translates into a longer duration before anastomotic connections are sufficient between the forehead flap and adjacent cheek skin to adequately sustain the flap once the pedicle is divided. For this reason, we recommend delaying detachment of covering flaps for 2 months following initial flap transfer in cases of total or near-total nasal reconstruction.

In most cases, we detach the interpolated covering flap before performing a contouring procedure. However, in this case, we left the pedicle of the forehead flap attached and performed two contouring procedures before pedicle division. The first procedure created a thinner covering flap for the entire nose. The second procedure created alar grooves. Maintaining the integrity of the flap's pedicle during these operations ensured the vascularity of the flap while achieving optimal flap contour as well as an extended interval before pedicle division without unduly prolonging the process of reconstruction. The total interval required to complete nasal reconstruction was approximately 5 months, excluding the minor office procedure that was performed 7 months later.

In cases of total and near-total nasal reconstruction, it is not always possible to construct the nose of ideal length. The limiting factor is the quantity of mucosa available for internal lining. As in the case presented, when a large portion of the nasal septum has been resected, the composite septal chondralmucosal flap used to line the lower vault may be of insufficient size to reach the ideal position for the nasal tip. In such instances, the constructed nose is short, and the tip is cephalically rotated. In the case presented the function and contour of the constructed nose are ideal, however the nose is foreshortened, and the tip is rotated cephalad.

26

Reconstruction of Ala, Cheek, and Upper Lip

Shan R. Baker

The patient was a 58-year-old woman who presented with a 2-year history of a growth on the skin of the right ala. She was in good health and had smoked $1\frac{1}{2}$ packs of cigarettes a day for 10 years. Examination of her nose revealed 1 cm of a slightly ulcerated skin lesion. Biopsy of the area revealed a basal cell carcinoma. Mohs' surgery was performed and resulted in a full-thickness loss of the entire ala. The defect extended to the medial cheek where a 2×1 cm loss of soft tissue was noted. In addition, a 2.0×1.5 cm skin defect of the adjacent upper lip was present (Fig. 26–1). This represented a complex facial defect involving three separate aesthetic regions: nose, cheek, and lip.

Full-thickness loss of the ala required replacement of lining, structural support, and external covering. Repair of the cheek required restoration of skin and subcutaneous tissue. The lip defect was primarily of skin and did not require replacement of muscle or mucosa. Keeping with the principle of repairing each portion of a defect involving multiple aesthetic regions with an independent covering flap, three separate skin flaps were used for repair. The defect of the lip was reconstructed with a rotation advancement cutaneous flap recruiting the remaining skin of the right lateral upper lip and oral commissure (Fig. 26–2). The boundaries of the flap remained within the aesthetic region of the upper lip. The flap was elevated in a plane immediately superficial to the obicularis muscle and advanced medially. The standing cutaneous deformity resulting from

the advancement of the flap was excised inferior to the lip defect and extended to the level of the vermilion.

The component of the defect involving the cheek was repaired with a 7.0×2.5 cm cutaneous advancement flap. The flap conveyed sufficient subcutaneous fat to fill the soft-tissue void in the region of the nasal facial sulcus. The flap was advanced to the level of the junction of the cheek with the nasal sidewall. The leading border of the flap was secured in position by sewing the cutaneous tissue to the periosteum of the ascending process of the maxilla with 4-0 polyglactin sutures. A standing cutaneous deformity developed inferiorly from advancement of the cheek flap. This facilitated closure of the donor wound from the lip flap because the standing cutaneous deformity presented in the area of the melolabial sulcus where the lip flap had been incised. The portion of the standing cutaneous deformity not required for a tension-free closure of the lip donor wound was excised and discarded.

Once the lip and cheek defects had been reconstructed satisfactorily, attention was given to repair of the ala. Techniques described in Chapters 11 and 14 were used to reconstruct the nose. First, a 4×3 cm ipsilateral septal mucoperichondrial hinge flap was incised and dissected. The incised borders of the mucosa remaining along the periphery of the donor site were carefully cauterized to control bleeding. The exposed septal cartilage was left in situ to heal by secondary intention. The mucosal flap hinged on the caudal septum was reflected laterally to provide lining for the ala

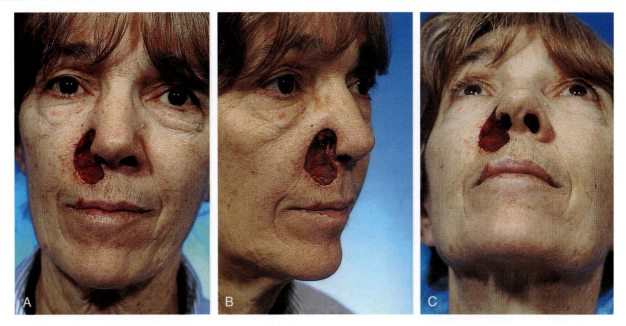

■ **Figure 26–1.** *A* to *C*, Full-thickness defect of ala. Defect involves medial cheek and upper lip.

(Fig. 26–3). Its margins were sutured to the margins of the mucosal defect with interrupted 5-0 polyglactin sutures. The distal border of the flap was left unencumbered so that it could eventually be sutured to the covering flap.

An auricular cartilage graft measuring 3 × 1 cm was harvested from the left ear with techniques described in Chapter 7. The graft was trimmed and sculpted so that it would precisely replicate the configuration and contour of the ala (see Fig. 26–3). At the superior border of the obicularis oris and the planned site for the alar base, a soft-tissue pocket was created to insert the lat-

eral aspect of the cartilage graft. It was secured in the pocket using 4-0 polyglactin sutures that passed from muscle to cartilage graft, then to subcutaneous tissues of the cheek flap. Joining the graft to the muscle of the upper lip and skin of the medial cheek assisted with stabilization of the graft and established the position of the alar base. The portion of the graft occupying the soft-tissue pocket served to provide an unyielding foundation for the alar base. The medial end of the graft was inserted into a pocket created in the nasal facet. The graft was scored to increase its convex contour. The superior medial border of the graft was sutured to

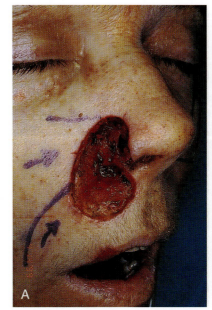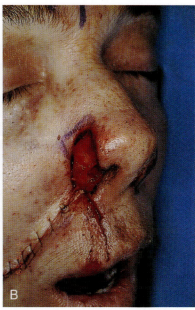

■ **Figure 26–2.** *A*, Rotation advancement (lip) and advancement (cheek) cutaneous flaps designed to repair lip and cheek defects. *B*, Flaps in place. Their standing cutaneous deformities were excised inferior to lip defect and in melolabial sulcus.

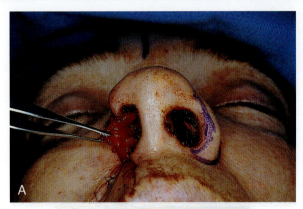

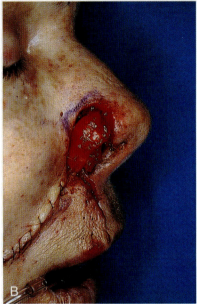

■ Figure 26–3. *A,* Ipsilateral septal mucoperichondrial hinge flap (held by forceps) used as alar lining flap. *B,* Auricular cartilage graft (in position) provides framework for ala.

Three weeks following the initial reconstructive procedures, the pedicle of the forehead flap was divided, and the flap was inset using surgical techniques described in Chapter 14. The proximal flap was trimmed and inset in the glabella after restoring the normal spacial relationship between the medial aspects of the eyebrows (Fig. 26–6). Because of the patient's history of tobacco, it was elected to delay detachment of the lining flap until the third surgical stage.

Two months following detachment of the pedicle of the forehead flap, a contouring procedure was performed to restore the alar groove and to destroy hair follicles transferred with the covering flap. Using surgical techniques described in Chapters 14 and 15, the flap was thinned, the hair follicles were cauterized, and the alar groove was constructed. The intranasal hinge flap was detached from the nasal septum (see Chapter 11). In addition, scar revisions were performed on portions of the scars of the forehead and cheek. Revision consisted only of elliptical excisions of scars and reapproximation of wound margins. Skin redundancy causing an inferior displacement of the vermilion of the right upper lip was excised along the vermiliocutaneous border.

Six months after the third surgical stage, other procedures were performed. These consisted of several Z-plasties on the cheek scar and a second contouring and depilation of the constructed ala. This was necessary because of mild nasal obstruction and persistence of hair follicles. The obstruction was also in part related to a synechium that had formed between the interior of the constructed ala and the nasal septum. The synech-

the caudal border of the lateral crus with figure-of-eight 5-0 polyglactin sutures described in Chapter 7. The septal mucoperiochondrial hinge flap was suspended to the cartilage graft by using mattress sutures that passed full-thickness through the cartilage graft and flap. The lining flap provided complete cover for the deep aspect of the graft. A template of the contralateral ala was created from foam rubber. It was reversed and used to design a paramedian forehead flap that served as the covering flap for construction of the ala (Fig. 26–4). Using surgical techniques described in Chapter 14, the forehead flap was transferred to the nose. Unfortunately, the presence of an inferior positioned anterior hairline necessitated including hair-bearing scalp in the flap. The flap was not aggressively depilated at the time of initial flap transfer because of the patient's history of tobacco use. The caudal border of the forehead flap was sutured to the caudal border of the lining flap (Fig. 26–5).

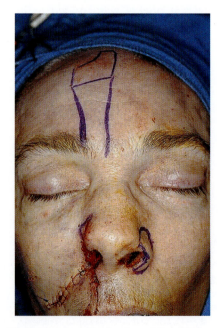

■ Figure 26–4. Paramedian forehead flap designed using a template of the contralateral ala.

ium was removed, and a silastic splint was placed between the two to prevent it from reforming.

Although the second contouring procedure and excision of the synechium improved the nasal airway, there was some persistent hair growth on the ala. The constructed nostril was smaller than its counterpart. To address these problems, a third depilation of the ala was performed. To reduce the size discrepancy of the nostrils, a full-thickness resection of the alar base was performed on the side contralateral to the constructed ala.

Discussion

The case represents a complex defect that was contiguous with three distinct aesthetic regions of the face. When a skin defect involves two or more facial aes-

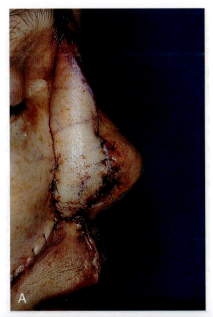

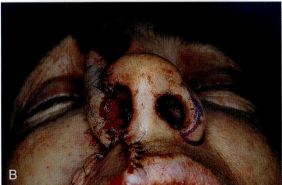

Figure 26–5. *A,* Forehead flap provides cover for reconstructed ala. *B,* Caudal border of forehead flap is sutured to caudal border of lining flap. Note slightly oversized nostril on reconstructed side.

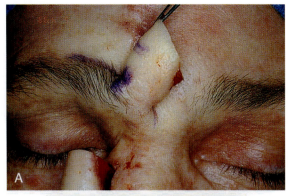

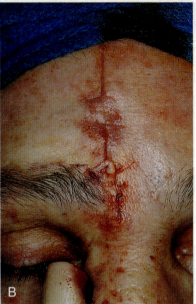

■ **Figure 26–6.** *A,* Detachment of forehead flap pedicle. *B,* Glabellar inset of pedicle.

thetic regions, Menick[1] showed that it is preferable to repair each unit with independent covering flaps. This principle has several advantages. It has the effect of dividing a large defect into smaller units, each of which may be reconstructed with smaller flaps harvested from a number of donor sites. Less tissue must be borrowed from a given area for repair when multiple flaps are used, compared with a single flap used to repair the entire wound. Using independent covering flaps for each facial region places many of the scars along the junction of aesthetic regions and maximizes scar camouflage. In the paranasal area, these junctional sites are concave. The greatest concave contour is the alar facial sulcus. By using independent flaps to cover defects of separate aesthetic regions, concave contours are better maintained and provide an area of shadow that helps to hide scars. Separate flaps for separate aesthetic regions often enable the surgeon to repair the portion of the defect occupying a region with skin from the same region. This is usually in the form of transposition

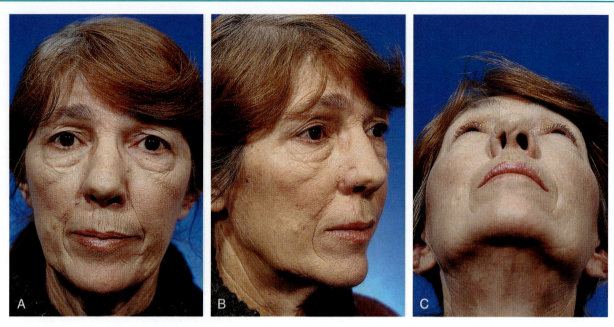

■ **Figure 26–7.** *A to C,* 2 years postoperative. In spite of asymmetry of nostrils, patient does not complain of nasal obstruction.

or advancement flaps that have nearly identical texture and color to those of the missing skin.

Large full-thickness defects of the ala and upper lip are best repaired in stages. The full-thickness lip defect is repaired first, and nasal reconstruction is postponed until the lip is healed. This approach enables a stable foundation for subsequent reconstruction of the nose. If the nose and lip are repaired simultaneously, it becomes more difficult to ensure proper positioning of the alar base. Scars resulting from the lip repair will contract and likely distort the constructed ala.

In the case presented, the component of the defect involving the lip was not full-thickness. The obicularis oris remained intact, and only skin and a minimal amount of soft tissue were missing. The persistent lip muscle in the vicinity of the missing ala provided sufficient native tissue for creating a soft-tissue pocket to serve as a receptacle for the auricular cartilage graft used as framework for the ala. It also served to stabilize the position of the constructed alar base.

A portion of the patient's defect occupied the upper melolabial fold, likely restricting the blood supply to any superiorly based melolabial cutaneous flap used to repair the nose. She also smoked tobacco. For these reasons, a paramedian forehead flap was selected as the covering flap for the ala in spite of the inferior position of the anterior hairline. Typical of most scalp hair transferred with a forehead flap, the hair proved to be recalcitrant to easy surgical depilation. Three surgical procedures were necessary to depilate the flap completely. The reasons for this frustrating phenomenon are discussed in Chapter 14.

In the case presented, the size of the reconstructed nostril was smaller than the contralateral side. This occurred in spite of initially constructing the nostril

slightly larger than its counterpart (see Fig. 26–5). We have observed that it is not always possible to predict the ultimate nostril size when reconstructing full-thickness alar defects. The larger the defect, the less predictable the outcome. Variations in scar contracture surrounding the covering and lining flaps and the variability of the intrinsic strength of the cartilage used for the alar framework play a role in the healing process and influence the nostril size. In addition to these factors, the formation of the synechium in the case presented may have enhanced the medial migration of the constructed ala. Before resection of the skin cancer, the patient was noted to have modestly large nostrils. This feature presents the surgeon with a greater challenge when attempting to restore symmetry between the constructed and native nostrils. When reconstruction is complete, and there is a discrepancy in nostril size, it may be helpful to reduce the nostril on the normal side by resecting a portion of the alar base. This is more readily accomplished without impairment of the nasal airway when the native nostril is large and there is flaring of the ala.

When reconstructing full-thickness alar defects, there is a tendency for the reconstructed nostril to be smaller than the contralateral nostril. This is due to the factors already discussed. As in this case, we construct a nostril slightly larger than the opposite normal side in an attempt to compensate for this phenomenon. Even with this effort, we are not always successful (Fig. 26–7).

Reference

1. Menick FJ: Facial reconstruction in regional units. Perspect Plast Surg 8:104, 1994.

27

Reconstruction of Nasal Dorsum, Sidewall, Cheek and Medial Orbit

Shan R. Baker

The patient was a 31-year-old female with a 2-year history of being treated for dacryocystitis of the left eye. A biopsy in the region of the lacrimal sac revealed an adenoid cystic carcinoma. Surgical resection of the tumor necessitated a medial maxillectomy and resection of the entire medial and inferior bony orbit and the medial canthal tendon. Portions of the medial aspect of the upper and lower eyelids were resected along with the medial periorbita and medial rectus muscle. A full-thickness resection of the bony dorsum and nasal sidewall was also performed. The anterior and posterior ethmoidal cells were removed (Fig. 27–1).

To provide soft-tissue cover of the medial cheek defect and bony support of the eye, a scapular osteocutaneous microsurgical flap was transferred to the defect 3 weeks following surgical resection of the neoplasm. A 4-cm segment of bone transferred with the flap was contoured to replace the floor and medial aspect of the bony orbit. The bone was secured with fixation plates to the remaining inferior bony orbital rim laterally and the frontal bone medially. The skin flap measured 5 × 4 cm and was used to replace the soft tissue and skin of the medial cheek and lateral nose (Fig. 27–2). The deep aspect of the flap exposed to the nasal passage and nasal pharynx was allowed to heal by secondary intention. The patient was treated with a complete course of external beam irradiation. Because of the loss of the medial rectus muscle, periorbita, and large portions of the bony orbit, the patient suffered enophthalmos, severe diplopia, and exposure keratitis. This necessitated a number of ophthalmologic surgical procedures, including two strabismus repairs, reconstruction of the lower eyelid, and medial suture tarsorrhaphy.

The patient was subsequently referred for reconstruction of the nose. When seen in consultation for nasal repair, the patient had a marked discrepancy of skin color and texture between the microsurgical flap and the facial skin. The region of the missing nasal sidewall and dorsum was covered by the flap. There was insufficient skin and soft tissue of the medial aspect of the inferior and superior orbit that caused ectropion of both eyelids. This condition was temporarily corrected with a medial suture tarsorrhaphy (Fig. 27–3).

It was elected to rehabilitate the medial orbit and eyelids to the best possible condition before considering nasal reconstruction. First, a 2.5 × 1.5 cm superiorly based cutaneous flap developed from the inferior aspect of the microsurgical flap was transferred beneath the medial aspect of the lower eyelid. This flap supplemented the lower eyelid skin and augmented the soft tissue covering the reconstructed bony orbital rim. The remaining portion of the microsurgical flap was con-

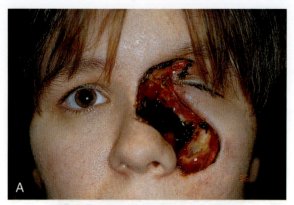

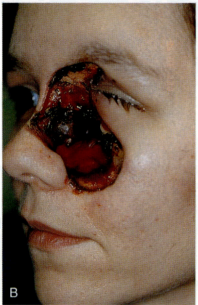

■ **Figure 27–1.** *A* and *B*, Full-thickness defect of nasal dorsum, sidewall, and medial maxilla and orbit.

toured by removing subcutaneous tissue from beneath the flap. The donor defect of the transposition flap was repaired with a 6 × 3 cm V-to-Y cheek advancement flap based on a subcutaneous pedicle (Fig. 27–4).

Nasal reconstruction was performed 3 months following restoration of the skin and soft tissue of the medial inferior orbit and contouring of the microsurgical flap. A cranial bone graft measuring 5.0 × 1.2 cm was obtained from the left parietal bone with techniques described in Chapter 8. The skin of the microsurgical flap occupying the aesthetic units of the nasal dorsum and left sidewall was removed (Fig. 27–5). A drill was used to contour the bone of the scapular flap in the area of the medial canthus. This provided space for reconstruction of the bony nasal sidewall with the cranial bone graft. The bone graft was divided into two pieces to provide a framework for the dorsum and sidewall of the nose. A plateau was created in the nasal process of the frontal bone to accommodate the dorsal bone graft. The dorsal graft was secured to the frontal bone with a

fixation plate and contoured with a drill before insertion of the second bone graft used to repair the nasal sidewall. The graft used for the sidewall was secured to the dorsal graft with a fixation plate (Fig. 27–6). The superior medial orbital skin and soft tissue were freed from the roof of the bony orbit to release an upper eyelid contracture, enabling the eyelid to descend sufficiently to cover the exposed cornea. This left a substantial donor site defect below the medial aspect of the left eyebrow. The scar tissue representing the medial canthus was secured to the posterior aspect of the nasal sidewall bone graft by a 4.0 polypropylene suture placed through holes drilled in the bone.

A template was fashioned that would provide sufficient skin to resurface the nasal dorsum, sidewall, and superior medial orbital defect. The template was used to design a right 10 × 5 cm irregularly shaped paramedian forehead flap (see Fig. 27–6). Using techniques described in Chapter 14, the flap was dissected and used to cover the bone grafts and replace the superior medial orbital skin. The forehead donor wound was partially closed by advancement of forehead skin after bilateral undermining in the subgaleal plane. Three weeks later, the pedicle of the forehead flap was divided, and the flap was inset. A portion of the proximal pedicle was returned to the forehead to restore the anatomical relationship of the medial aspect of the eyebrows. The transposition of soft tissue and skin from the microsurgical flap to the medial aspect of the inferior orbit and from the forehead flap to the superior medial orbit proved sufficient to correct the ectropion of the eyelids and enabled the subsequent removal of the suture tarsorrhaphy.

Eight months after nasal reconstruction, the portion of the forehead flap covering the nose was contoured by removing subcutaneous tissue. Three Z-plasties (as described in Chapter 14) were performed between the skin of the forehead flap and native nasal skin along the inferior border of the flap. The forehead scar was revised by excising the epithelial surface of the scar. The surrounding skin margins were then widely undermined in the subgaleal plane and advanced over the deeper portion of the scar left in situ (see Chapter 15). The cheek scars were dermabraded.

Five months later the scapular bone used to reconstruct the superior medial bony orbital rim was augmented with hydroxyapatite. This enhanced the contour of the region and provided additional support to the soft tissue of the superior medial orbit. The nose and microsurgical flap were dermabraided to improve the skin color match between forehead and native nasal skin and between microsurgical flap and native cheek skin.

The patient's last reconstructive procedure was performed 10 months later. Due to surgical resection of the superior medial orbital skin and soft tissue and the use of a right paramedian forehead flap to repair the nose,

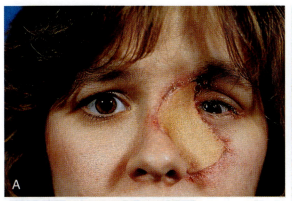
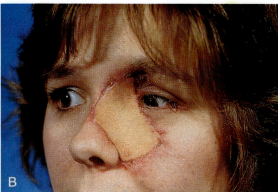
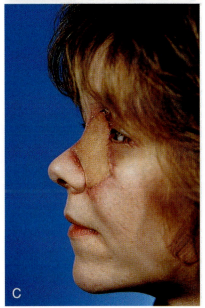

■ **Figure 27–2.** *A* to *C*, Scapular osteocutaneous microsurgical flap used to provide soft tissue and skin for cover and bone for structural support. Deep aspect of flap exposed to nasal cavity left to heal by secondary intention.

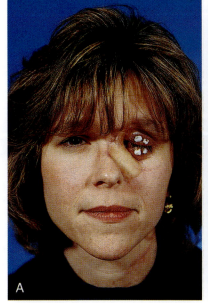
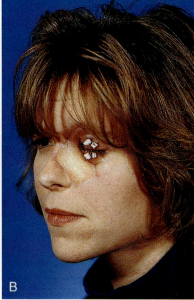

■ **Figure 27–3.** *A* and *B*, Insufficient skin and soft-tissue replacement of medial aspect of orbit caused ectropion of upper and lower eyelids, necessitating medial suture tarsorrhaphy.

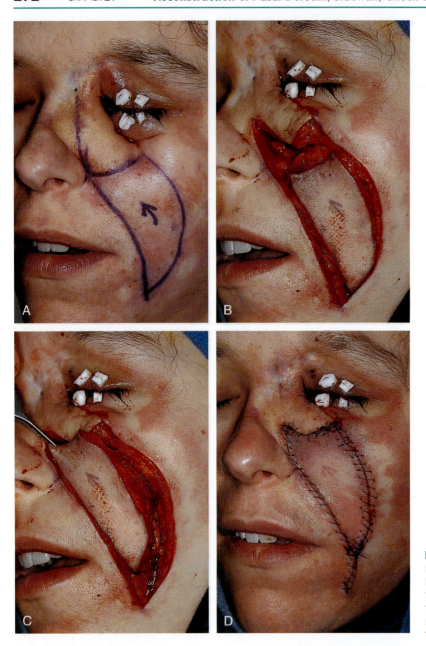

Figure 27–4. *A to D,* Superiorly based transposition flap used to augment inferior medial orbit with skin and soft tissue. Donor wound of transposition flap repaired with large V-to-Y cutaneous advancement flap based on subcutaneous pedicle.

there was asymmetry in the position of the medial aspect of the eyebrows. The level of the right eyebrow was inferior to the left. To correct this, a right direct eyebrow lift was performed. There was also a 4 × 3 cm depressed contour involving the skin surrounding the medial aspect of the left eyebrow. A depression of lesser severity extended superiorly to involve the lower two-thirds of the left forehead. The entire depression was corrected by inserting a 4 × 3 cm expanded polytetrafluoroethylene implant beneath the skin through a limited incision placed in a scar resulting from the surgical resection (Fig. 27–7).

Discussion

Full-thickness defects that involve the nose and significant portions of the cheek are reconstructed in stages. The early surgical stages are directed toward repair of the cheek to provide a stable foundation for subsequent reconstruction of the nose. The concept of first restoring the foundation on which to place the constructed nose before initiating nasal reconstruction is used whenever a sizable full-thickness defect of the

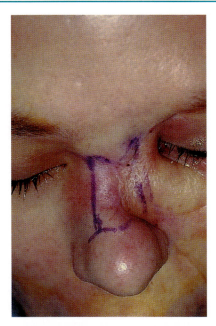

■ **Figure 27–5.** Skin (indicated by blue outline) of microsurgical flap occupying aesthetic units of nasal dorsum and left sidewall was removed. Deep tissue of flap left in situ to provide vascularized recipient site for bone grafts.

cheek or lip is associated with a full-thickness nasal defect. For example, when there is a full-thickness loss of the nose and adjacent upper lip, it is prudent to delay reconstruction of the nose until the lip is repaired and scars have contracted to their maximum propensity (see discussion in Chapter 26).

The advantage of reconstructing the full-thickness

cheek and medial orbital defect prior to attempting repair of the nose is clearly evident in this case. Once cheek wounds had healed sufficiently to account for the majority of wound contraction (3 months), nasal reconstruction could proceed with assurance that the region of the nasal facial sulcus would remain a solid platform for subsequent construction of the nose. A paramedian forehead flap serving as a covering flap for the nose was sutured to the skin of the microsurgical flap with assurance that migration of the nasal facial sulcus would not occur. In this case, reconstruction of the cheek before the nose also offered the additional advantage of providing a method of repairing the lining defect of the nasal cavity.

In the case presented, the microsurgical flap offered sufficient soft tissue to restore the medial cheek and sufficient bone to assist with support of the eye. The flap also served as a temporary cover for the nasal defect. The deep aspect of the microsurgical flap covering the bony nasal and ethmoid sinus defect was allowed to heal by secondary intention. Epithelium along the margins of the mucosal defect will migrate over exposed subcutaneous tissue and eventually form an epithelial cover over the deep portion of the flap exposed to the nasal cavity. Only the skin of the microsurgical flap covering the nose was removed during nasal reconstruction. The deeper soft tissue was left in situ to provide lining for the nose and a vascularized soft-tissue recipient site for the bone grafts.

The paramedian forehead flap used as covering for the nasal repair was unusual because a portion of the flap was designed to replace a skin and soft-tissue deficiency of the superior medial orbit. This deficiency re-

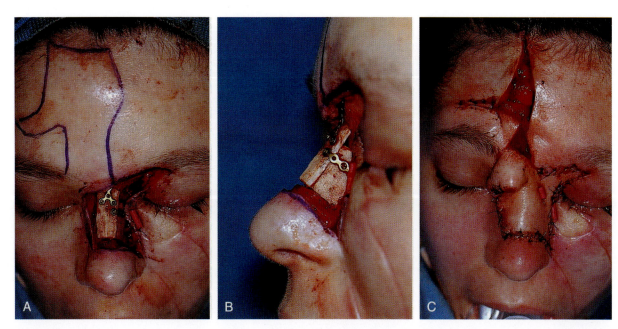

■ **Figure 27–6.** *A to C,* Cranial bone grafts used to provide structural support for bony dorsum and left sidewall. Irregular shaped paramedian forehead flap used to cover bone grafts and replace skin and soft tissue of superior medial orbit.

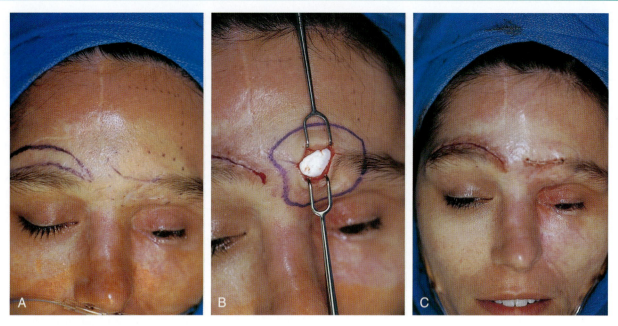

■ **Figure 27–7.** *A,* Right direct eyebrow lift outlined. *B,* Implant used to correct depressed contour can be seen through access incision. Dark blue marking represents size and configuration of implant. *C,* Incisions closed.

sulted from tumor resection. Unfortunately, the microsurgical flap was not of sufficient size to completely restore this portion of the resection, and the patient subsequently developed retraction of the upper eyelid. In general, when reconstructing defects of the nose that extend to adjacent facial aesthetic regions, each region is repaired with separate covering flaps to provide maximum scar camouflage and contour regularity. However, in this case the only source of tissue available to replace the infrabrow skin and soft tissue of the medial orbit was the forehead. For this reason, the paramedian forehead flap was designed to resurface the nasal dorsum, left sidewall, and superior medial orbit. The portion of the forehead flap used for the orbit facilitated the release of an upper eyelid contracture, restoring a normal position to the upper eyelid. This in turn provided greater cover of the cornea by the eyelid and, together with the transposition flap to the lower eyelid,

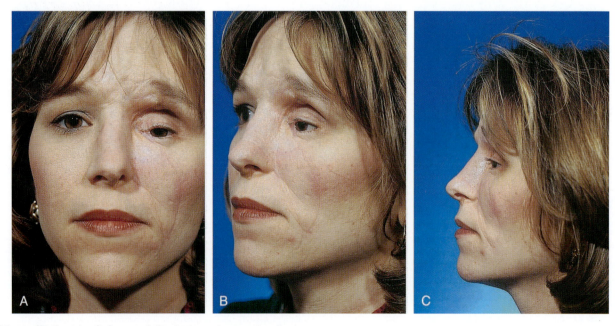

■ **Figure 27–8.** *A* to *C,* 2 years following nasal reconstruction.

enabled the elimination of the medial suture tarsorrhaphy.

Reconstruction of the nose was a relatively simple project compared with that of the cheek and eyelids. Cranial bone grafts harvested and grafted using techniques described in Chapter 8 provided structural support. A paramedian forehead flap provided cover for the repair. Refinements of the covering flap included contouring, Z-plasties of the scar along the inferior border of the flap, and subsequent dermabrasion. These techniques are discussed in Chapter 14 and 15.

The donor wound resulting from the forehead flap could not be completely closed, and a portion of the wound was left to heal by secondary intention. Forehead scars resulting from this type of healing often produce scars that are unobtrusive near the anterior hairline. However, more inferiorly, a wound healing by secondary intention can result in a scar that has an atrophic shiny appearance that is more visually apparent. Revision of these scars usually results in an improved appearance. The preferred method of scar revision is as follows. An incision is made along the borders of the scar to the level of the subdermis. All of the epidermis covering the scar is sharply dissected off the underlying scar tissue, which is left in situ. The incision is deepened around the periphery of the scar to the level of the periosteum. A wide subgaleal dissection is performed to mobilize the forehead skin on either side of the scar. The skin on either side of the wound is advanced toward the other so that their borders can be approximated, covering the tissue left in the deeper aspect of the scar. The skin borders can usually be approximated without excessive wound closure tension if the forehead skin has been sufficiently undermined. Healing results in a narrow scar much improved over the appearance of the original scar.

Preserving the deeper portion of the scar aids in filling the depressed contour that is associated with the atrophic scar resulting from secondary intention healing. Scars of this nature are usually revised 3 to 6 months after transfer of the forehead flap. This time allows the remaining forehead skin to stretch as the scar contracts during maturation. Scar contraction has the same effect as prolonged tissue expansion, restoring additional skin to the forehead. Upon excision of the atrophic scar and undermining of the forehead skin, the wound can be approximated primarily and without excessive wound closure tension. This provides a narrow, nearly imperceptible, scar.

Although restoration of the nose required standard procedures, this case represents a complex and difficult reconstructive challenge. In such cases, a number of surgical procedures are necessary, sequenced in a fashion to allow proper healing of the preceding surgery. The goal is to restore the patient to a level where function is not severely impaired and reconstructed facial features are as near to their original appearance as possible (Fig. 27–8).

Index

Note: Page numbers followed by the letter f refer to figures; those followed by the letter t refer to tables.